Praise for
THE FIRST CELL

"An incisive critique-cum-memoir." —*Nature*

"Raza, a Columbia University professor of medicine and practicing oncologist, offers a passionate account of how humans grapple with the scourge of cancer....Showing that compassion is just as important for cancer patients as the drugs administered to them, Raza's deeply personal work brings understanding and empathy to the fore in a way that a purely scientific explication never could."
—*Publishers Weekly* (Starred)

"With elegant literary references and a compassion that deeply personalizes her interactions with patients and families, [Raza] engages readers in a commitment to finding a better way. Intelligence, empathy, and optimism inform the argument for new research on cancer that could obviate the suffering prevalent today."
—*Kirkus* (Starred)

"An affecting, fascinating, timely, and uncompromisingly honest look at where we stand in treating the most fearsome disease in most people's worry list."
—Steven Pinker, author of *Enlightenment Now*

"Azra Raza's *The First Cell* is both a chronicle of her journey as a doctor and a scientist, and a 'call to action' to change the fundamental paradigm in our effort to prevent, treat, and cure cancer. Raza provides deep and moving insights into the shifting lives of her patients as they traverse their own journeys through illness, while never losing sight of the larger landscape—the vast scientific, medical, and strategic arena—of cancer science and therapy. Raza writes with searing honesty about our failures, with exhilarating verve about our successes, and with boundless empathy about the sanctity of the patients who endure the brunt of therapy. Her own experience with her husband's illness and death runs through the book like a red line, marking her courage and dignity as cancer enters her own family and devastates her life. The result is an elegantly conceived, powerfully written, and far-reaching tome that will change the conversation around cancer for decades to come."

—Siddhartha Mukherjee, author of *The Emperor of All Maladies*

"We are accustomed to a narrative of war in books by cancer researchers. The doctors are generals on the barricades alongside their soldier patients. Progress is slow, but the battle is gradually being won. This book tells another story. The drugs that are declared successes offer only a few weeks of painful extension of life. The best clinicians are usually thrown back on the primitive combination of cut, poison, and burn that as students, they thought they would look back on as an embarrassment. Bespoke genetic treatments have significant limitations. Azra Raza breaks out of the official story to tell a new one. She's not fighting a war. She's negotiating with a resilient and dynamic enemy. She wants to change the terms of engagement. No more fighting at the endgame, but hunting down the first deviant cells. This book is a passion project, a personal story, a scientific proposal, and quite simply one of the most compelling books you'll read. It breaks out of the standard narrative. It invents a whole new one. It works. By the end you'll want to sign on to her revolution."

—Sherry Turkle, author of *Reclaiming Conversation*

"When the history of cancer is eventually written, Azra Raza's book will be one of the touchstones that illuminated the path to victory."

—Amanda Foreman, author of *The Duchess*

"With command and clarity, Azra Raza indicts the cancer industry with such force that it begs the question: Are we really winning the cancer war? *The First Cell* is an intricately woven, often lyrical, tapestry of anecdote and authority that returns the suffering patient to the foreground of medical innovation. Raza expertly illustrates the complex choreography of cancer's nefarious dance, and her fascinating proposal will surely thrust cancer therapy from the 20th to the 21st century."

—Tina Brown

"A beautifully written book from a leading cancer expert who is also a caring, committed clinician."

—Peter D. Kramer, author of *Against Depression*

"As a cancer survivor, I can testify that Azra Raza's call to action for more research on early detection is vitally important. In a world driven by profit, this book is by a doctor who thinks about the patient first."

—Ruchira Gupta, journalist and activist

"Azra Raza is famed as a titan in the field of oncology. Perhaps less well-known is that she is a sensitive and passionate writer as well. In *The First Cell* she combines the scientific and the human, medicine and the arts, to give us a unique view into something that touches all of our lives—offering us reasons for hope, and reasons also for sorrow."

—Mohsin Hamid, author of *Exit West*

"Unraveling myth and metaphor surrounding the disease with unrelenting acuity and sharing the pathos of lives that have been slashed of years and months and shorn of hope and promise by cancer, Dr. Raza reveals a world that has of yet been inaccessible to those who mourn humanity's lack of progress against the disease while being simultaneously baffled by it. Here is a masterful rendition of how an emphasis on curing cancer, instead of working to detect its first venomous breath, has exacted a terrible price in human lives, including that of her very own husband, Harvey. *The First Cell* is an intertwining of literature and life, science and cutting-edge cancer research, that demands a radical transformation in the way we humans understand the most tragic killer of our time. Through her poignant story-telling and the strength of a scientific vision built on decades of hard-wrought lessons gleaned from her work as a clinician and research scholar, Dr. Raza presents an arresting account that challenges our core understanding of cancer and cure."

—Rafia Zakaria, author of *Veil*

"With wisdom distilled from more than three decades of clinical practice, the sensibilities of a poet, and a deep compassion for her fellow humans, Dr. Azra Raza provides a compelling argument that a key way forward in improving patient outcomes is early diagnosis and treatment, before cancer has become much too complex for any therapy to overcome."

—David Steensma, Attending Physician at the
Dana-Farber Cancer Institute and Associate
Professor at Harvard Medical School

"*The First Cell* is the rare book that brings both a personal and scientific experience of cancer together. It questions the profiteering that floods our environment with carcinogens in the first place, and also those that profit from treating it. Azra Raza puts our focus where it should be: on prevention and early detection."

—Gloria Steinem

THE
FIRST
CELL

THE
FIRST
CELL

And the Human Costs of
Pursuing Cancer to the Last

AZRA RAZA

BASIC BOOKS
New York

Basic Books
Hachette Book Group
1290 Avenue of the Americas, New York, NY 10104
www.basicbooks.com

Printed in the United States of America
First Trade Paperback Edition: December 2020

Published by Basic Books, an imprint of Perseus Books, LLC, a subsidiary of Hachette Book Group, Inc. The Basic Books name and logo is a trademark of the Hachette Book Group.

The Hachette Speakers Bureau provides a wide range of authors for speaking events. To find out more, go to www.hachettespeakersbureau.com or call (866) 376-6591.

The publisher is not responsible for websites (or their content) that are not owned by the publisher.
Additional copyright/credits information is on page 327. Print book interior design by Linda Mark.

The Library of Congress has cataloged the hardcover edition as follows:
Names: Raza, Azra, author.
Title: The first cell : and the human costs of pursuing cancer to the last / Azra Raza.
Description: New York : Basic Books, 2019 | Includes bibliographical references and index.
Identifiers: LCCN 2019016257 (print) | LCCN 2019018259 (ebook) | ISBN 9781541699502 (ebook) | ISBN 9781541699526 (hardcover)
Subjects: | MESH: Neoplasms—therapy | Medical Oncology | Neoplasms—prevention & control | Personal Narrative
Classification: LCC RC263 (ebook) | LCC RC263 (print) | NLM QZ 21 | DDC 616.99/4—dc23
LC record available at https://lccn.loc.gov/2019016257

ISBNs: 978-1-5416-9952-6 (hardcover); 978-1-5416-9950-2 (ebook); 978-1-5416-9951-9 (paperback)

LSC-C

Printing 1, 2020

To Sheherzad

Khurshid-e-Jahan Taab Ki Zau Tere Sharar Mein
Abad Hai Ek Taza Jahan Tere Hunar Mein
—Allama Iqbal

The spark in you is a radiant sun
A new world lives in your talent

And to my siblings
Amera, Atiya, Tasnim, Javed, Sughra, and Abbas

In honor of what the G7 share: the deep love of each other
and of Syed Ali Raza and Begum Zaheer Fatima,
and memories of the best of times at Gulistan e Raza—
the secure, warm, and fun home in our beloved Karachi

کاوش کا دل کرے ہے تقاضا کہ ہے ہنوز
ناخن پہ قرض اس گرہ نیم باز کا

Kaavish ka dil karay hay taqaaza kay hay hunoz
Nakhun pe qarz uss girah e neem baaz ka

—GHALIB

The heart demands greater exertion into inquiry, for yet
Our fingernails owe a debt to the half-undone knots

The work of the eyes is done. Go now and do the
heart-work on the images imprisoned within you.

—RAINER MARIA RILKE

Contents

CANCER AND ITS DISCONTENTS

IN THE EARLY SPRING OF 1998, MY HUSBAND, HARVEY PREISLER, was diagnosed with cancer. The following year, we planned to take our five-year-old daughter, Sheherzad, and my brother Javed's two children visiting from Pakistan, Musa and Batool, eight and twelve, to San Francisco for a highly anticipated vacation. We had already postponed the trip twice before, but it could be delayed no longer. The children were eager, and given Harvey's disfiguring facial edema and the enlarging nodes, some form of aggressive treatment—sure to require us to stay put in the city for months—was now imminent. Before any of that happened, he felt strongly that the family needed to get out of the sweltering heat of Chicago for a vacation, even if for just a week.

Our flight to San Francisco was on a bright, clear summer morning. Having arrived at the gate a good ninety minutes before our departure, we split up; Harvey sat down in the boarding area while I chased the children around O'Hare. We got something to eat at the food court and then returned to the gate.

I was shocked by what I saw. Harvey sat, looking dazed, as streams of sweat poured from his body, making little puddles under his elbows on the armrests of the chair and under his knees on the floor. He was beet red. Tributaries of glistening perspiration filled the lines in his handsome face, making it appear startlingly young. He looked at me with hushed anxiety. I sent Batool running for the nearest café to get me a handful of napkins. I dabbed Harvey's face and arms, wiping the chair and floor. There was no respite. The sweat came in torrential waves. His T-shirt and shorts were entirely soaked and dripping. The children stood around trying not to look, their faces ashen. It was a good fifteen minutes before the deluge subsided. I walked to the gift shop and purchased a fresh pair of pants and shirt. Without saying a word, little eight-year-old Musa stepped forward, quietly took the package from me, and gently escorted a bewildered Harvey to the restroom.

Being oncologists, both Harvey and I understood precisely what the sweating meant. Known as a B-symptom, it is a well-recognized manifestation of many cancers, especially lymphomas, and it is not a good sign. B-symptoms are associated with a more advanced, more aggressive disease with a poorer prognosis. I suggested we cancel the trip and return home, but Harvey, not willing to disappoint the children yet again, insisted on going ahead.

The first twenty-four hours in San Francisco were filled with apprehension as we drove the children around the Crooked Street and the harbor, not knowing what to expect, fearing the worst. Nothing much happened. Harvey began to relax. Then, in the middle of the third night, I woke up with a start. Water dripped steadily on my face. Harvey's arm was arched over my head and running like a faucet. This time, we not only had to change his clothing, we had to call housekeeping to replace the soaking-wet sheets.

By the time we returned to O'Hare a week later, Harvey had developed another bizarre syndrome associated with many cancers. His left wrist suddenly blew up to twice its normal size. Despite the extra-strength Tylenol I had given him, he was writhing in agony as we climbed into the car to go home. It took twenty-four hours of cold packs and heavy-duty analgesics to control the excruciating pain. The next few days were some of the most tormented. He experienced regular episodes of drenching sweats, once or sometimes twice during the night, requiring fresh bedsheets and clothing changes.

As swelling subsided in one joint, it popped up elsewhere without warning. Fresh lesions began with a tingling, burning sensation, becoming bright red and sizzling hot within hours. Nomadic lymphoma cells meandered autonomously, rudderless. Edema regressed from the face only to reappear in his joints. Lymph nodes in the neck and armpits swelled one day and receded the next, followed by a sudden enlargement of the spleen. Itinerant cells segregated, dispersed, re-collected, vanished, regrouped. They wandered the body with a studied carelessness, entering and leaving organs at will, disgruntled, edgy, exploring possible niches in various organs, rejecting some, settling in others. Horrified, helpless, we watched the drama unfold, Harvey from inside, I from the outside. The lymphoma marched on its aimless, monomaniacal journey into irresolution with a motiveless malignity.

Cancer is what I had been treating for two decades, yet until I shared a bed with a cancer patient, I had no idea how unbearably painful a disease it could be.

It was the summer of our discontent.

Cancer and its discontents.

FROM LAST TO FIRST

I COULD NOT HAVE WRITTEN THIS BOOK WHEN I WAS THIRTY YEARS old. It is not because of any great discoveries I have made or research papers I have published since. It is because of the experience the intervening decades have given me as I cared for thousands of cancer patients and accompanied many to their deaths. Because the disease I treat is generally fatal, solace seems contrived, personal academic success egregious. My surroundings may not have changed much, but my perceptions have. I have learned to reexamine things I took for granted, to seek comfort in odd places. I have learned new things about what I thought I already knew: like the difference between illness and disease; between what it means to cure and to heal; between what it means to feel no pain and to feel well; about the harrowing nature of keeping appointments one never made. In clinic, in scientific meetings, I have felt like a fraud, a posturing intellectual phony. The complexity of another's illness has made my own life appear simpler; in the march to death, I have begun to catalog the tragedies of survival. From time to time, I even feel buoyed without reprieve.

I treat and study a bone marrow preleukemic condition known as myelodysplastic syndromes (MDS) as well as acute myeloid leukemia (AML), which develops in a third of MDS patients. The treatment landscape for AML has not evolved much in fifty years, nor has it for most of the common types of cancers. With minor variations, a protocol of surgery, chemotherapy, and radiation—the slash-poison-burn approach to treating cancer—remains unchanged. It is an embarrassment. Equally embarrassing is the arrogant denial of that embarrassment. Technologic advances and the cure of cancer in animal models are loudly proclaimed as if those successes have had anything to do with treating the disease in humans. Improvement in survival of cancer patients measured in weeks is regularly referred to as a "game changer." To make rosy pronouncements is profoundly unfair to patients. No one is winning the war on cancer. It is mostly hype, the same rhetoric from the same self-important voices for the past half a century.

Cancer treatment was primitive just a century ago. Historians will say the same about our practices fifty years from now. We boast of magnificent godlike technologic advances, editing the genome efficiently, turning genes on and off at will—yet cancer treatment, for the most part, remains Paleolithic in comparison. The issue is not so much that there has been little progress in cancer research. The question is why there is so little improvement in treatment. Why can't we make use of the millions of research papers published in the past fifty years claiming huge successes in understanding the biology of cancer? For four decades, I have been hearing the same glowing predictions about the magic treatment just around the corner, resulting from a better understanding of oncogenes, tumor suppressor genes, the human genome and transcriptome, the immune system, or choking off blood supply to tumors. Most have fallen flat when brought to the bedside. The gaping disconnect between knowledge about cancer biology and the capacity to use this knowledge to benefit patients is staggering.

How we speak of cancer is primitive, too. In these past decades, I have attended thousands of academic lectures and listened to countless public talks on YouTube by cancer researchers. The latter almost all begin with descriptions of how the speaker's passion for research started in youth, recount the history of their subsequent hard work and occasional setbacks, followed by their eventual personal success, the reason they own the podium. By the end of the talk, every oncologist relates at least one patient success story, providing an optimistic, bright summary of definite progress, small and incremental but progress nonetheless, and ends with the promise of even greater imminent success. *Stay positive* is the refrain, as if it were a sin to voice the intense pain and suffering of cancer patients. Why are we so afraid to tell the stories of the majority who die? Why keep promoting the positive anecdote? Why all this mollycoddling? Treating the public like fragile, vulnerable, oversensitive, easily hurt, anxious adolescents needing protection from stressful details is unfair, shortsighted, and in the long run, counterproductive for everyone involved.

A society and culture obsessed with winning views the death of cancer patients as a failure and therefore a subject best avoided. Dying is not a failure. Denying death is. The Western mind—portrayed, at least, by the classical literary canon—has not always been in denial. The depiction of suffering in Greek tragedy was meant to produce a paradoxical catharsis in its audience. Seeing their worst nightmares enacted openly onstage, debating the consequence of actions, and identifying with the characters in the play could dispel the fear of pain and death. Real-life situations presented in highly exaggerated forms underscore the deep-seated sources for inner anxieties and insecurities. Cancer stories, unlike Greek tragedies, need no exaggeration to depict the drama of pain and grueling decisions. Insights come from reading both types of stories for those who imagine changing places with others, empathizing with their deadly challenges.

The stories invoke in us a profound sense of wonder, a cleansing of the cobwebs obscuring the complexity of life, unraveling unexpected interludes of beauty, witnessing small acts of heroism in seemingly impossible situations, inspiring a deeper appreciation of all things good: *There is no love of life without despair of life,* Albert Camus once wrote. Clarity comes from role-playing. By learning from the experience of others, we can interpret our own lives better, choose a different death, record our wishes in advance. In his essay "Letter from a Region in My Mind," James Baldwin clarifies our shared destiny with startling eloquence:

> Life is tragic simply because the earth turns and the sun inexorably rises and sets, and one day, for each of us, the sun will go down for the last time. Perhaps the whole root of our trouble, the human trouble, is that we will sacrifice all the beauty of our lives, will imprison ourselves in totems, taboos, crosses, blood sacrifices, steeples, mosques, races, armies, flags, nations in order to deny the fact of death, which is the only fact we have. It seems to me that one ought to rejoice in the *fact* of death—ought to decide, indeed, to *earn* one's death by confronting with passion the conundrum of life. One is responsible to life: It is the small beacon in that terrifying darkness from which we come and to which we shall return. One must negotiate this passage as nobly as possible, for the sake of those who are coming after us.

As it is, too few of us have any idea of how to prepare for it or what to do when it strikes.

I see thirty to forty patients every week, yet it felt surreal telling the handsome, tanned, forty-three-year-old Henry W., father of three young children, who was used to playing tennis regularly, whose wife, Rose, was an artist, that the reason he developed spontaneous bruising while on vacation in Bermuda is because he has AML. A bone marrow test showed that the leukemia had arisen in the background of profound dysplasia. The presence of multiply damaged chromosomes and a mutation in the p53 gene, also known as TP53, marked his case as a particularly virulent one, impossible to control. His only chance of survival was to attempt remission of the leukemia with intensive rounds of chemotherapy first, and if successful, followed immediately by a bone marrow transplant. The couple's innocent, beguiling reactions followed the expected cycles: swinging between disbelief and horror to finding strength in distractions like researching the disease, looking for second opinions, exploring the latest medical options available, checking his siblings' blood types in anticipation of the transplant.

Sitting across from me in the exam room, after a particularly gruesome conversation about the gravity of Henry's condition on their second visit, Rose said before leaving that she and her husband could not decide how or what to tell their three children, ranging from ages five to ten, who had sensed something was wrong and dreaded the worst. Children instinctively register parental anxiety, and they grade tension; like birds, they hear the infrasounds of approaching disaster. Following dinner the night before, when the children had settled in the family room with ice cream, Rose found an opportunity to start a conversation. She began by saying that because Dad had to receive frequent treatments for a blood disease, they would be spending a lot of time in the hospital. Grandma W. would be with them most evenings. She said it would also be a good idea for Dad to avoid infection and eat healthy things. The two boys sat staring, frozen with fear, the elder one looking like he was about to pass out. They did not want to hear any details. Rose could not continue. Henry choked up. Their five-year-old daughter broke the awkward silence. She walked to the trash can and dropped her ice cream cone, calmly saying, "I will not eat dessert until Dad can."

Before Henry could start the intensive chemotherapy requiring four to six weeks of hospitalization, he was admitted to the hospital with a high temperature, resulting in violent, shaking chills and intense sweating. A million-dollar workup failed to reveal any specific cause. He started three antibiotics intravenously, along with antifungals and antiviral therapies. The fever of unknown origin raged on, unabated. He was seen by the transplant team, and several potential matches were identified. First, we had to reduce the number of leukemia cells in Henry's bone marrow from 80 percent to less than 5 percent or the transplant would not be of any benefit. As the leukemia surged, chemotherapy was reluctantly initiated despite the spiking temperatures. His marrow emptied out of all blood-forming cells, resulting in dangerously low blood counts. He spent the next three weeks in a virtual fog, weakened by the double whammy of high-dose chemotherapy and potentially lethal sepsis. Then, things slowly improved. After six interminable weeks of hospitalization, he went home, only to return three weeks later with shaking chills and fever. The leukemia had come roaring back. From diagnosis to death, it took less than six months. Henry had received the same combination of two chemotherapy drugs I have been using since 1977.

The cancer winter continues.

◌∾◌

TREATING CANCER AS one disease is like treating Africa as one country. Even in the same patient, it is not the same disease at two sites or at two different points in time. Vicious and self-obsessed, it learns to grow faster and become stronger, smarter, and more dangerous with each successive division. It is a perfect example of intelligence at a molecular level, able to perceive its environment and take actions that maximize its chances of survival. A feedback loop, using past performance to improve its efficiency, forms the basis of its seemingly purposeful behavior. It learns to divide more vigorously with time, invading new spaces, mutating to turn the expression of pertinent genes off and on, enhancing its fitness to the landscape, optimizing seed-soil cooperation. We see this metamorphosis in front of our eyes when treatment causes regression of the tumor in one area just as fresh lesions crop up in another, bearing a novel genotype, selected precisely because of their refractoriness to the administered therapy; as mini-Frankensteins, they emerge like ghosts from the machine, bent upon destroying their maker.

The disease is fantastically complex. More fantastic is the reductionist conceit that targeting a single genetic abnormality with a single drug will be curative. This "magic bullet" concept became especially entrenched because of a couple of early successes—in the case of chronic myeloid leukemia, a chromosomal translocation in the malignant cell codes for an abnormal hybrid protein targetable with a drug, imatinib mesylate, with dramatic results. Acute promyelocytic leukemia, a particularly deadly disease, is also driven by a single abnormality. It is now curable with vitamin A. These two success stories seemed to confirm a paradigm: cancer results from a genetic mutation that can be cured with a drug.

Unfortunately, most common cancers have proved to be more complex, with many more biologic aberrations driving the malignant phenotype. The trafficking of cancer cells is more labyrinthine, tangled, knotty, and impenetrably convoluted than the London Underground. The cell continually transforms itself, covering generations of its natural life span in mere hours, ditching genes and entire chromosomes, acquiring new mutations, revving organelles, deforming proteins, neutralizing death signals, forging ahead deliriously, driven by the unrelenting engine of malice, bursting its hot contents on unsuspecting organs, impregnating them with its potent malignant seed, callously moving on. Cancer rules over the host with despotic autocracy.

To develop treatment strategies for so dense a disease by attempting to duplicate its complexity in tissue culture cell lines or animal models has been an unmitigated disaster. The failure rate for drugs brought into clinical trials using such preclinical drug-testing platforms is 95 percent. The 5 percent of drugs that reach approval might as well have failed, since they prolong survival of patients by no more than a few months at best. Since 2005, 70 percent of approved drugs have shown zero improvement in survival rates while up to 70 percent have been actually harmful to patients.

These conceptual errors are due to cause more harm tomorrow than they do today. Based on available data, some 18 million new cancer cases were diagnosed worldwide in 2018, with about half as many dying of their cancers. The American Cancer Society reports that the global burden will grow to 21.7 million new cancer cases and 13 million cancer deaths by 2030 as the worldwide population grows and ages. A frequently cited statistic shows that the death rate from cancer declined in the United States by 20 percent between 1980 and 2014. There were 240 deaths per 100,000 in 1980 while only 192 deaths per 100,000 in 2014. However, this decrease is not due to improved treatments but mostly to early diagnosis and a decline in smoking. There has been a disturbing increase in cancer deaths from specific malignancies, both across the United States and in delineated pockets. Liver cancer deaths have increased by 88 percent nationwide from 1980 to 2014. Deadly breast cancers in women, prostate cancers in men, as well as mortality from cancers of the pancreas, colon, and rectum escalated among low socioeconomic groups and in impoverished regions with a high incidence of obesity. And even as lymphomas have steadily claimed a death rate of 8 per 100,000 across the United States, small pockets in Ohio, West Virginia, and Kentucky experienced an increase in deaths by up to 74 percent.

And then there is the financial issue. Tarceva, a drug that extends the survival of pancreatic cancer patients by twelve days, costs $26,000. An eighteen-week course of cetuximab for lung cancer costs $80,000. Among the 9.5 million new cancer cases diagnosed during a fourteen-year period in America, almost half (42.4 percent) had lost all their life savings within two-plus years. Overall, cancer care cost $125 billion in 2010 and is likely to be $156 billion by 2020. And these are just billings to patients and insurers and does not include the infusion of money from other sources like philanthropies, private organizations, nonprofit funding institutions, universities, industry, and the FDA. A literature search reveals that more than 3 million papers have been published to date on cancer, the PubMed database showing 3,843,208 publications with 165,567 in 2018 alone. A good 70 percent of what is reported is not reproducible.

The consensus today is that prevention is preferable to treatment. Yet actions to make this happen are obscenely lagging behind. In the meantime, precious lives are lost, resources wasted. As oncologists, we are charged with providing, from diagnosis to death, care to our cancer patients that enhances their quality of life, reduces pain and suffering.

Are we accomplishing that, and if not, then why not, and what can be done to improve the outlook for future patients? Are we truly appreciating the deep tragedy of cancer at an intimate, individual level, the profound devastation of families, cancer's social and financial impact, its searing psychologic traumas? Above all, are we doing the best we can with available options, or should we be questioning some of the draconian measures we are practicing? How good are the solutions we offer if we constantly have to ask ourselves whether the cancer or the treatment we prescribe will kill the patient? Which of the two is worse? Using chemotherapy, immune therapy, and stem cell transplant to cure cancer, as someone has aptly observed, is like beating the dog with a baseball bat to get rid of its fleas. Why is this the best we can offer?

⌘

HOPES OF FINDING better drugs using the existing discovery platforms or using even more artificial systems of genetically engineered animals are as realistic as dissecting the brain and expecting to discover consciousness. After fifty years of developing cancer drugs this way, is it time to reassess the preclinical model?

No.

It is time to abandon the strategy altogether. Jeremiads alone are pointless unless a new strategy accompanies the lamentation.

The new strategy is to stop chasing after the last cancer cell and focus on eliminating the first. Better still, prevent the appearance of the first cancer cell by finding its earliest footprints.

To begin the ending, we must end the beginning. Prevention will be the only compassionate, universally applicable cure.

It is not prevention through lifestyle changes. Individuals with pristine eating and exercising habits get cancer because cancer-causing mutations accumulate as natural consequences of reproduction and aging of cells. The new strategy must go beyond early detection as practiced currently through mammograms and other routine screening tests. The prevention I am talking about is through identification and eradication of transformed cancerous cells at their inception, before they have had a chance to organize into a bona fide malignant, incurable disease. This may seem an unattainable, utopian dream, but it is achievable in a reasonable time. We are already using sophisticated technology to detect the residues of disease that linger after treatment, the last cancer cell. Can we not reverse the order of things and use the tests to detect the first?

I started focusing on a study of preleukemia, MDS, thirty-five years ago for this reason. It was clear to me even back in 1984 that AML is too complicated and difficult a disease to cure in my lifetime. I pinned my hopes on studying the preleukemic stage, findings ways to prevent it from evolving to AML. I have stuck to this strategy for all these years. Among a handful of researchers with the same mind-set is Bert Vogelstein at Johns Hopkins University, who studied the transition of benign adenomas into malignant colon cancers and eventually came to the same conclusion—the best strategy is prevention and early detection. His team is leading the charge in breast, colon, pancreas, and lung cancers; they are using "liquid biopsies" to look for very early biomarkers of malignancy in bodily fluids. Vogelstein has repeatedly pointed out that 30–40 percent of all cancers can be cured today by implementing techniques to detect early markers of cancer, such as somatic DNA driver mutations; epigenetic changes; cancer-specific RNA and proteins; cancer-specific metabolites in the plasma, sputum, urine, and stools of these individuals; and by employing molecular imaging techniques. The sensitivity can be increased from roughly 40 percent to 80 percent for gynecologic cancers simply by looking for cancer-derived DNA markers in Pap smears. Fifty years from now, Vogelstein says, cancer deaths could be down by 75 percent just through prevention, early detection, and development of newer strategies to deal with early- rather than late-stage disease.

Once my mind was made up to try to detect the first leukemia cells in an MDS patient and target their destruction at the very inception, the next challenge was a practical one. I needed leukemia cells to study. This provided the impetus for banking samples any time I performed a bone marrow biopsy on my patients. Thus began the MDS-AML Tissue Repository. This repository is the most concrete, tangible proof of my lifelong commitment to study cancer at its earliest stage, to find the first cell and to eliminate the scourge at initiation. Dating back to 1984, it is now the oldest MDS and AML repository in the world collected by a single physician. Not a single cell has been contributed by another oncologist. Today, the repository contains some sixty thousand samples from thousands of patients.

Every vial in those freezers invokes a poignant memory; every test tube tells a story. Only I am a witness to the pain each patient—some of them more than a dozen times over the course of their illness—endured to undergo this procedure. That makes everything deeply personal for me, sacred. Some of those vials in the freezers contain parts of patients that can be thawed back to life in lab dishes decades after the patients are no more. Including Harvey. How can I afford to let any of those patients down?

❧

I CAN ALMOST hear some objections surfacing in the minds of my oncology and scientific colleagues.

The first objection will likely be that I am ignoring the 68 percent of all cancers we are managing to cure today. My answer is that most of it was achieved several decades ago with the surgery-chemoradiation therapies. Recent advances relate primarily to improvement in cancer mortality due to early detection, not meaningful advances in the treatment of metastatic cancers. An exciting exception, and one worth applauding wholeheartedly, is the introduction of novel immune therapies. Two fine scientists, James P. Allison and Tasuku Honjo, won the Nobel Prize in 2018 for their pioneering work in this field. As a result of their groundbreaking work, many hopeless lung cancer, melanoma, lymphoma, and acute lymphoblastic leukemia patients are living years beyond their predicted survival, and a few are even cured. It is great, but the immune approaches are not universally curative and, at present, help very few patients. At a minimum, the cellular therapies are financially draining; at worst, they may cause very severe side effects because of their superefficient killing. The sudden simultaneous deaths of billions of cancer cells in a person with a very high tumor burden cause life-threatening toxicities, as cytokine storms damage the liver and lungs while the kidneys choke on cellular debris. Finally, a small but definite fraction of treated patients, ranging between 7 and 30 percent, experience inexplicable resurgence and paradoxical hyperprogression of their tumors. All these side effects could possibly be avoided if the same therapy is instituted when the tumor burden is low. Indeed, harnessing the body's own natural killers to eliminate the first cancer cells will be the ideal treatment in the future.

Another constant refrain I hear from practicing oncologists goes something like this: "In the last twenty-five years, a shift toward better survival is seen in many cancers. Breast and prostate cancer and chronic myeloid and chronic lymphocytic leukemia have truly become diseases that patients live with and not die from. Even in lung cancer, which was the most depressing malignancy for decades, there is a trend toward survival improvement, albeit at great expense. There are at least ten to twelve targetable mutations. An additional 20–25 percent of patients respond to immunotherapy." I have no disagreement with this assessment. Of course there has been progress in many areas. It reminds me of something that a beloved Raza family friend, the late Syed V. S. Kashmiri, a fantastic immunologist and scientist in his own right, once said to my youngest brother: "Abbas, if one day, the sun rose in the west, practically the whole world would stop and stare. But there is a handful of people who watched it rise in the east every day and wondered why. These are the people who change the world." I quote Kashmiri Sahib because we, too, have been taking much for granted. We often talk about our patients only registering the positive parts of conversations. As oncologists, we are doing the same by focusing on the minority of our patients who benefit for limited durations. The time has come for us to think about the majority who don't, but who suffer the ghastly toxicities of therapies and end up losing their life savings in the process.

I can likewise anticipate criticism from the scientists cataloging paradigm-shifting progress in the molecular and genetic understanding of cancer pathology resulting from animal studies or in vitro tissue cultures. I agree that these modalities are the basis for deep insights into the biology of cancer and must continue. Nevertheless, as you will soon discover, these tools come in for ringing condemnation in this book. In no way am I advocating that we abandon such invaluable research tools. My problem is using these systems for oncologic drug development where they have proved of little benefit to the patients. Of course, individual researchers and oncologists who are trapped in a system cannot be held responsible because they would lose research grants or be sued for malpractice and negligence if they don't follow the prescribed guidelines. I know because I am one of them. Every bit of criticism applies as much to me as to any researcher or oncologist reading the book. My criticism is directed not at us but at the system we have unwittingly evolved and the culture we have unintentionally created collectively both in clinical practice and basic cancer research.

Finally, and most importantly, both oncologists and basic scientists might feel that I am too pessimistic, not just in my view of the past but also of the future. This, too, is a patently false conclusion. In fact, while being realistic about the past and present, I am exceedingly optimistic about the future of cancer treatment. The pessimism you might sense in the coming pages is not because I have a fatalistic or nihilistic attitude. Rather, it is an expression of deep frustration at the status quo. Too many lives are being lost because of our own unshakable hubris, convinced as we are that we possess the power to untangle the intricacies of as complex a disease as cancer. It is like saying we will cure aging. It may happen, but not any time soon. As you reach the end of this book, you will be sharing my hope for a much brighter outcome for future cancer patients. It will happen because we will have learned to avoid cancer's tragic, end-stage pain and suffering altogether by nipping it in the bud. I predict a radical shift in all of health care in the coming decades. Early detection of neurologic, metabolic, cardiac, and oncologic diseases will naturally follow once we implement sensors designed to gauge disease-caused perturbations years ahead of their actual clinical appearances. This is how over the next few years, effective, evidence-based preventive modalities will be developed, refined, and perfected.

⚮

ALTHOUGH ISSUES OF science are critical to this book, its true raison d'être is to improve the outcome for individuals negotiating cancer's capricious, pernicious challenges. I hope this book will be a source of empowerment—rather than discouragement—for cancer patients at several levels. For one, as we will see, not every gloomy prognosis comes to pass. For another, the fact that thousands of oncologists and researchers are working day and night to find better solutions for cancer is a powerful truth, as well. On a daily basis, I witness the astonishing, selfless devotion to patients displayed by my fellow oncologists in a hundred ways, great and small, just like the basic science researchers who work tirelessly to devise new experiments to test their hypotheses, reach out selflessly to collaborate and help us understand the inner happenings of cancer at a molecular level. Their dedication to cancer patients is humbling and inspiring. Most importantly, the book should assure any cancer patient reading it that they are not alone. We are in this conversation together. Every one of us has a fifty-fifty chance of being in their shoes tomorrow. The stories of men and women, young and old, facing grim choices reflect our collective challenges, give a voice to our anxieties as a species as well as to our vulnerabilities, our frailties.

Some fortunate individuals with cancer survive to tell their stories. In this book, a few of my patients agreed to do precisely that. Their humanity is on full display in their fierce desire to live, to celebrate life, even as they face life-threatening illnesses. Almost all of them rejected anonymity. Instead of signing their stories with a soup of alphabets or case numbers, they chose to provide their real names, even their pictures. They *want* to be identified. They want you to know they are living, breathing individuals. They want their voices heard. They walk you through their private hells, but then they also share with you their Joycean spirit: "To live, to err, to fall, to triumph, to re-create life out of life." Above all, it is their palpable desire to live just a little longer at all costs that leaps from the pages. They are the reason why we, the oncologists, obsessively, zealously, fanatically, pursue implausible treatment options—exploring wild possibilities, not giving up, not letting them give up. They provide the helium for our sagging spirits.

Many more, however, have died. When the decisions and actions that lead up to those deaths are not reexamined carefully, questioned, challenged, the indifference—our silence—kills patients again and again. My role in this examination shifts across multiple dimensions. I am variously a treating oncologist; a wife and then a cancer widow; a friend; an observer; a remote consultant; a basic scientist; a clinical researcher. I question the recommendations of experts, the choices that families made. I marvel at the innocence and hopefulness of the patients as they agonized their way through one excruciating experimental trial after another. Above all, I question my own decisions. Were they based on hard facts, or were they uncomfortable choices based on inadequate data derived from incompetently designed studies? If I could not provide a better life to my patients, could I have provided a better death? Can I improve upon my communication finesse? How do I acquire the skills missing from my tool kit for interacting more compassionately with my patients at a deeper human level? Isn't that why I became a doctor in the first place? Candid discourse humanizes both the patients and their oncologists. The aim is to proffer new ideas, make all of us rethink, question ourselves, challenge norms, and take a hard look at our rigid systems, our medieval institutions, through the prism of profoundly human issues affecting patients, families, survivors, oncologists, basic researchers.

Ultimately, I ask, if any of those involved—friends, families, patients, doctors—were to cast a backward glance, knowing what they know now, having had time to think, digest, and live with the loss, what decisions would they alter? A clear picture can only emerge with retrospection, recalling snippets of conversation, nagging details, hopeless choices. The sharp vision, the clairvoyance of grief, present from the first moment but suppressed, trickles into consciousness gradually. Honesty finally becomes possible on both sides as talking to families years later allows me to give my candid interpretation because they are finally ready to hear it. The process of retrospection forces us to relive the trauma, awaken repressed memories. The goal is not to revel in suffering but to liberate us from the past, prepare us to do better in the future.

As long as there is a single Henry W. dying a swift, brutal death, there can be no disagreement about whether great or little progress has occurred in cancer research and treatment. Let us, first and foremost, accept with all humility that our job remains unfinished. I would go further and say, let us accept that the traditional ways of doing most things are sclerotic. My insistent focus on the granularity of individual pain and suffering in the pages that follow is to highlight the urgent need for change, to force us, as individuals and as a society, to cast off the manacles of dogma and tradition. The burden of this book is to redraw the scientific route radically, to redirect our intellectual, technologic, physical, and emotional faculties away from fundamentally flawed models of adding a few months to survival; instead, to conceive and strive for the substance of things hoped for, a real cure through early detection and prevention. To go from last to first.

There is one and only one goal for all of us—to ensure that all our intellectual efforts are directed toward the relief of humanity's suffering. Suffering is what I see on a daily basis and what I chronicle in *The First Cell*. And where human suffering is concerned, scientific and emotional, medical and poetic impulses merge effortlessly and become inseparable. This synthesis, representing a rival paradigm of cancer research and treatment, even of writing about it, this dialogue of compassion, this science of empathy, of care and concern, can liberate us from the confident complacency of assumed righteousness in the way things are done, liberate us from the mental cages we have inadvertently imprisoned ourselves in. Our lives are at stake. Our future is at stake. Let new technology and new ideas rearrange our laboratories and our psyches, break the stalemate. Let us assume responsibility and seize the opportunities. Let us deconstruct what has become an indifferent science and reconstruct it through the prism of human anguish.

> *Kaun seh pai ga laikin meri aankhoun ke azab*
> *Kis ko yay hausla hoga kay hamaisha dekhay*
> *Apni palkoun ki saleeboun se utartay huay khwab*
> *Jin ki kirchioun ki chubhbhan roh mein buss jaati hay*
> *Zindagi, Zindagi bhar key liyay kur lati hay*

> —Ahmad Faraz, "Eye Bank"

> Who will be able to bear though
> the ruin my eyes have seen
> Who will be so brave
> keep their eyes always open
> Even as chimeras roll down
> the branches of their lashes
> Even as shrapnel twists
> and encamps in the breath
> Even as life cries out
> for the rest of life

> —Translated from Urdu by
> Anjuli Fatima Raza Kolb

| # OMAR

The Nobleness of Life
Is to Do Thus

There's a special providence in the fall of a sparrow.
If it be now, 'tis not to come; if it be not to come, it will be now;
if it be not now, yet it will come: the readiness is all.

—Shakespeare, *Hamlet*, act 5, scene 2

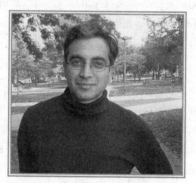

I ONLY SAW OMAR TWO OR THREE TIMES WITHOUT NAHEED, HIS mother, in the roughly sixteen months of our acquaintance in New York. It is hard for me to think of them separately. From the first message I received from Omar in the summer of 2007 to my last glimpse of him as he lay dying with his mother curled up next to him in bed, I was exquisitely aware of the unique privilege it was to be witnessing this sublime relationship. Of course, love is never quantifiable. The friendship alone that existed between Omar and Naheed would require new heavens and new earths to accommodate it.

arz o sama kahan tiri vus.at ko pa sakey
mera hi dil hai vo ki jahan tu sama sakey

—KHWAJA MIR DARD

The sky and all the planets could not comprehend your expanse
Only my heart has the largeness to embrace the anguish

Naheed brought her two sons to meet me in September of 2007, shortly after I had moved to New York. Omar, the thirty-eight-year-old elder son, a graduate of Oxford and Columbia, had been diagnosed with a highly malignant osteogenic sarcoma of the left shoulder.

They had come for dinner. Omar had received a round of aggressive chemotherapy a few days before, and his mouth was a battlefield of raw ulcers, abraded mucosa, bleeding gums. As we sat down to an elaborate meal with family and a few close friends, Omar calmly produced a bottle containing some sort of a bland, soothing drink and sipped away as if it were an exclusively prepared gourmet meal, all the while entertaining us with his signature brilliant quips and observations. Such was his class, such his chic.

I can divide my association with Omar into three distinct phases. The first phase starting long-distance in the early summer of 2007 was all business: we were preoccupied with questions of what hospital he should choose, which surgeon; whether he should seek a second opinion in Boston; whether he should receive one combination of chemotherapy or another.

The second phase came when he started the dreaded but inevitable slash-poison-burn cycles. Omar underwent radical surgery first, where surgeons tried to remove the tumor in its entirety. Reports from the excised mass unfortunately showed that cancer had already spilled into the veins. This was essentially a death sentence. In an attempt to eradicate the microscopic tumor cells, aggressive rounds of chemotherapies and radiation therapies were initiated. He settled more or less into a routine of sorts, punctuated by periods of pancytopenia, or a decrease in the number of blood cells; an intense susceptibility to infections; excoriated mouth; an occasional hospitalization due to sepsis; and finally, a brief period of respite, only to be followed by more of the same.

He suffered horrible toxicities from each treatment and derived little benefit. The tumor continued to grow. One week, a nodule sprouted in the lung, where it appeared surreptitiously on the CT scan. Another morning, a tender, red lump appeared on the wrist.

Once during this time, I asked Naheed in front of Omar why she did not go back to Karachi for a few days. Her mother was ailing, and Naheed needed to fetch her own things, as she was now planning to stay for the long haul, at least until Omar's chemotherapy ended. "He will not let me go," she simply said. I looked at Omar. It was true. He could not bear to let her out of his sight. "Azra apa, [*apa* and *aps* are terms of respect accorded an older woman]," he said, "if a mother is around, nothing bad can happen to her child." So Naheed, who had come for a few days to New York, ended up staying for eighteen months, spending practically 90 percent of her waking time either with Omar or working on something related to him.

Surprisingly, this second phase, perhaps the most exhausting for any normal individual, proved to be the most productive for Omar. He was teaching at John Jay College; he was analyzing current events; he was teeming with original ideas; he was writing profusely. Above all, he was confident and optimistic. He was newly married.

He never lost the life of the mind. He came to dinner at my place in May 2008, when Richard Dawkins was visiting. Naheed had brought her fabulous book, *Kashmiri Shawl,* as a present for Richard, who was thrilled to take it home to his wife, a fellow aficionado. Omar had prepared a series of questions to ask and had a long chat with Richard. In early June, Omar called me one evening to say that, as opposed to someone who has come up with a list of the hundred books one must read before dying, he had compiled a list of a hundred books that one must read in order to live. Would I be interested in going over the list with him? My friend Sara Suleri Goodyear, professor in the English department at Yale, was staying with me at the time. We were both delighted at this idea and arranged for Omar to come over for dinner with his list. That evening turned out to be exceptionally stimulating. Sara and I offered our remarks on the titles that Omar rolled out with a twinkle in his eyes. Most of our own personal favorites appeared on his list—from Homer, Plato, Aristotle, Herodotus, Thucydides, and Virgil to the Old and New Testaments, the Bhagavad Gita, and the Quran to Machiavelli, Omar Khayyam, and Aesop's Fables. He listed Augustine, Cervantes, Dostoevsky, Tolstoy, Ibsen, Flaubert, Proust, Lampedusa, Ishiguro, Rushdie, Adam Smith, Darwin, Hawking, Stilgitz, Pinker, and Bertrand Russell to Feynman, Kuhn, and Diamond. The entire list can be seen in the article I wrote about him for 3 Quarks Daily. After he left, Sara and I talked late into the night about Omar. We marveled that someone so captivated by life, so engaged, so erudite, so *young*, could demonstrate such equanimity in the face of almost certain death.

The third phase of my acquaintance with Omar began around September 2008. He was now on a slippery slope and knew it. Despite multiple surgeries to remove metastatic lesions, including parts of both lungs, he continued to experience recurrences at distant sites. On the day we came together to celebrate his fortieth birthday, he was diagnosed with a large mass on the arm even while receiving chemotherapy. This was not good news.

Omar's family responded. Naheed, his best friend, Noor, and his devoted, inspiring, and lovely wife, Mursi, brought him to see Dr. Gerald Rosen, a well-known bone and soft-tissue sarcoma expert at St. Vincent's Comprehensive Cancer Center. Gerry advised a second round of radical surgery to remove practically half his shoulder, arm, and chest, hoping that would excise a wide margin around the primary tumor, which Gerry felt strongly was the principle origin of the malignant cells. Gerry offered to arrange with surgeons he knew to undertake the risky and extensive surgery, insisting that this was absolutely essential. With Omar's tumor, as with most solid tumors, Gerry felt that if it couldn't be cut out, the battle was already lost. The surgical team at the treating hospital was not in favor of this, and Omar was torn. The four came to my office after their visit with Gerry. Omar pointedly asked my opinion, and I was blunt with him. "The radical surgery Gerry is recommending is an enormous risk, but it is the only lifesaving measure. You are young, and the odds are high that you will get through it fine. Give yourself a chance and go for the surgery." The alternative was an experimental trial. Under the best of circumstances, as I told Omar, trial drugs would prolong his life by a few months. Surgery represented the only possibility of a cure, even if it was fraught with potential catastrophes. But if he wanted to pursue an experimental trial, I told him, I promised to get him any drug he wanted. Omar listened calmly and finally said he would think about what I had said.

Informing Omar's thinking were his two siblings, who had been working valiantly throughout to save their brother's life. They searched incessantly for news of any novel approaches to therapy or announcements of clinical trials. Sara, Omar's sister, came to see him with her adorable little boy, and Omar was immensely cheered up by their visit. (One of the loveliest things about Omar was that while he was interested in big things, he knew how to be genuinely happy in small ways.) He brought Sara over for dinner one evening. I was astounded by the detailed questions Sara asked me about Omar's situation, the choices available to him, his immediate and long-term prognosis. His brother, Farid, was completing his doctoral dissertation at Brown, but he nonetheless spent every moment he could spare with Omar. Farid accompanied Omar to his medical appointments whenever he was in town and stayed with him at the hospital when Omar was an inpatient. One evening as they were leaving my home, I was greatly touched to see Farid quietly adjust the sling on Omar's arm and help him into his coat without a word from Omar, who continued talking to me the entire time.

Although deeply involved, Omar's family as well as his friends completely respected Omar's independence and supported him unconditionally whether they agreed with his decisions or not. They stood resolutely by him and faced the tragic choices with a fortitude that reminded me on more than one occasion of the famous line from Faiz Sahib: *"Jo aye aye ke hum dil kushada rakhtay hain"* (Let whatever is in store come; our hearts are capacious).

In the end, Omar decided against the radical surgery that Dr. Rosen had recommended. He called me a couple of days later to ask my help in getting him enrolled in an experimental trial. He subsequently began one at Montefiore Medical Center and seemed in an unusually good mood when he and Mursi came for lunch at my place in November. By early January, however, the trial had failed, and he was exploring other possibilities with his usual vigor and velocity. We were all frantically searching. He became fixated on a drug called dasatinib, which was being tried in his type of sarcoma, although he was reluctant to participate in another experimental trial because it would restrict his ability to try other therapies. I promised to obtain a compassionate exemption for him from the makers of the drug and wrote a single subject protocol requesting the drug for him.

Omar had now lived through seven major surgeries—removal of practically half the shoulder followed by removal of parts of the right lung and then the left. He had received round after round of toxic chemotherapies with bouts of radiation treatments in between. He then enrolled in experimental trials with zero benefit. Meanwhile, the tumors kept popping up in new parts of his body.

⌘

OMAR'S PREDICAMENT HIGHLIGHTS how spectacularly we are failing to treat cancer.

His treating oncologists and I knew that the chemotherapy or experimental drugs he received following the failure of the original surgery had zero chance of curing him. If palliation was all we could offer postoperatively, what was a better option—to treat or not to treat? Was it cruel to Omar and his family to keep suggesting new drugs, which would give him a few additional weeks at best, when the writing was on the wall? It's not clear they ever registered how short term any benefits would be. Omar and his family fully believed that, if a drug were FDA approved or at least in FDA-approved trials, there would be lifesaving benefits to offset the pain of any side effects. Did they really comprehend the fact that any survival benefit would be measurable in weeks?

The expectations of patients are compounded by the action of regulators. It takes ten to twelve years to bring a new cancer drug into the market at a prohibitive cost of anywhere from $500 million to $2.6 billion. Extensive intellectual and financial resources as well as time are invested in conducting preclinical research to identify potential new therapies for cancer, but these rarely translate into any real benefit for the patients. Only 3–5 percent of cancer patients participate in experimental trials; of these, only 3.8 percent of the participants in phase 1 trials between 1991 and 2002 achieved an objective clinical response. The results for phase 2 and 3 trials are not much better.

Recognizing the unmet need in oncology and pressured by advocacy groups and cancer patients, the FDA is willing to approve an agent if it can prolong survival by a mere 2.5 months over existing treatments. Even with this low bar for approval, only 5 percent of drugs make it to market. Cancer has the lowest success rate among twenty-one disease indications. Those few drugs that are approved might as well have failed; once they are administered in non-trial settings, the results are no better than those that were not approved. This is partly because of how trials are conducted. Subjects participating in experimental protocols are handpicked and generally in reasonable physical shape. They have to pass strict eligibility criteria, including a good performance status, normally functioning heart, lungs, liver, and kidneys, and be free of any serious comorbid condition. Most cancer patients are more decrepit, suffering from additional comorbidities. Whatever little advantage is achieved in prolonging survival under the rigorously supervised clinical trial settings is lost once the drug is approved and used freely by practicing oncologists to treat unselected patients.

Over the twelve-year period from 2002 to 2014, seventy-two new anticancer drugs gained FDA approval; they prolonged survival by 2.1 months. Of eighty-six cancer therapies for solid tumors approved between 2006 and 2017, the median gain in overall survival was 2.45 months. Of the cancer drugs approved during the past two decades, 70 percent of them were at best useless, showing no measurable survival benefit. Between 30 and 70 percent of the drugs may actually be harmful to patients. A study published in the *British Medical Journal* showed that thirty-nine of sixty-eight cancer drugs approved by the European regulators between 2009 and 2013 showed no improvement in survival or quality of life over existing treatment, placebo, or in combinations with other agents. My own specialty, MDS, is a case in point. There are two approved strategies to treat MDS. One drug, lenalidomide (Revlimid), is restricted for a subset of patients, roughly 10 percent, whose MDS cells have a deletion in the long arm of chromosome 5. For the remaining 90 percent, one of two approved drugs, azacitidine (Vidaza) or decitabine (Dacogen), are recommended. With either drug, the chance of improving anemia in low-risk MDS, to the point at which transfusions would no longer be needed, is approximately 20 percent. There is currently no way to preselect the 20 percent of patients likely to respond. This means 80 percent will receive chemotherapy for five to seven days every month for a minimum of six months with little or no benefit but with all attendant toxicities and at prohibitive financial expense. In responding patients, the drug administration must continue for as long as there is no progression in the disease. Responders are not cured; the median duration of response is ten months, and an occasional patient continues in remission for years.

So what advice should an oncologist give to a patient faced with these options? In a larger sense, the choices we make for our patients are made by people we never meet. Even if I felt differently, I could not make a truly independent decision. Other experts have devised formal criteria for best practices, and any nonconformity could leave the deviant open to legal challenges. Driven by internal forces, we seek refuge in emulation. Responsibility is assumed collectively by a group of key opinion leaders, or KOLs, in the field. The group takes into account all the existing scientific literature and a fair summary of innumerable clinical trials to eventually distill the experience into a broad set of principles. The guidelines that emerge are at the heart of evidence-based medicine, and the wider community of oncologists subsequently uses these to classify, stage, and treat their cancer patients, evaluating the results of their treatment in a uniform and universally interpretable language.

This is a good thing. Indeed, evidence-based medicine is essential. But it is not sufficient by itself when caring for individual patients. No matter how large or statistically significant the data are from which the universal rules are derived, application of population-based insights to specific patients remains very challenging. The typical experimental trial with a 30 percent response rate is really telling us that if a hundred patients with similar clinical and biologic characteristics were treated with the drug, thirty will likely respond. For an individual patient today, we have no way of knowing whether they are one of the 30 percent who respond or the 70 percent who don't. Besides, how meaningful is the response? If the median duration of response is, say, ten months, then of the thirty patients who responded, fifteen will lose the response before ten months, and fifteen will continue to benefit beyond that. A few of those will be long-term responders. The disease will come back. This rule applies to even the most successful targeted therapies today with only rare exceptions. They offer improvement in survival by a few months over supportive care. Nevertheless, when I'm faced with an elderly patient with lower-risk MDS without deletion of chromosome 5, receiving two units of blood every two to three weeks, the KOLs say I should give the FDA-approved treatment, despite its 20 percent chance of a limited-duration response. And when faced with a patient like Omar, should experimental trials be offered if the treatment is of no survival benefit? Again, the KOLs say yes.

Imagine now, with these data in hand, you are sitting across the desk from Omar. It is impossible to use the best evidence-based medicine derived from large populations to make decisions about him as an individual. There is embarrassingly little information to predict the most likely outcome for Omar. If he were one of the fortunate ones, then we hoped he would be that rare long-term responder. We had to give it a shot. Nothing ventured, nothing gained.

The oncologists believed that by treating Omar with experimental drugs and chemoradiation therapy, they at least offered him a chance of response, no matter what the odds. But the problem isn't simply that the drugs he was given ultimately didn't help him—the problem was with the advice he got, too. It's possible the advice we gave him wasn't realistic or explicit enough—perhaps we should have suggested he spend whatever time he had left enjoying life rather than vomiting his guts out after each round of chemotherapy and living on revolting, tasteless liquids because of the raw carbuncles that studded his throat. He could have spent at least a little time traveling with his new wife, visiting friends in England and his family in Pakistan and Bangladesh. Instead, Omar was a perpetual captive; either he was receiving one kind of therapy or another or suffering their side effects, which, beside the vomiting and the ravaged mouth, included very low blood counts and a highly suppressed immune system, landing him in the hospital regularly with bouts of infections.

Was it really the best solution to do nothing? If we had withheld treatment, the tumors would have grown rapidly and caused tremendous pain as well. Which would be less excruciating? Subjecting patients to painful toxicities of futile treatments with their enormous attendant physical, financial, emotional, and psychological burdens is challenging. Would palliation of the pain with local control of growing tumor masses have been any less painful? Did we ever give Omar the choice of no treatment at all? And should we have? The past is some guide. The toxicities of chemotherapy and radiation therapy are well recognized today, whereas it has become rare to see the ravages of unconstrained cancer. Stephen Hall, in his excellent book *A Commotion in the Blood*, describes the last stages of a highly malignant sarcoma in a young girl at the end of the nineteenth century:

> The endgame in cancer is never pretty, less so in an era where doctors chased rather than managed the less ghastly symptoms. The breast tumors had become the size of goose eggs, the abdominal tumor even larger; the length of her body from head to toe was stippled by small tumors that Coley likened to buckshot or split peas. Last came the vomiting, several times a day, though she had no solid food; soon, she was regurgitating copious amounts of blood. "The attacks occurred almost hourly," Coley noted, "and were very exhausting to the patient in her extremely weak condition." Elizabeth Dashiell remained conscious of this horrific piracy of her eighteen-year-old body until very nearly the end, when finally, mercifully, she died at home in New Jersey at 7:00 a.m. on January 23, 1891.

Not only is such an uncontrolled death horrible, hopes are squandered on chasing cures that can't be found. But then, unexpected benefit can also occur, even after ten years of repeated failures, if the right drug is given. The challenge is how to match the right drug to the right patient from the start.

One patient of mine, Philip Kolman, suffering from a lower-risk MDS, was essentially giving himself up for dead. In his own telling, "One day in early 2017, my Florida doctor told me that he had nothing left to give me. My transfusions were becoming very frequent, two or three units of blood a week. He said that I should contact everyone I knew to see if there was a [research] program available for me." In stark contrast to Omar and his siblings, Kolman says, "I accepted the news with the understanding that I didn't have much time left, and I started to make final arrangements." Among them was to write to me.

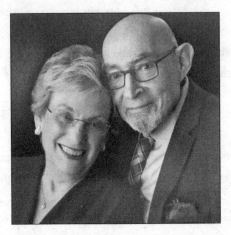

Although he was prepared to lie down, I was not; I told him to fly to New York for tests for a new research program. Once he was in, his need for transfusions quickly dropped from every week to every four to five weeks; his condition worsened a bit before stabilizing at a transfusion every two to three weeks. "I'm now waiting for the next drug to come along with its promise of a new beginning and hope."

◈

WEEKS BEFORE HIS death, I visited Omar at home on his fortieth birthday. He was quite the dandy, and that evening, he had taken care to dress up. He wore a formal black jacket and beautifully fitting trousers. With an impossible innocence, he took me aside. He had something to show me: a rock-hard reddish growth that had appeared out of nowhere on his arm in the preceding forty-eight hours. With an indefatigable will to live, the exceptionally intelligent young man stared intently at his arm and asked me whether I thought it meant the return of the sarcoma. He hoped I would say no, that it was an infection. It was the one time during the course of my time with Omar that I felt physically ill— and I was not even his family. It wounded me to think of how Mursi and Kamal, Sara and Farid, and most of all Naheed would take the cancer's resurgence. I could not bear to stay at the party. Despite Naheed's remonstrations, I left within minutes, and before I could reach the subway, I was retching on the sidewalk.

My husband, Harvey Preisler, was directing the Rush University Cancer Center in Chicago when, at fifty-seven years of age, he received the diagnosis of cancer. He had personally supervised my training in oncology. One rule he emphasized was not to become too close to patients. I am not certain that I have followed his advice as faithfully as he wanted me to. He appalled me when he said, "You are going to take care of me."

"But, Harvey," I objected, "all my life, you are the one who insisted that I could no longer remain objective if my feelings clouded my clinical decisions."

He simply said, "Sorry, I only trust your judgment."

In the subsequent five years, we looked at countless blood reports, MRIs, and CAT scans together, staring at the growing masses in his abdomen, the persistent fungal infection spreading menacingly in the lungs. Harvey knew precisely what those images meant. He was not someone looking for false hope. He was not a man easily duped. Yet he would invariably turn to me and ask, "So what do you think, Az?" He needed to suspend his judgment and looked to me to decide how he should feel. I took infinite care never to break his spirit.

Julie Yip-Williams, who blogged about her colon cancer and died on March 19, 2018, at age forty-two, said, "Cancer crushes hope, leaving a wasteland of grief, depression, despair and a sense of unending futility. Hope is a funny thing, though. It seems to have a life and will of its own that I cannot control through the sheer force of my mind. It is irrepressible, its very existence inextricably tied to our very spirit, its flame, no matter how weak, not extinguishable."

What were Omar's choices? Succumb to hopelessness and despair, face the terrified looks of his wife and mother who followed his every move, or pin his hopes on the oncologists pushing the limits of modern medical offerings? With cancer, it is rarely a matter of either-or; there is seldom a choice between hope and despair. Patients face both simultaneously, or serially. Omar did, too, with a stoic's sobriety combined with an unflagging optimism of will.

∞

OMAR'S EXPERIENCES, AND Philip's, point to some devastating concerns about the state of cancer research today.

A common semantic distortion relates to the description of an ineffective therapy as "the patient failed the drug" instead of the other way around. The drugs, not the patients, arrive at the bedside for clinical trials when confidence in their success is 5 percent at best. The preclinical lab data used to identify the potential benefits of a drug cannot predict what will actually work in a clinical setting. We were forced to use trial and error both in Omar's case and Philip's, instead of being able to identify sooner what could or could not work for each, at great financial and personal cost. What are we doing wrong? Why have we failed to translate the scientific advances of high-profile publications into improved outcome for our patients?

It is high time to question the current paradigm of research. There are bright spots—many subsets of patients, even with aggressive tumors, have been successfully treated with drugs developed using the present approaches: chronic myeloid leukemia, most childhood malignancies, and some forms of adult bone marrow and lymphoid cancers. We shall see why. But we shall also see that the exceptions exist among a litany of failures. These failures are systemic. The vast majority of researchers are studying diseases they never see, in animals who don't get them spontaneously, or in test tubes where the "cancer" must be artificially created and maintained. Such contrived data bear little resemblance to the actual tumors, yet these "models" are the ones turned over to industry for further clinical development. This approach to drug development, the exceptions notwithstanding, has been stupendously unhelpful. How did we get here?

IN JANUARY 1912, Alexis Carrel, soon to be a Nobel laureate for work in surgery, removed cells from the heart of a chicken embryo, plated them on a dish in his laboratory, and, to the great surprise of the scientific community, kept them alive and growing robustly for the next three decades. The cells thrived as long as they were fed the right cocktail of nutrients, and Carrel's miraculous culture led to the conclusion that living cells have the potential for immortality. Unfortunately, no one else could replicate Carrel's results—in general, investigators could maintain cells in culture, but no one could demonstrate the continuity of survival for weeks, let alone decades—nor explain what enabled them to survive in Carrel's flasks.

The question whether cells possess the potential for immortality remained unresolved until 1960, when Leonard Hayflick provided the answer. Through a complex series of experiments, Hayflick succeeded in routinely growing cells in culture for long periods, but not forever. Cells are not immortal. They age and they die. If external forces do not kill them first, Hayflick found that, after roughly forty-five divisions—known today as the *Hayflick limit*—cells follow one of two paths. Either they eventually dial down their activities to the bare minimum necessary for viability, curl up, and enter a period of senescence, or they commit suicide. Carrel, Hayflick argued, could not have been culturing his original cells all those years. Instead, the nutrient solution Carrel used daily to feed the cultures most likely contained viable embryonic stem cells, which seeded and grew on their own.

The Hayflick limit, accepted as a golden rule of biology, has proved to be true for normal cells ever since. Cancer cells, however, are different. One tumor took off in the laboratory and achieved immortality. On February 8, 1951, a cervical cancer was removed from Henrietta Lacks and brought to the laboratory of George Otto Gey. HeLa cells, labeled using the first two letters of the patient's first and last names, began to thrive in culture, giving rise to the first human tissue culture "cell line." Acting almost as if they were a monstrous superorganism, HeLa cells have steamrollered their way from test tubes to animals, gulping cocktails of nutritious chemicals, floating in flasks and cutting jagged paths across methylcellulose-coated petri dishes, climbing, creeping, fanning, and expanding perpetually for six decades. They metamorphosed; compared to the normal human cell's chromosome number of 46, their chromosome number varies between 70 and 164. HeLa cells are unique in their ability to survive under the most challenging environmental conditions, carving out a space for themselves with unmatched velocity, be it in inorganic flasks or in mice.

To date, some forty thousand pounds of HeLa cells have been grown, studied, molecularly dissected, genetically reprogrammed, used as teaching tools for graduate students, formed the backbone of elaborate, major grant proposals, and otherwise spread throughout science. This orgy has led to an embarrassment of riches for the researchers, earning for them thousands of patents covering diseases ranging from polio to cancer. Ironically, this unexpected gift, an enormous boon for researchers, exchanged hands and laboratories, crossed oceans and continents, all without the knowledge or consent of Ms. Lacks, who died eight months after the original tumor was plucked from her pelvis. (Rebecca Skloot skillfully recounts the scandalous drama of HeLa cells, involving interactions of race and research, greed, business, and bioethical issues, in her 2010 best-selling book, *The Immortal Life of Henrietta Lacks*.)

The consistent, predictable growth and behavior of HeLa cells provided researchers with an opportunity to experiment, including tests of the efficacy of a number of agents, on a reproducible in vitro model. The success with HeLa led to the broader discovery that, with practice, skill, and a little luck, malignant cells from a variety of tumors could be induced to grow continuously in the laboratory. This in turn gave birth to development of additional cell lines, and researchers flooded the field with a deluge of experiments conducted on all types of cancers.

Many such experiments examined the effects of potential anticancer agents on these tissue culture cell lines with the hopes of developing reliable methods to predict responsiveness. The question was, how faithful are cell lines to their ancestry? Partially so. The success of a tumor in a human (or any other animal) depends on many factors, including how well it has managed to subvert the tissues in which it exists to support its growth at the expense of normal cells surrounding it. Cell lines are created by removing tumor cells from this natural habitat, forcing them to adapt to a new, and hostile, environment. The journey from an organ to plastic containers results in the creation of almost a new species of cells that diverge wildly from their parents in morphology, genotype, phenotype, and biologic behavior. The artificially grown cells can only replicate some but not all the characteristics of the cells from which they originated. As a rule, for example, they don't grow in perpetuity. To survive for any length of time, however, additional transformative changes occur, affecting not just the raw material of genome but also the expression of genes, so that before long, cells in vitro bear little resemblance to the parent from which they originated. For one thing, the doubling time of cultured cells is much faster. In fact, they are selected for long-term passages in the lab precisely because of their ability to divide rapidly and grow furiously. Cultured cancer cells also have a very different relationship with oxygen. In the body, cancer cells exist with low levels of oxygen, whereas those in the lab come to require significantly higher oxygen levels—up to ten times as high.

In addition to acquired genetic mutations, another issue with cultured cells relates to expression of genes as messenger RNAs. The sum of all transcripts representing expression at the RNA level is called the *transcriptome.* When gene expression profiles of various cell lines derived from different cancers were studied, the transcriptomes of the cell lines resembled each other more than they did the cells of organs from which they were derived.

Compounding the issues was the discovery that some of the fastest-growing cultured cells regularly find their way into adjacent plates, even under the most stringent of lab protocols. The first hint of trouble came as early as the 1970s, when chromosomal studies of cell lines derived from a variety of cancers showed that all appeared contaminated with HeLa cells, which turned out to be the Mother of All Contaminants.

Drugs tested on these cell lines could reliably predict response in the cell lines. The in vitro test showed no predictive value when brought to the bedside. HeLa cells accurately predicted the efficacy of drugs for HeLa cells. Not humans. Despite their utility for genetic and scientific experiments, cells cultured in vitro could not be relied on for drug development.

At that point, it might have been logical to give up the idea of in vitro modeling attempts for drug development. Instead, more artificiality was introduced into the preclinical model. Although it appeared that cell lines grown in animal models instead of plastic dishes were more comparable to cancers thriving in humans, it was not clear what the precise in vivo requirements were for hospitable and—importantly—comparable growth. The infinite complexity of a human body was neither comprehensible nor reproducible. Instead, researchers sought to hijack the body of a surrogate to grow these tumor cell lines. Enter the mouse model.

∽

ON THE MORNING of May 3, 1998, my husband, Harvey, having been diagnosed with cancer in March, looked over his coffee mug and handed me the *New York Times*. HOPE IN THE LAB, a headline shouted. A CAUTIOUS AWE GREETS DRUGS THAT ERADICATE TUMORS IN MICE. The gobsmacking opening line of the article read: "Within a year, if all goes well, the first cancer patient will be injected with two new drugs that can eradicate any type of cancer, with no obvious side effects and no drug resistance—in mice. Some cancer researchers say the drugs are the most exciting treatment that they have ever seen." Richard D. Klausner, the director of the National Cancer Institute, was quoted calling the work "the single most exciting thing on the horizon." Jim

Watson, the Nobelist for discovering the structure of DNA, said, "Judah is going to cure cancer in two years." Judah Folkman himself, the researcher at the heart of the story, was more cautious; as the article's author, Gina Kolata, put it, "All he knows, Dr. Folkman said, is that 'If you have cancer and you are a mouse, we can take good care of you.'"

Harvey and I had lived through many cycles of frenzy in our professional life caused by laboratory triumphs of drugs followed by dashed hopes in humans. Now our relationship was more personal. Harvey expressed skepticism, yet a cancer patient's wistful anticipation had propelled him to ask me what I thought in the first place. The basic premise of the strategy was exciting and the animal data deeply compelling. Both drugs acted by cutting off the blood supply of tumors, causing starvation, growth arrest, and eventual regression without producing any toxicity. Thanks to the *New York Times* report, the sensational story leaped from the confines of a research laboratory in Boston to make headlines in newspapers and television broadcasts across the nation. Cancer patients pleaded with their oncologists, desperate to get the drugs, imploring to be selected for clinical trials, ready to travel anywhere needed. The stock price of the company EntreMed, which produced the drugs, shot up fivefold in one morning, soaring from twelve dollars to eighty-five dollars. I got in touch with Dr. Folkman, who was exceptionally responsive and kind. He invited me to a daylong scientific conference in Boston where all the data along with clinical trial plans were to be presented. I registered for the meeting and came back greatly encouraged about the possibility of rapid translational success. Within a short time, word got out: however spectacularly the drugs worked in mice, they failed spectacularly in humans.

Although mice and human lineages diverged about eighty-five million years ago, humans have been recording observations related to physiologic traits in mice since the dawn of civilization. The systematic practice to understand human ontogeny through a study of anatomy and physiology in animal models dates back to ancient Greece, and as Aristotelian methodology traveled along the ancient trade routes, animal models became the preferred research tool of Arab and later European physicians.

Domestication of a variety of mice as pets occurred in China and Japan in the eighteenth century, eventually leading to the development and creation of modern laboratory mice. While Victorian England was busy trading in "fancy" mice, the use of animal models had become the established method to conduct biologic studies by the beginning of the twentieth century. Theories of Mendelian inheritance were investigated through mating programs in mice, and genetic mapping was well under way as early as 1915. A variety of approaches was pursued in developing mouse models for cancer research, and as is true for every model, each had its advantages and its limitations. Approximately 97 percent of human genes have homologues in the mouse genome, for example—a clear advantage versus other laboratory organisms. But the nucleotide sequences of mouse and human genomes are only about 50 percent identical.

Many of these differences are directly owed to the dissimilarities in the environment in which the two species evolved. The major dissimilarities between mice and humans relate to factors such as the life cycle of mice. They reach sexual maturity at six to eight weeks, gestate a litter of five to eight pups in less than three weeks, and live only about three years. Mice have a metabolic rate seven times greater than humans. Since drugs in mouse models are very rapidly metabolized, the amount used in mice and humans is very different. The dosage of drugs is reduced drastically when used in clinical trials. The immune system in mice evolved to combat earthborn pathogens, whereas most of our challenges come from airborne pathogens. This stark difference in the immune systems is reflected in the cell types circulating in the blood of the two species. Humans have 70 percent neutrophils and 30 percent lymphocytes, while mice have 10 percent neutrophils and 90 percent lymphocytes in the blood. Besides these glaring differences, one of the biggest challenges in using mice as the in vivo host to human tumor cells is that, unlike a human with cancer, the target lab mice are healthy. To accept transplanted human cells without having a mouse's body reject them as foreign bodies, the immune system of the recipient mouse has to be destroyed first. Such immunocompromised mice could hardly represent the in vivo environment of the human body in which cancer cells thrive. Yet scientists fully expected the behavior of these cells to help them identify useful drugs for patients.

The idea of using an animal to provide the vital growth environment for tumor cells led to the birth of today's most frequently used cell line–derived xenografts (CDX). Tissue culture cell lines were injected into mice with the intent of creating a more reliable model for cancer therapeutics. Use of animal models as preclinical platforms for cancer drug development began in earnest with the mouse-in-mouse grafted tumors during the 1960s. Such models produced by transplanting a given mouse tumor yielded early successes in that several cytotoxic chemotherapies like procarbazine and vincristine were identified and proved useful in the treatment of a host of cancers. That does not say much for the efficiency of the CDX model per se because cytotoxic drugs kill cells indiscriminately, be they normal or cancerous. This is why they are so toxic when administered to patients. The same results would likely be seen in less elaborately constructed, cheaper cell culture systems. Nevertheless, CDX became the model of choice for all kinds of drug development. Responses to cytotoxic drugs ranged between 25 and 70 percent among different cancer types. The NCI invested generously in producing between six and nine cell lines each, derived from a number of common tumor types, hoping that this would cover the variability seen in efficacy. This led to the creation of the NCI-60 panel, comprising sixty cell lines derived from nine types of cancers, which was then handed over to investigators for the development of CDX models.

They failed uniformly as far as drug development was concerned.

In reality, such models for drug development represent an irresponsible and serious waste of shrinking research resources, and not just in oncology. Sepsis, burns, and trauma in animals were all investigated as models for the inflammatory changes associated with those phenomena in humans. There was no correlation. Indeed, every one of the 150 treatments for sepsis brought to the bedside of acutely ill humans because of their success in treating mice was a staggering catastrophe.

Humans do not benefit but are harmed by misleading animal testing, especially when it comes to predicting the efficacy of targeted therapies. These are drugs developed to attack individual and specific cancer-driving proteins. The targeted therapies identified through CDX models have an abysmal success rate of 5–7 percent when brought into clinical practice. This includes the agents developed to target genetic mutations such as BRAF, EGFR, HER2, and a few others. When occasional drugs appear to work in both humans and the in vitro models, it is not because of similarities in the biology of the diseases but because the drugs happen to be general cytotoxic agents. Timothy Johnson, a physician, told the *Boston Globe* during the height of the enthusiasm for Folkman's work that "my own medical perspective is that animal cancer research should be regarded as the scientific equivalent of gossip—with about the same chance of turning out to be true, i.e. truly effective in humans. Some gossip turns out to be true, but most of it does not . . . and gossip can cause great anguish for those affected, in this case millions of desperate cancer patients worldwide." He was right.

As various in vitro and CDX efforts failed, focus then turned to improving quality of the cancerous seed rather than the soil in which it was planted. Instead of using cultured cell lines as starting points for creating a preclinical in vivo CDX model, freshly obtained human tumors were implanted in animals, at times, even matching organ to organ; cancer cells from human pancreas implanted in mouse pancreas. These patient-derived xenografts (PDX) models could serve as "avatars" for individual patients to test a variety of drugs against their tumor cells directly as they grew in vivo in a mouse. Once again, the NCI invested large sums of money in producing and handing out one hundred PDXs to investigators for research.

Unfortunately, the technique didn't always work. In one instance, a laboratory company pursuing this research was able to culture tumors for only half of the 1,163 people who sought their help. The researchers ultimately found only 92 patients who received treatments based on testing in the PDX models, although they did find that the PDX predictions were accurate 87 percent of the time. How practical this approach would be is questionable since it can take six weeks or more for the tumor to grow in the mouse and be ready for appropriate testing against a series of drugs.

But, the above notwithstanding, there are strong signs that PDX is, generally, not going to be predictive, again owing to adaptations for the implanted tumor to its new environment. To study how the genome of the tumor changed through multiple rounds of transplantation in mice, more than one thousand PDXs representing twenty-four types of cancers were studied. Implanted tumors evolved differently from their parent cells. While glioblastomas gain extra copies of chromosome 7 in humans, the PDX model of the tumor lost them over time. The National Cancer Institute tested twelve anticancer drugs—that were already being successfully used to treat humans—on PDX mice growing forty-eight different kinds of human cancers. In 63 percent of cases, the drugs failed. Even worse, according to a report in *Nature* on the study, researchers at the NCI concluded that other compounds that might work in humans were never tested on the erroneous belief that if they couldn't help PDX mice, they couldn't help humans either. But from my perspective, even if the models worked as well as we had hoped they would, the fundamental problem would still remain—very few effective anticancer treatments exist, so the predictions made through these models are more likely to be useful in what to avoid rather than what to give the patient. I cannot stress this enough times; scientists need to stop making more and more artificial mouse models and tissue culture cell lines for cancer drug development. These resources can and should be invested in better pursuits.

No one, however, willingly surrenders their pet projects, no matter how far they have drifted from the original intent, as long as they can maintain their grip on grants and power. A repetitive triangular pattern characterizes the scientific culture, similar to the *kyklos,* the recurrent cycles of government, described by the Greeks, of democracy, aristocracy, and monarchy along with their degenerate forms—ochlocracy, oligarchy, and tyranny. What begins as a perfectly sensible democratic state of affairs transmutes into an oligarchy when a small group of privileged individuals exercising control over institutions and organizations handing out perquisites succeed in dominating the field. The democratic-to-oligarchic shift gives rise over time to a "hereditary aristocracy" in which newly minted key opinion leaders, with the blessing of their scientific mentors, inherit the exclusive power to define rules, monopolize grant-funding powers, and reward each other with perks the field has to offer. Adding a final insult to injury, these little arrogant cliques manage to hijack the entire narrative in a field.

I met a young male researcher recently whose ego was so dense, light would bend around him. He presented a seminar at Columbia University, where he described mouse models carrying a mutated gene associated with MDS. He also presented data that administering a drug that inhibited activity of the protein, not the mutated protein, was curing whatever disease he had inflicted upon the mice (it certainly was not anything even close to human MDS). When I asked him what gave him any confidence that the results of the drug therapy he showed in mice would have value for humans, he scoffed, "Sorry, Azra, mouse models are not going away." That was already two years ago. I am sure he has cured a lot more mice since then. I am also sure he has received grants to continue this work. His coresearcher at the same institution started a recent lecture with a slide comparing survival curves of AML patients for each decade from 1970 to the present. The graph showed essentially zero improvement. He then used words I have been hearing for forty years describing how he was going to understand the intricate molecular mechanisms inside AML cells and then devise ways not to kill them but to modify their behavior so they no longer remained malignant. This is precisely the problem. It is as if the past forty years have not existed. Freshly minted brilliant young scientists arriving in waves, confidently proclaiming their plans to convert cancer into a chronic disease that patients can live with and not die from. On what basis? Indeed, there are unimagined novel technologies now that did not exist a few decades ago, but the complexity of cancer remains beyond their reach. To think otherwise is unrealistic and a victory of hope over experience.

Clinical researchers are busy trying to open new experimental trials, and basic researchers are worrying over the next grant they need to write. The only way to unmask the magnitude of bizarreness is to find a new and improved way of doing things, a way not just marginally better but quantum leaps better. This is precisely what oncology needs right now. If we'd kept trying to improve upon the typewriter, we would never have invented the word processor. Toying with or repairing old models of treating cancer will yield incremental advances at best. The cancer problem requires a radically different approach. We should not be aiming for weeks of improved survival. Our goals should be higher. The public needs to see how far we have drifted from the original aims as oncologists and researchers and at what cost to the patient.

Everyone needs to pause and think about what they are doing and why. Young researchers and all oncologists must think differently, to question dogma, to reject the deep-rooted archaic traditions, to discard the existing, inadequate research models and boldly use the emerging technologies to explore exciting new strategies to solve the cancer problem. Only a new way of thinking and doing will shift the paradigm and get the practitioners to discard their old ways. *All* researchers need to pay attention to technologic aspects emerging within and outside of their own disciplines, developing a broader strategy to address the complexity of cancer by using inclusive, pluralistic approaches rather than relying solely on reductionist strategies. Young researchers need to practice consilience, learning from and cooperating with experts in disparate fields to solve the biologic and technologic hurdles. The traditional strategy of treating cancer reached its maximum potential several decades ago. Dying for a Cure, a British advocacy group, bemoans that "at the current rate of progress it would take 1,778 years at least before we saw a 20-year survival improvement for all 200 types of cancer!"

For the next quantum leap, fundamentally different strategies have to be developed. The two immediate steps should be a shift from studying animals to studying humans and a shift from chasing after the last cancer cell to developing the means to detect the first cancer cell. Develop the technology, invent, create, collaborate, reach out across disciplines, harness all your intellectual and emotional faculties, and keep reminding yourself that your first and last duty is to the cancer patients.

Scientists continue to perpetuate various incarnations of the mouse model, changing the seed or the soil, tinkering with the immune system, knocking genes in and out to refine the mouse's ability to recapitulate the human disease for the same reason why oncologists cannot give up on trying one barely effective drug after another in patients. Each is a captive of the system that demands great exactitude in details while bypassing the fidelity of the fundamental proposition. Scientists are busy questioning the number of controls or drug doses in an experiment rather than looking to see why there is a 5 percent success rate for drugs developed through their preclinical platform. Oncologists spend most of their time balancing electrolytes rather than balancing the patient's unrealistic expectations. Both suspend judgment faced by a system that prescribes algorithms and demands algorithms; scientists cannot expect grant funding unless their experimental design includes an animal model, and oncologists follow guidelines provided by key opinion leaders or they are opening themselves to legal challenges. Oncologists let the key opinion leaders decide how they treat patients, and scientists let their mentors set the agenda. Oncologists have no better options to offer their patients, and scientists have no alternative to a mouse model for the kind of experiments they must perform to gain any detailed understanding of biologic phenomena. Both fail to question the basic premise, whether it relates to scientists using a profoundly flawed mouse model to develop drugs with a negligible chance of producing benefit, or oncologists administering costly and invariably toxic drugs expected at best to prolong survival of their patients by a few weeks. Both do what they do because this is all that is available for them to do. Both are looking for car keys not where they dropped them at night but under the lamppost because it is light there.

When I gave grand rounds at Columbia University recently, pointing out some of these issues, Ed Gelmann, my colleague and previous director of the division, said, "Azra, before the young people in the room slit their wrists, please tell them what they should be doing with their careers until a better cancer treatment is discovered."

My message to the young oncologists is that until you find a cure, make sure you are upholding the fundamental rule of medicine: primum non nocere—first, do no harm. Each physician evolves a unique clinical style of dealing with patients, but the one that never fails is spending more time with them. A surprising amount of success, as someone once said, comes from just showing up, and as Yogi Berra famously pronounced, "You can observe a lot by just watching."

Medicine is the most social of sciences, demanding heightened communication skills. Patients are anxious, distracted, knowing they have a fixed allotted time with their doctors. Disease, pain, and fear are disorienting. Often, patients cannot verbalize their deep anxieties without a prompt. Facing a "doorknob" doctor, whose one hand is always on the handle, they have no time to communicate their worries and expectations, their preferences. They are sensitive to the body language of their physicians, but their own bodies speak through a far more eloquent language. Instead of always reaching into the medicine shelves, doctors need to start reaching into the shelves containing books written in this corporeal language. They should consult their own libraries where the great works of fiction will teach them to link semiotics with the scientific, to interpret the human experience of disease, the illness part, written in the patients' notational system of nonverbal communication complete with its own unique syntax, semantics, and pragmatics.

Finding a new molecular signaling pathway in the cancer cell is great, of course, and it will earn you awards, acknowledgment in the field, and the respect of your peers. Trying to heal patients when they are dying from lack of treatment will not earn you gold medals or appear on your CV, but it will make you a better doctor and a finer human being, bring more peace to your own inner life, help you accept your own set of afflictions that life will inevitably hurl your way. Engaging in a narrative of humility; decoding the signs and symptoms of illness with empathy; and understanding that despite varied nationalities, each one of us has only one unique home—our bodies—will enrich interaction and help both sides accept and deal with the elusive, paradoxical, pernicious disease. The widely accepted 1964 version of the Hippocratic Oath succinctly encapsulates these practices: "I will apply, for the benefit of the sick, all measures [that] are required, avoiding those twin traps of overtreatment and therapeutic nihilism. I will remember that there is art to medicine as well as science, and that warmth, sympathy, and understanding may outweigh the surgeon's knife or the chemist's drug."

There is a very beautiful *sher* (couplet) by the great Urdu poet Ghalib:

Taufeeq ba andaza e himmat hay azal se
Aankhoun mein hay wu qatra jo gauhar na hua tha

From infinity, accomplishment rests on endurance
Rain's triumph lies in becoming a tear and not a pearl

The myth in Urdu poetry is that only the first few raindrops from the very first rains of the season have a chance of becoming a pearl if they land inside a clam. In this couplet, Ghalib provides consolation to raindrops that missed being the first of the season and therefore have no chance of becoming a pearl. He reminds them that they cannot become a pearl, but now they have the possibility of becoming a tear that comes out of the eyes of a lover. The cure part is the pearl; healing is the tear. You can do both.

When Philip Kolman wrote me, so, too, did his wife, Marsha, complimenting me generously on being an exceptional doctor. I wish I felt like an exceptional oncologist. Most days, I feel like a complete failure. However, Marsha's letter clearly points out what the patients and families need from their physicians. "I have sat in many doctors' offices over the years with Philip. I can only think of you and one other doctor that did not make me feel I was invisible while discussing medical issues," she wrote. "What is most impressive is not feeling you have to be a detached, unemotional doctor. You can be clear and professional but also show us your emotional human side."

Marsha's letter made me think about how and why our medical culture has evolved in such an anomalous manner that patients are surprised by finding an emotionally engaged physician. That should be the rule rather than the exception. It reminded me of the time when my daughter was a premed undergraduate student, and a very successful physician friend, over for dinner, proceeded to compliment her rather obliquely, "Sheherzad, I am so happy to see that you are considering medicine for your future profession. A great choice! As a doctor, you will never be without a job, no matter what part of the world you are in, you will gain instant respect, even from strangers, and of course you can make as much money as you want." To which Sheherzad sweetly replied, "But my parents always told me that the only reason to go into medicine is to reduce the suffering of fellow humans."

We have become a health-care system highly skilled in pursuing a cure but not healing, dealing with acute emergencies yet alarmingly lacking in simple acts of empathic communication. Today, physicians caring for hospitalized cases spend less than 20 percent of their time on direct interaction with patients and 80 percent or more on bureaucratic nightmares of dealing with electronic records, making chart rounds, checking test results, viewing x-rays and scans, and performing inane administrative duties. In the outpatient setting, there is intense pressure to see as many patients as possible within the allotted time. The crushing piles of nonmedical work crammed into too little time makes overworked, emotionally stressed, physically challenged doctors become physicians they themselves detest. Most physicians today feel dissatisfied with much of what they do, and they yearn for the chance to spend more time with their patients. Defined in the strictest Aristotelian manner, happiness is the pursuit of excellence, or living up to one's potential. Our job as teachers and mentors is to facilitate compassionate interaction between the young physicians and those they are charged to care for, encouraging them to meditate thoughtfully upon the drama of human distress and sorrow they witness. The reality is far from this: *ought* is definitely not *is*. Caught in the deluge of morale-sapping, monotonous, demeaning, tedious, menial scut work, the pursuit of anything other than sleep is unthinkable for young physicians. Before pointing a finger at them, we need to ask ourselves as a society whether we have created the conditions so they have the opportunity to become the best versions of themselves or not.

∞

APPROXIMATELY 90 PERCENT of patients who die of cancer die because their disease is advanced—metastasized. This situation has changed little in the past fifty years as newer strategies have failed to benefit patients with metastatic disease. When novel treatments are tested on monotonous populations of biologically uniform cells, be they grown as cell lines in plates or in animal models, spectacular responses can be achieved regularly. They fail as spectacularly at the bedside because cancer is immeasurably heterogeneous, infinitely evolving, perpetually mutating in the human body. What accounts for this disastrous failure? First and foremost, it is a consistent denial on our part to appreciate the dense and profound complexity of our foe and our insistence that we can use a reductionist approach to break down the problem to a single culprit gene or signaling pathway that can be easily targeted. In this chapter, we have seen that this approach might work in all types of laboratory experiments but not in actual patients. In the next chapter, we will see why, by examining the root cause of cancer.

⟨∿⟩

THE DRUG DASATINIB that Omar so badly wanted was approved for him on a compassionate basis in record time. Before I could actually deliver it to him, however, I received the fateful call from Naheed. It was Tuesday night, January 20, 2009, and I was having dinner at home with my friend Mona Khalidi. "Omar is having difficulty breathing, so I thought I would let you know." I could not swallow another bite after that call. Mona was very disturbed to see my state. "Is something wrong?" Yes indeed. Something is terribly wrong when a parent is watching her child die. "The response to a greeting from a younger person in Arabic is often, 'May you live to bury me,'" Mona said. Alas, for my friend Naheed, this was not to be.

I arrived at Omar's place to find him propped up in bed, severely short of breath. Kamal, his beloved father, sat ashen-faced in the living room; Naheed and his friend Noor were fussing around Omar while Mursi, ever the most loving wife and efficient caregiver, was taking detailed instructions from the home health-care nurse at the dining table for the administration of sublingual morphine.

Despite the shortness of breath, Omar was his usual self, wearing a pink Lacoste shirt. He never lost his sense of style. As soon as he saw me, he asked about the dasatinib. I told him we got it, and he gave the brightest smile, which lit up the room. He proceeded to recount the great time he had had watching the swearing-in ceremony of Mr. Obama. "Now," he said to me, "please tell me a good joke." I promptly recounted the apocryphal story going around. Mrs. Clinton, piqued by a snide remark about her husband's administration, turned on the reporter and said through a steely grin, "So. Please remind me exactly what you did not like about my husband's eight years in office? The peace or the prosperity?" Omar let out a hearty laugh at that and then wanted Mursi to come and change him into pajamas. He insisted on getting up to go to the bathroom even as Mursi tried to get him to stay in bed. That was the last time he would get out of bed. He was given more oral medications after that and sublingual morphine, and slowly he slipped into a sleep of sorts. His breathing became more and more labored.

I thought he should be admitted for intravenous morphine, but Mursi said his wish was to meet the end at home. In that case, I wanted them to bring a morphine pump for him; the nurse said it could not be done until the next day, as such elaborate arrangements take time. This would prove the only time in the space of sixteen months that I saw Naheed lose her cool.

"What kind of a system is this, Azra? We have paid for everything all along, and we are prepared to pay cash for whatever they want now. Why aren't pharmacies, which are supposedly open twenty-four hours a day, able to provide him with morphine now? It's money they always worry about in this country, isn't it? Tell them I will give them all the cash they want. *Azra, tell them!* Get them to bring morphine for him now!"

"Let us go for a little walk," I suggested. I forced her to come down, and we stood outside the building on Riverside Drive in the freezing January night, and she smoked, her face impassive. Eventually, she turned and looked me in the eyes and asked me how long it would be now. I could not meet her gaze for long. "Do you want me to be brutally honest?"

"Yes," she said, staring blankly at the sidewalk.

"It could take several days, but I don't think he will last this night."

She looked away and kept smoking.

We came upstairs silently. Half an hour later, she asked me to sit on the sofa with her in the living room. "Okay," she said, "now describe to me in detail what to expect when the end comes." I did. Slowly and deliberately. After a while, she went and lay down next to him. Thus

I found them several hours later as I went in to say goodbye. A few hours later, around 5:30 a.m., I got her call. She simply said Omar had stopped breathing.

∞

I REMEMBERED THE first time he had come to my apartment in New York when Omar had shown such astonishing composure as we ate an elaborate meal and he calmly braced himself to swallow the tasteless protein shake. His lips puckered ever so slightly as the liquid painfully swirled its way through denuded mucosal gashes in his mouth. *"The aesthetic is to reach poise,"* as Mahmud Darwish quoted Edward Said. In that moment, with that one movement of his mouth, one innocuous sip, months before the end, I knew that Omar owned the aesthetic.

∞

MARK ANTONY IN *Antony and Cleopatra,* act, 1 scene 1, says, "Let Rome in Tiber melt, and the wide arch / Of the rang'd empire fall! Here is my space / Kingdoms are clay; our dungy earth alike / Feeds beast as man / The nobleness of life is to do thus." Indeed, the nobleness of life is to do exactly what both Omar and Naheed did during the scoundrel times they faced together. I salute them both and feel the richer for knowing them.

Maqam e shauq teray qudsiun kay bass ka naheen
Unhee ka kaam hay yay jin kay hauslay hain ziyad

—ALLAMA IQBAL

Striving toward ultimate consummation is not the purview of angels
Only those with vast reserves of valor dare venture

| # PER

Sandpiles and Cancer

IN 2001, I READ MARK BUCHANAN'S WONDERFUL BOOK *UBIQUITY* and became introduced to the "sandpile" game devised by physicists Per Bak, Chao Tang, and Kurt Wiesenfeld, and the concept of critical states. Bak, Tang, and Wiesenfeld created a computer model of grains of sand falling one at a time in a pile; as the pile grows and becomes unstable, a single grain of sand can set off an avalanche. The grain of sand that sets off the avalanche is no different from the other grains already in the pile. Rather, what changes is that the pile becomes increasingly hypersensitive and unstable as the grains fall, forming a peculiar self-organized system that gets pushed away from equilibrium, prone to sudden and cataclysmic changes. This state is called a *critical state,* and it seems to develop in the sandpile on its own, without the need for any external organizing force. This is not just true of sandpiles; self-organized criticality has been found to underlie events as disparate as earthquakes, forest fires, stock market crashes, and mass extinction of species.

Not long after I read the book, I was thinking about the application of these universal laws to cancer—especially the parallels between self-organization in sandpiles and the initiation of leukemia through self-organization in bone marrow cells—when I received a call from a cancer patient who wanted to consult with me from London. His name was Per Bak, and he had been diagnosed with MDS.

Since he was too sick to be transferred to the United States, I referred Per to my colleagues in London, where he underwent both chemotherapy and ultimately a bone marrow transplant. Following interminable and depressing weeks for Per in the hospital, I finally received the good news that he was improving.

There were many days when Per would call me with his latest results or ask me to help interpret what the hematologists had told him. After our professional consultation was over, we frequently ended up discussing critical states and a related concept, known as *power laws*. Many things became clear to me for the first time during these trans-Atlantic conversations with Per. What if we imagined the grains of sand as cells and the pile as the body? With time, the body acquires many changes due to the unintended consequences of aging and becomes unstable, more prone to disastrous avalanches resulting from the same innocuous activities of the cells that in the past did nothing to disturb the pile. Exploration of the potential causes for initiation, expansion, spread, and lethal behavior of the disease from this perspective would require that more or at least equal attention be paid to the soil in which the seed of cancer thrives. This would represent a radical shift of our focus from concentrating on the properties of the diseased cells to examining the health of the entire body. A disheartening fact that nags me constantly is that despite spending more than $500 billion on cancer since 1971, which amounts to $50 billion per year or $20,000 per cancer patient who died in the past forty years, we were—and are still—uncertain about the roots of cancer. Perhaps involving brilliant minds like that of Per Bak, who belong to entirely different disciplines, would bring new insights into our field?

⟋⟋⟍

WHAT CAUSES CANCER?

In his poem, "Miss Gee," W. H. Auden offered a scathing criticism of the prevailing view of cancer in the 1930s where society associated the disease with a failing of the individual.

Doctor Thomas sat over his dinner,
Though his wife was waiting to ring,
Rolling his bread into pellets;
Said, 'Cancer's a funny thing.

'Nobody knows what the cause is,
Though some pretend they do;
It's like some hidden assassin
Waiting to strike at you.

'Childless women get it.
And men when they retire;
It's as if there had to be some outlet
For their foiled creative fire.'

It is not exactly childless women and retired men who get cancer; today, one in two men and one in three women will get it. Many of my patients look puzzled by their diagnosis, as did Doctor Thomas, not because of the state of their creative fire but because of how they lived; these people never smoked or drank, and they exercised regularly. Take, for example, Suketu Mehta, the author of the fantastic book *Maximum City*. He became my friend not long after I moved to New York City. One evening in 2009, I received an unexpected call from Suketu. He sounded shaken. "Azra, I have just been diagnosed with lung cancer. How is this happening? I am forty-five years old. I have never even smoked." After a night of chili with his partner and their families, Suketu had woken with a fluttering in his chest. Worried by memories of his uncle, who died at thirty-four of heart disease, he went to see his doctor. She gave him an EKG. "Your heart is fine," she told him. "The fluttering is probably nothing more than heartburn. But let's get you a chest x-ray, just in case."

And there it was: a two-inch spot over my lung, the earliest stage of a malignant tumor. I've never smoked, so I never would have been checked for this. By the time I developed symptoms, it would have been too late: 85 percent of people diagnosed with lung cancer die within six months.

Cancer is what happens when some part of ourselves wants to live forever. The body is more a confederation of cells agreeing to act in concert than a single organism. When a cell refuses to die and transmits that obdurate life force to its neighbors, we get cancer—death brought on by the striving for immortality.

Where does such agreement, the pursuit of immortality, come from? Is cancer related to our lifestyle, exposure to toxins, what we eat, or where we live, or is it a random event? Is it a consequence of aging? In the memorable phrasing of the science writer Wayt Gibbs, anyone seeking "a workable theory of cancer has to explain both why it is predominantly a disease of old age and why we do not all die from it. A 70 year old is roughly 100 times as likely to be diagnosed with a malignancy as a 19 year old is. Yet most people make it to old age without getting cancer."

Cancer begins with genes. Genes, made up of DNA, coiled and packed into chromosomes during mitosis, carry the code for proteins. DNA is first copied into RNA, which serves as a template for protein synthesis by the cell. Proteins carry out cellular functions. Each time a cell divides, it must faithfully double its DNA, to parcel it out equally to the two daughter cells. Because three billion base pairs need rapid replication, errors or mutations occur. Mutations are continuously edited, repaired, and corrected by built-in cellular mechanisms. If repair is not possible, and the mutation is in a vital gene, the cell is forced to commit suicide. If the mutation is in a gene not vital for the cell, it can persist and be passed on to the next generation. Most DNA mutations are inconsequential—their resulting proteins are either insubstantially changed or not changed at all. If, however, the error affects genes whose function is to either promote or arrest growth, a cell can be driven into wildly irregular paths of unstoppable proliferation: cancer.

Essentially, cancer-initiating events can be triggered by a factor internal to the individual, such as increasing age or a genetic predisposition, or by something external to the individual, such as DNA-damaging environmental toxins, tobacco, alcohol, ultraviolet radiation, or pathogens. Pathogens as etiologic agents for malignancy might seem surprising, but roughly 20 percent of cancers worldwide are caused by viruses or bacteria. For example, in 1977, adult T cell lymphoma was described among the Japanese population and later, human T cell lymphotropic virus-1 (HTLV-1), discovered in the laboratory of Robert Gallo, was shown to be the cause. HTLV-1 can cause many nonmalignant, morbid and fatal diseases like uveitis or myelopathy, but its cancer-causing or oncogenic potential is dramatic. Other viruses considered as causative agents in cancer include papilloma viruses (associated with several types of cancers, most notably, cancer of the cervix), Epstein-Barr virus (Burkitt's lymphoma, some forms of nasopharyngeal and stomach cancers), the hepatitis B and C viruses (liver cancer), and human herpes virus-8 (HHV-8 associated with Kaposi's sarcoma). Helicobacter pylori is the first and only bacterium directly associated with cancer (gastric cancer and gastric lymphoma).

The pathogens listed above cause cancer in a manner similar to the way smoking causes lung cancer. Both initiate changes in a cell that free it to launch into endless cycles of division, unchecked by normal growth-inhibiting impulses, acquiring a life of its own, evolving and metamorphosing into a killer machine with a lawless, mutinous, riotous independence. Lung cancer does not disappear when the patient stops smoking because the harm done by smoking was only the initiating event. No matter what the triggering event—smoking, a virus, or toxic exposure—ultimately, the prevalent view is that a genetic change must happen *within* the cell if there is to be cancer.

What type of genetic change? In cancerous cells, one can find mutations that seem to shut down genes protective against cancer and to trigger those that seem to cause it. One can also find a condition known as *aneuploidy,* or a change in the chromosomal makeup of cells. There could be extra copies of chromosomes, or chromosomes could be missing, or they could be broken. In short, the causes seem to involve either genetics—what genes are there—or cytogenetics—what the chromosomes are like, or both. And then there's the questions I was discussing with Per Bak: whether each change could be like a grain of sand, and cancer the point when the pile suddenly collapses. Could the anarchic insurrection staged by cancer, the nihilistic mobocracy, be the result of external factors forcing the cells into mutiny?

◌◌

BORN IN 1879 in Baltimore, Peyton Rous was keenly interested in biology from an early age. He graduated from Johns Hopkins University in 1905 with an MD, and from 1909 to his death in 1970 at ninety years of age, he was attached to the Rockefeller Institute in New York. Rous was working as a pathologist in 1910 when a farmer brought him a Barred Plymouth Rock fowl with a lump in its breast. Rous diagnosed this as a sarcoma and proceeded to study it further in his lab. He transplanted the malignant cells from the primary tumor into other animals. When he transplanted them into unrelated animals, nothing happened. When he transplanted them into related animals, however, fresh tumors not only appeared, they became increasingly more aggressive, more invasive, with subsequent passages. "It is a spindle-celled sarcoma of a hen," Rous wrote in his report, "which thus far has been propagated to the fourth generation. This was accomplished by the use of fowls of pure blood from the small, intimately related stock in which the growth occurred. Market bought fowls of the same variety have shown themselves insusceptible, as have fowls of mixed breed, pigeons and guinea-pigs."

Cancer could be transmitted from one animal to another, but the question about the causative agent remained. Rous began by mincing the tumor in saline and passing it through a filter so fine that it trapped cells and any other particles as small as bacteria. He injected the filtered extract into related healthy fowl. New tumors appeared. Because both cancer cells and bacteria had been filtered from the extract, Rous concluded that something smaller than a bacterium, a virus, was the cause of sarcoma. With this observation began the field of tumor virology. The Rous sarcoma virus (RSV) was later classified as an RNA virus because of its RNA genome and subsequently as a retrovirus after the discovery of how RNA could be reverse-transcribed into DNA. RSV became the first known cancer-causing virus.

Initially, Rous's discovery, which would eventually earn Rous a Nobel Prize half a century later, went unacknowledged, unstudied, ignored. At the time when Rous reported his findings, cancer was not a widely examined, popularly studied subject, and neither were viruses. What's more, it was hard for scientists of the time to imagine how a tumor in birds could have any relevance for humans. Rous himself doubted the significance of his findings and abandoned cancer research. But then in 1930, a second cancer-causing virus surfaced, when Richard Thorpe showed the papilloma virus to be the cause of warts in rabbits. It was now hard to ignore Rous's work, and the discovery of a second cancer-related virus rekindled interest in RSV. The newfound attention restored confidence in Peyton Rous, who returned to studying cancer. Subsequently, cancer-causing viruses were discovered in many other animals, including mice, cats, and primates. In 1964, Epstein-Barr virus was shown to be the causative agent of a type of lymphoma in humans. The race was on to find new oncogenic viruses and the mechanism by which they induced cancerous behavior in cells.

RSV reliably transmitted sarcoma in inbred animal models. Once molecular techniques became available, the study of RSV began in earnest. Mutations were artificially induced in its genome, and a strain was developed that continued to replicate but failed to cause cancer. When Peter Duesberg and Peter Vogt compared the two strains of cancer-causing and non-cancer-causing RSV, they found that the former had two subunits of RNA, a large and a small one, while the latter contained only the smaller one. The larger piece of RNA was the ultimate driver of the malignant phenotype. The first cancer-causing gene, or oncogene, had been identified. It was named *src* because it caused a sarcoma. Once the transforming activity of a virus was shown to depend upon the oncogene it was carrying, additional oncogenes were discovered in rapid succession in cancers affecting birds and mammals. The joke in the 1980s was to name an A-list cancer researcher who had not yet discovered an oncogene.

A wise person once said that an important discovery in science should not be followed by an exclamation mark but by a semicolon, as science is always a continuous process. Certainly the story of oncogenes became more exciting when two scientists, Mike Bishop and Harold Varmus, showed that the src oncogene, with minor variations, was also present in human cells. The gene was likely picked up from human cells by the RSV retrovirus during its natural life cycle. Now there were two oncogenes with minor differences—the RSV viral version called *v-src* and the human cellular version called *c-src*. The proteins made by v-src and c-src control fundamental functions of cell proliferation and death. Because the c-src in human cells was not directly associated with existing cancer, it is considered a proto-oncogene. Proto-oncogenes acting normally serve to promote cell division. They can become dysfunctional in one of two ways—by a mutation that changes the behavior of the gene, causing it to drive cell division in the absence of normal growth signals, or because the regulation of the proto-oncogene becomes abnormal, leading to excessive copies of the gene—and so its own regulatory proteins—being made. Either way, the result is the runaway tissue growth characteristic of cancer.

Cancer can also result when growth-arresting signals are lacking. The genes responsible for arresting the growth of tissues are known as *tumor suppressor genes* (TSG). The TSG p53 is the most important member of this class. Its function is to constantly survey the cell for any sign of DNA damage. Upon detecting an unrepaired piece of DNA or abnormal growth signal, p53 forces the cell to either repair itself urgently or commit suicide, thereby preventing cancerous behavior of the cell. TSG p53 is known as the *guardian of the genome*. It activates proteins that put brakes on cell division. It is our most prominent intracellular defender against cancer. In order to make it past this policeman of the cell cycle, cancer cells need to subdue the normal surveillance function of p53. Mutations in the gene lead to production of an abnormal p53 protein incapable of performing the vital cell-wide supervision and induction of programmed cell death. This failure results in unchecked growth of the cell. Indeed, p53 is the most commonly mutated gene in many types of cancers.

Germ line mutations in tumor suppressor genes also lead to cancer susceptibility. Li-Fraumeni syndrome (LFS) is a hereditary disease in which 100 percent of affected individuals end up with cancer. Half of them develop a malignancy before thirty years of age and all by seventy years. Cancers of the blood, brain, breast, bones, gonads, adrenals, and GI tract are the most common. Mutations in p53 are present in 70 percent of LFS cases, while the remaining 30 percent show mutations in another tumor suppressor gene called *CHEK2*.

Aruna and Sam Gambhir found out about Li-Fraumeni syndrome through an unspeakable personal tragedy. Their brilliant fourteen-year-old son, Milan, was lake-tubing when he struck his head and suffered a concussion. The treating doctor ordered a CT scan of his head to rule out intracranial bleeding, but no one could have imagined that this simple act of imaging could damage a cell sufficiently to cause brain cancer. Milan died at the age of sixteen from one of the most aggressive, ruthless killers known to mankind: glioblastoma multiforme, which has a five-year survival of less than 5 percent. Sam Gambhir's entire professional life had been spent finding ways of detecting cancer early. The previous year, in fact, he had successfully competed for a $10 million grant to detect early signs of cancer. Milan himself had worked with researchers in the Canary Center at Stanford University to develop a wearable ultrasonic wristband for early detection of recurrent cancer using a sophisticated microbubbles technology. In a crushing, ironic twist, Sam—who chairs the Department of Radiology at Stanford University—watched as the first films revealing the large intracranial mass in his son's brain emerged from the CT machine after Milan presented to the emergency room with a seizure.

Aruna Gambhir had already weathered two bouts with breast cancer. Milan's wristband idea was a direct inspiration from realizing that it was early detection of breast cancer that saved his mother's life. Mother and son underwent genetic testing after Milan's diagnosis, and both showed the presence of an inherited p53 mutation. "It's possible that he developed this tumor from the CT scan radiation," says Sam Gambhir. "When you carry this p53 mutation, you are much more susceptible to radiation. In a normal person, a CT scan wouldn't be a big deal. But in someone with this mutation, it likely increases their chances of cancer. We will never know for sure."

The functional integrity of p53 is associated with cancer prognosis as well. In MDS, for example, when patients present with damage to multiple chromosomes, the cancer genome has been considered highly unstable with a resultant poor prognosis for the patients. Studies show that if the complexity of cytogenetic damage is accompanied by a p53 mutation, the prognosis is indeed quite poor, but if there is no p53 mutation, then patients can live for many years without disease progression despite having many damaged chromosomes. The primary driver is the mutation in p53 and not the damaged chromosomes. On the other hand, MDS patients who present with an isolated deletion in the long arm of chromosome 5 (deletion 5q) are supposed to have a good prognosis—a stable, slowly progressive disease with a long survival. But one in five such patients with ostensibly low-risk disease shows mutations in p53, and they tend to advance to acute leukemia rapidly. This is why any information relating to a possible bad prognosis in patients with complex cytogenetics or good prognosis in patients with deletion 5 is incomplete until p53 mutational status is known. Genetics trumps cytogenetics.

There is another curious aspect of p53 that has come to light recently. Chances of spontaneous mutations increase each time a cell divides. Because larger animals have more cells, it would appear to stand to reason that they should have more mutations, and so, more cancer. Yet the opposite is true; the incidence of cancer in humans is lower than in mice and higher than in whales. Elephants hardly ever get cancer. This conundrum is known as Peto's paradox, named after the epidemiologist Richard Peto. It poses the question of why the incidence of cancer does not increase with increasing numbers of cells in an organism. Peto speculated that intrinsic biologic mechanisms operating within the cells of an expanding and aging animal protect them from cancer. That seems to be right.

Large body size is important because it improves fitness and assures longer life by avoiding predators. There are eleven placental mammalian orders in the animal kingdom, and ten of them have acquired large body sizes, along with a number of different strategies to avoid cancer. One mechanism discovered recently is that elephants have twenty copies of p53. Just as proto-oncogenes can become oncogenes by increasing their copy number, a higher copy number of p53 can prevent cancer altogether. The discovery prompted excitement; can we become the elephants in the room and begin the ending of the cancer saga by inserting multiple copies of p53 into our genomes? Such redundancy would mean both more gene transcripts and protection against any one copy of the gene being disabled by random mutations. As scientists tinkered with this idea in the lab, they ended up with mice whose cells showed a hyperactive p53. The mice were resistant to developing cancer if exposed to DNA-damaging agents that normally induce malignancy. The discovery was very exciting. Unfortunately, the trade-off was less so. The p53 hyperactive mice aged rapidly, and within months, they looked very old, and their life spans shrank by 30 percent. The mechanism of this rapid aging turned out to be stimulation of the hormone responsible for cell proliferation called *insulin-like growth factor 1,* or *IGF-1,* which is controlled in turn by p53. Amplified IGF-1 signaling accelerated the entry of cells into senescence. And senescence, as we have seen before, is closely linked to aging. In short, if there is no p53, the cell becomes cancerous; if there is overactive p53, the cell ages and dies prematurely.

The story does not end here, because there is yet another remarkable twist in the saga: p53 is kept in check by its controller, called *Mdm2*. As soon as p53 is switched on, it activates Mdm2 to assure its simultaneous degradation, thereby preventing its accumulation and overactivity. Artificially suppressing Mdm2 activity in turn would be expected to enhance p53's activity. To study this effect, Mdm2 knockout (KO) mice were created that lacked the controller entirely. When a drug to stimulate p53 was administered to these KO mice, the results were nothing short of catastrophic. The mice essentially melted away due to massive, uncontrolled suicidal death of cells all over the body. The unintended consequences of tinkering with the p53 gene are brilliantly described in Sue Armstrong's eminently readable book *p53: The Gene That Cracked the Cancer Code.*

To make the story of p53 even more complicated, in 2002, another group reported the generation of mice with extra copies of p53. These "Super p53" mice were protected from cancer and did not age prematurely, probably reflecting the fact that p53 was under normal regulatory control.

But p53 is also not the only answer to the issue of large animals and cancer. Whales don't get cancer, but unlike elephants, even the gigantic bowhead whale—with a life span of over two hundred years—shows no extra copies of the tumor suppressor gene p53. One way to prevent cancer in large animals is by slowing down metabolism and reducing the production of DNA-damaging reactive oxygen species. Another, seen in naked mole rats, is activation of a different tumor-suppressing pathway signaling through hyaluronic acid.

Little of this has shown us how to avoid cancer in humans. But comparative biologic studies are certainly adding enormously to the body of knowledge that, one day, is sure to be extremely helpful for all animals on the planet and should continue.

WHETHER MUTATIONS TRIGGER the activity of oncogenes or alter the function of suppressor genes, statistical analyses conducted by Bert Vogelstein and Cristian Tomasetti indeed show that the number of times an organ's stem cells divide determines how prone the organ is to cancer. In thirty-two different types of cancers, 66 percent of the mutations that drive the malignant process—which are known as *founder mutations*—were due to DNA replication errors.

Work done by Vogelstein's group on colorectal cancer also showed the rate at which the mutations arise and which mutations actually tip a cell into cancer. Colorectal cancer develops slowly, transitioning through the three distinct phases of initiation, expansion, and metastasis, often taking two to three decades to reach the full-blown form that we see in advanced cases. Immortalization of the cell is most commonly due to acquisition of somatic mutations in the DNA. Some of these can be hereditary, while others are induced by environmental factors (much like benzene-caused mutations leading to secondary MDS and AML). But the vast majority of DNA mutations arise due to internal processes of the cell. An average of three copying errors occur with each round of DNA replication. In addition, mutations arise due to the quantum effects of base pairing between the two strands of DNA in a chromosome; mistakes induced by DNA polymerase, the enzyme that enables DNA molecules to copy themselves; metabolic DNA damage from reactive oxygen species; and hydrolytic deamination, which has the effect of converting DNA bases into different forms. All contribute significantly to DNA damage. Usually, there is one or very few driver mutations in vital genes that tip the cell into a malignant state. There are approximately 140 so-called driver genes, affecting just about a dozen major signaling pathways involved in the cell's proliferation, differentiation, and normal functions that are responsible for the cancer phenotype. Genes that determine cellular fate and survival constitute about 90 percent of these while 5–10 percent control the rate of mutations of all genes. The most familiar of the last group are BRCA1 and BRCA2 genes where an inherited mutation leads to vastly increased risk of many types of cancers, especially those of breast and ovaries.

Such driver mutations might seem obvious targets for treatment, and they are in children, as the malignant cells in a child's cancer are otherwise naive to the many "passenger mutations" that cells acquire over the course of decades. Cancer cells generally show one or two founder mutations but produce a scattering of daughter cells, each of which has acquired a different set of passenger mutations. A passenger mutation does not directly affect proliferative function, but by hitch-hiking along the founder mutation, it can affect clonal expansion. As cancers grow, they evolve, continuously acquiring additional mutations and genetic diversity, so that an ecosystem of clones is produced bearing the original founder and a variety of additional passenger mutations.

Expansion of a clone depends upon the fitness landscape between its genetic architecture and the microenvironment. A primary tumor in the stomach would have a very different soil to negotiate compared to one of its daughter cells that home in the liver as a metastasis. The founder mutations would be the same in the clones of cells growing in the stomach and the liver, yet their behavior and responsiveness to therapy would depend on the sum of passenger mutations and local signals in the soil. A drug targeting the founder mutation could get rid of the dominant clone of cells producing even dramatic tumor re-gressions, but the subclones waiting on the sidelines with a different genetic profile would eventually acquire a growth advantage and cause relapse. No—they cause relapse with a vengeance, because by defini-tion, these are clones selected for survival precisely because they were resistant to therapy.

There are several questions that arise from the above conclusion. The first relates to prevention. If cancer always results from a cell's in-trinsic typo and has nothing to do with factors outside of the cell, such as the environment, then no amount of lifestyle changes would make a difference. However, this is not the case since we do see lifestyles affecting cancer incidence. For lung tumors, for example, DNA copying errors accounted for only 35 percent of the mutations while environmental factors accounted for 65 percent. A second question is, if a mutation can happen any time a cell is preparing to multiply, then why is it that cancers are more common in older age? Here Per Bak's work and life come back into focus. MDS, which Per was suffering from, results both from factors intrinsic to the cell and the microenvironment surrounding the cell that appears to be full of inflammatory changes. Perhaps the only seed that can survive in such a toxic environment is a cell with a genetic mutation that has caused it to escape the normal growth-controlling signals. What possible changes in the microenvironment of the human body would increase the chances of a cell carrying a mutation to survive at the expense of normal cells? After reading about the phenomenon of self-organized criticality, I began to wonder about events *preceding* the intracellular gene-chromosome catastrophe causing a malignant transformation. The system could have already become unstable, poised for an avalanche at the least disturbance.

⁙

THE DISTURBANCE IN an unstable system poised for catastrophe may come from aneuploidy, a biological reality that challenges the current gene-centric obsession of cancer researchers. Humans inherit two sets of twenty-three chromosomes, one from each parent. A cell has aneuploidy if it contains fewer or more than those forty-six chromosomes. Aneuploidy arises during cell division due to unequal segregation of chromosomes with one daughter cell acquiring more and the other fewer than forty-six. What causes aneuploidy? Mutations in genes, especially those regulating repair of damaged DNA in a cell, can cause chromosomal instability and subsequent aneuploidy. As far back as 1902, the German scientist Theodor Boveri observed that if sea urchin eggs were aneuploid, embryos showed abnormal development. He proposed that having the incorrect chromosome number predisposed a cell toward cancer. Cells with aneuploidy produce abnormal amounts of proteins because of the number of functioning genes, interfering with vital proliferation and death signals. Roughly 90 percent of solid tumors and 75 percent of liquid cancers manifest aneuploidy.

Both genetic mutations and aneuploidy are hallmarks of malignancy, but the relative importance of each as the primeval cause of cancer has been a subject of debate for decades. One side argues that aneuploidy comes first, and genetic mutations arise because of chromosome breaks, while the other suggests a driver role for genetic mutations with aneuploidy as the downstream consequence.

In 2017, researchers at Cold Spring Harbor conducted an experiment in which they cultured two groups of cells side by side. One had the normal number of chromosomes, and the other had one additional chromosome. The aneuploid cells grew slowly at the start, but eventually, a sudden burst of growth occurred and, almost overnight, they began dividing rapidly. As cells multiplied, more and more abnormalities appeared in their chromosome number. The lab dish seemed to recapitulate events in the body, where a primary tumor grows sluggishly for a while, abruptly bursting into metastases with newfound aggression. Cells with aneuploidy had a survival advantage over cells with a normal chromosome number. They also displayed genetic instability as aneuploidy sequentially worsened in daughter cells, some having more and some fewer chromosomes than the parent cells.

Could the initial slow growth represent a phase of self-organization with the system persistently moving toward entropy, the population becoming increasingly more unstable just like sandpiles, ultimately reaching the state of self-organized criticality when any event could tip the system? Just as the last grain of sand causing collapse in a sandpile is no different from other grains, the cell causing a cataclysmic change may not be very different from others in the plate. The whole plate of cells becomes hypersensitive and unstable, prone to cataclysmic changes. In this setting, even a minor copying error in the DNA, a passenger mutation picked up as the cells divided, which otherwise would be of little consequence, could tip the system.

⚭

ON A BEAUTIFUL morning in early 2000, Harvey, Sheherzad, and I were enjoying a particularly spectacular sunrise over Lake Michigan from our living room window. Our apartment in Chicago overlooked Lakeshore Drive and Lincoln Park Zoo and provided a panoramic view of the city from the John Hancock building to the Sears Tower. Harvey was in a great mood. It was a happy morning as Sheherzad ran around, ecstatic at seeing her parents looking relaxed for a change. Harvey asked me if there was something special I wanted to do. He looked rested and well, so I made the impossible demand. Would he come with me for a jog by the lake? We used to love running together, but Harvey had not ventured out in months. His eyes lit up, and he said, "Why not?"

We had barely reached the Peggy Notebaert Nature Museum, a couple of blocks from our building, when Harvey slowed down.

"What's wrong?" I asked.

"I'm not sure, but I feel I can't breathe properly," he replied.

We stopped and rested for a bit and tried again. Another block and the same thing again. We returned home. He started to get shorter of breath as the day wore on. I suggested we go to the ER, but he refused. I gave him Sheherzad's nebulizer, and it helped him for a while. We spent an anxious day at home. Harvey went to lie down in the bedroom, watching the Ken Burns series on the Civil War. He became so engrossed that my periodic intrusions to check up on how he was feeling became annoying. I tried to leave him alone.

By now, Sheherzad was used to sudden cancellations of our best-laid plans and did not blink when I told her we would be eating at home. We went to bed early. At 4:00 a.m., Harvey woke me up, saying he needed help. He was sweating and looked like he was about to pass out, struggling to catch his breath. I wanted to call 911, but he asked me to drive him instead because the ambulance would take us to the nearest ER, while he wanted to reach Rush University hospital, where we worked. With the help of the housekeeper, I got him dressed and into the car. I had called the hospital in advance, and as we drove up, the crew was waiting with a wheelchair at the door. Harvey was intubated within minutes and placed on a ventilator.

It took days to get him off the machine. Following an exhaustive workup, including a bronchoscopy, no cause for the pulmonary issue was revealed. A diagnosis of adult-onset asthma was finally given, and he was eventually discharged on high-dose steroids and bronchodilators. Was this sudden onset of a brutal asthmatic attack in any way related to his lymphoma? In the absence of a history of lung problems, an association had to be considered, but a definitive answer was not possible. It was only a year later that the asthma was retroactively rediagnosed as a paraneoplastic manifestation of his primary cancer.

The ferocity of the brutal symptoms Harvey experienced resulted from a combat between lymphoma and a misdirected immune system, burning and blasting its way through his ravaged body in episodes that would last a few days or sometimes weeks, followed by an eerie calm, leaving him spent and exhausted in a way that no physical activity could possibly do. In November of 1999, we were in Manhattan for a brief meeting. We were staying at the Plaza, and Harvey had been excited to take Sheherzad to the Central Park Zoo. As he began to dress the next morning, he abruptly sat down and clutched his left calf. "Must be a cramp," he said. By now, I assigned everything he experienced to the lymphoma, and he would lose his patience with me because he did not want to be constantly reminded of the diagnosis. By the time we landed back in Chicago, he was visibly limping. I forced him to see the internist. An ultrasound revealed deep-vein thrombosis, or DVT, in the calf. The universal verdict between his oncologist, pulmonologist, rheumatologist, and endocrinologist was that the DVT, night sweats, and migratory polyarthritis, even the asthma diagnosed the year before, were interconnected. Harvey's symptoms could have been because of the lymphoma traveling throughout the body, causing local reactions extending from skin to lungs. But the same sorts of symptoms are seen with solid tumors confined to their organs of origin. How do we explain these?

Paraneoplastic syndromes can sometimes be the first presenting symptom of an unsuspected malignancy. They can affect any system or organ. They are tissue agnostic. David Ansari described the history of our knowledge of these syndromes by tracing the curious association between pancreatic cancer and thromboses.

The Manchester surgeon Charles White first demonstrated in 1784 that "milk leg" was not caused by retained milk or lochia, but rather by obstructing clots in the veins. In 1847, the German Rudolph [*sic*] Virchow [1821–1902] observed that venous thrombi often migrated to the lungs. In 1865, the French physician Armand Trousseau [1801–1867] described that migratory venous thromboses occurring during the course of his own pancreatic cancer. It has after that for a long time been considered a "truth" that carcinoma of the pancreas has an inherent and unique ability to induce a hypercoagulable diathesis that leads to clinically significant thrombosis. This has, however, later on been challenged and there have been voices stating that the relationship between cancer of the pancreas and thromboembolic disorders should be de-emphasized since it is neither unique nor especially in association with pancreatic carcinoma, and since it may be almost as frequently encountered in other visceral malignancies.

Harvey's experience was also one of the many reminders that whatever the cause, cancer as a disease is more than a tumor confined to one organ. If not the primary tumor itself, then the immune reactions to cancer in the body can affect any system with cryptic, unanticipated displays, sometimes more painful than the tumor itself. Elimination of the underlying cancer is the only permanent treatment option. All other attempts are palliative and symptomatic to reduce pain and inflammation.

Night sweats are reminiscent of infectious episodes and suggest involvement of the immune system and the release of cytokines, a type of protein vital to the body's way of responding to and fighting cancer. The body knows something is wrong. It mounts a ferocious immune reaction. Cancer cells escape the wrath by either expressing a signal on their surface that says, "Don't eat me," or cloaking the signal that says, "Eat me." The immune response ends up causing more harm by damaging normal tissues instead of eliminating the cancer cells. The immune system is not always subdued in cancer patients but rather overactive, and it sometimes manifests both over- and underactivity.

Harvey's life-threatening problems resulted from a weakened response of the immune system to repeated bouts of infections that landed him in the hospital several times a month during the last year of his life. He was given regular infusions of intravenous immunoglobulins to boost his immunity. At the same time, with the distressing night sweats and intensely painful polyarthritis, he manifested signs of an overactive, erratic immune response to the lymphoma. It is difficult to reconcile the ideas of a simultaneously underactive and overactive immune response. One possibility is that the cancer is masquerading as friend, fooling the immune system, but only partially. Another idea is that the syndromes result from chemicals and proteins secreted by the tumors and carried around the body via blood, setting up reactions in susceptible tissues. The converse is also possible in that the cancer itself arose because of a flawed immune system in the first place. And if cancer is a consequence, then what systemic changes in the body made the environment more hospitable to the survival of a mutated, transformed, malignant cell? Could it be the inflammatory response of an overreactive immune system?

A reductionist approach is the driving force for advances in the biomedical field, but at the expense of devaluing individual experience.

Cancer, the disease in individual cases, can be a multi-organ illness even as the malignant cells remain confined to an organ. Only in its earliest manifestations is it defined by, or limited to, the properties of its individual components. The cause of remote, far-flung, body-wide effects of cancer cannot be traced back to the malfunction of individual malignant cells alone. Rather, single entities interacting with each other and with host defenses produce unpredictable complex behaviors as a collective. Immune cells seem not to recognize the cancer as alien and fail to eliminate it. But they can't seem to ignore the cancer either, at least in some patients. The fired-up, activated immune system misses its real target, hurting the host more than the cancer. Depending upon what becomes the target of the immune attack, a bizarre panoply of paraneoplastic syndromes are experienced by patients. It is more like two states of water manifesting an unexpected emergent property. Upon freezing, water becomes ice. There is no change in the molecular components of water in liquid or solid form, so what accounts for the slipperiness of ice? The sum of individual parts cannot explain the complexity that emerges from the whole. Paraneoplastic syndromes seemed like an emergent property of cancer.

A comprehensive exploration of these complex issues requires more than sequencing the genome of tumors to identify causative mutations. Cancer can only be transplanted artificially into healthy animals whose immune system is destroyed. As a result, all the accompanying reactions of the body, the counterpunch resulting in a misdirected immune response, the system-wide reaction to the presence of malignancy, the whole array of paraneoplastic syndromes are entirely absent in animal models. Who has cataloged the B-symptoms of joint pains and night sweats in mice?

◌

CANCER INCIDENCE INCREASES with age, although the two processes—aging and cancer—are biologically almost the opposite of each other.

As cells age, they don't necessarily die; they enter a state of suspended animation called *senescence,* where they halt proliferation, minimize metabolic activity and energy consumption, and no longer perform any useful function, but continue to produce waste products as a natural consequence of being alive.

When cells hit the Hayflick limit, they go into senescence or die. The clock that keeps track of the number of divisions are stretches of DNA on the ends of each chromosome known as *telomeres,* which shorten every time a cell divides. Most cancers avoid senescence or death by producing an enzyme called *telomerase,* which can rebuild the lost DNA. Three scientists—Elizabeth Blackburn, Carol Greider, and Jack Szostak—shared the 2009 Nobel Prize in Medicine and Physiology for their discovery of how chromosomes are protected by telomeres and how telomere DNA is restored by telomerase.

Older age is associated with shortened telomeres and accumulating senescent cells. The problem with these senescent cells is that by maintaining minimal biologic activity to stay alive, they continue to produce waste products without performing any useful function. The "trash" removal system of the body works overtime to remove the debris of not just functioning, dividing cells vital for the body but also these freeloaders. In addition, the senescent cells produce proteins that cause chronic inflammation. The resulting toxic environment is perfect for hosting and promoting growth of mutated cells and is a significant contributor to both cancer and other age-related diseases. The mutated seed finds a hospitable soil in an aging body.

Aging causes inflammation. Cancer cells thrive in an inflammatory soil. And of course, as we've seen, with aging also comes a collection of DNA mutations, their number increasing exponentially with age.

Surprisingly, there are otherwise healthy individuals—over the age of sixty, usually—with no sign of any disease, walking around with anywhere from 2 to 20 percent of their blood cells derived from a clone carrying mutations in genes associated with highly malignant diseases like MDS and AML. This situation where there is no clinically apparent abnormality in the blood counts or identifiable marrow disease but in which disease-related mutations are nonetheless present in blood and marrow cells is called *clonal hematopoiesis of indeterminate potential,* or *CHIP.* The long name suggests that there is a group or clone of cells carrying a mutation known to be associated with serious pathology, but in the absence of low blood counts, its potential to cause disease is indeterminate. Incidence of CHIP increases by every decade of life. Up to 20 percent of individuals in their sixties and 50 percent of individuals in their eighties have CHIP. CHIP turned out to have a very low incidence of progressing to MDS (about 1 percent) but is associated with other illnesses like cardiovascular disease and strokes, especially in those cases where no apparent risk factor for cerebrovascular disease was easily identifiable. Few centenarians show CHIP. If you dream of hitting a hundred, make sure you don't have CHIP.

In addition to senescent cells, accumulation of mutated DNA segments, increasing debris, and a pro-inflammatory microenvironment in the elderly, a spatial reorganization of the bone marrow with increasing age may also disturb the normal physiologically graded cell-cell signaling. Activities of cells are, at least partially, under the control of their microenvironment or the stromal cells through chemical and neural signals. The dose of the signal is critical, and, to some extent, depends on the physical distance between the two cells. With increasing age, a great deal of actual tissue is lost as cells reach their proliferative limit and die. In a healthy adult, roughly half the marrow is occupied by blood-producing cells, and the other half is empty space filled with fat. With increasing age, this fifty-fifty fat-to-cells ratio changes so that it is common to find a seventy-year-old individual with 70 percent of the space in the marrow filled with fat. Such fat increases the distance between effector and target cells. Even a slight decrease in the inhibitory signal dosage would result in a proliferative advantage for the target, distanced from its controlling stromal cell. If such a target cell also has accumulated mutations, it would gradually lead to an unchecked expansion of the clone. As this abnormal situation continues unchecked, the marrow can eventually become predominantly "monoclonal" or populated by the daughters of one cell. This monoclonal population could also be marked by specific and identifiable genetic mutations, the most common CHIP-associated ones affecting TET2, DNMT3A, and ASXL1 genes.

Monoclonality, however, does not mean that a malignant transformation in one of the daughter cells is imminent. Rather, monoclonality may predispose the cells to the development of malignancy. As the clone continues to expand rapidly, the number of monoclonal cells grows, and the system may begin to move away from equilibrium and toward self-organization and a critical state. Could the reorganization of cells residing under an abnormal architecture in the marrow be governed by the same rules as self-organization in sandpiles? Once a critical state has been achieved, the system would be prone to sudden and cataclysmic changes. Support for this comes from several observations. For example, practically every malignant cell in patients with chronic myeloid leukemia is marked by a translocation between chromosomes 9 and 22, which is known as the *Philadelphia chromosome* in honor of the city where the discovery was made. Some years ago, it was demonstrated that clonal expansion and a monoclonal state preceded the appearance of the Philadelphia chromosome.

The incidence of monoclonality increases in direct proportion to advancing age; as many as 40 percent of females over age sixty show monoclonal-born marrow function. Not only are almost all cancers monoclonal, but their precursor state, called *dysplasia,* is also monoclonal. Normal cells start to look dysplastic in abnormal environments. Thus, dysplastic states affecting the bone marrow, cervix, liver, esophagus, and stomach are all monoclonal, and the dysplastic morphology suggests an abnormal soil or microenvironment. Once a system follows critical-state universality, it is impossible to predict the course it is going to have.

AGING IS THE most potent carcinogen because it creates encounters between all the phenomena that cause cancer. Nora Ephron, with her wry wit and laser-sharp observations, famously advised women to start hiding their necks once they turned forty-three. "Our faces are lies and our necks are the truth. You have to cut open a redwood tree to see how old it is, but you wouldn't if it had a neck." When I look in the mirror these days, I often wonder, if these are the changes on the outside, what havoc is being wreaked by aging inside my body? A lot, it seems. At least four major areas of profound biologic alterations turn the aged body into a hotbed where malignant cells can thrive. I call it the MIST of aging. First are *mutations.* In addition to heredity and exposure to toxic environments, each new round of DNA replication as a cell divides causes fresh copying errors. Cellular metabolism also causes DNA damage. Mutations from these sources add up over time. The second is the *immune* system's increasing inefficiency. All bodily processes become more decrepit with age, causing the immune system to falter and miss eliminating a cancer cell at its very inception. Third is an increase in the number of *senescent* cells with age. Senescence by itself is anticancer because the cell stops dividing. However, it is carcinogenic for other cells because it is still metabolically active, producing waste material that accumulates, causing the natural habitat of cells to turn toxic. This inflammatory microenvironment provides the ideal soil for the abnormal cancer seed. Finally, there is the problem of *tissue* loss with age, dramatically visible on the face and neck but equally disfiguring internally. Tissue depletion leads to geographic reorganization in organs such as the bone marrow with resulting spatial renegotiation between cells whose activity depends upon precise physiologic gradations of chemical signaling. These four factors descend like a mist that cloaks the elderly in the possibility of cancer. Where in Per's model, a grain of sand is eventually enough to tip the system into an avalanche, the bodies of the elderly are engulfed in a swarm of them.

Every carcinogen—whether the inheritance of a genetic predisposition, or changes due to aging, or exposure to toxic agents or pathogens—

gives rise to mutations in oncogenes and/or tumor suppressor genes. Theoretically, this should simplify the search for solutions aimed at targeting the genetic mutations. The problem is the nonstatic nature of the changes. With each division cycle, the cancer cells sustain new mutations. The emergent complexity of cancer in adults is because of this constellation of hundreds of small cuts acting together and is the reason why cancer in the elderly is harder to treat than in children. In the elderly, the assortment of mutations is not the same even in subsequent generations of cancer cells within the same individual, let alone in two different individuals. In the young, there is no time to have accumulated DNA replication errors; cancer arises from the malfunctioning of a major gene- or nodal-signaling pathway, which immortalizes the cell into a perpetual cycle of proliferation at the expense of maturation. Attacking a single target has a higher chance of being effective than trying to overcome the cumulative dysfunction of many proteins operating in a toxic, proinflammatory microenvironment. This happened in the case of chronic myeloid leukemia, but even there, the drugs proved effective only during the stable, chronic phase of the disease, not when the acute, blastic phase evolves. Finally, the interaction of cancer cells with the immune system results in a panoply of disparate, painful, and life-threatening signs and symptoms grouped under the broad term of *paraneoplastic syndromes.* Biologic studies spanning half a century should be sufficient to illustrate the unsolvable nature of carcinogenesis for a long time to come. In the next chapter, application of this knowledge to design individualized approaches to treatment will be examined and results of such precision medicine initiatives discussed.

∞

PER BAK'S TRAGIC story evolved a continent away, at a great remove from me—I only learned the details through phone calls and e-mails. And yet, it acquired a great significance for me. I was advising him about handling some of the exact same issues related to end-of-life decisions that Harvey and I were facing. The parallels were surreal: two brilliant, energetic, driven, focused men at the peak of their productive careers with megaplans for the ensuing decades, abruptly shown the finish line. Both had young children who they would not live to see become adults, graduate from college, marry, give them grandchildren.

Many a night, I woke up to see Harvey sitting perfectly motionless at the edge of the bed with his back to me, deep in thought, for what felt like interminable hours. What does time mean to people who are running out of it? An inexplicable, intuitive reticence restrained me from interrupting the trafficking in his mind. How does a man hearing the footsteps of death approach closer every day negotiate the themes of dying, loss, pain, grief, the withering sense of waste, the unbearable, crushing sadness of things that will be left undone? How could it be otherwise? Cancer chipping away at the body relentlessly in slow, steady, excruciating blows; the lucid, sharp, coherent mind forced to reside in an aching, skeletal corpus, documenting each ignominy with sensorial precision. In those dark Chicago nights, we were two tormented souls caught in our own private hells, frozen into rigid postures; his vertical immobility matched by my horizontal stillness. Both were afraid to acknowledge that the other was awake because that would invite language to intrude. Verbalizing a fraction of what we were suffering, objectifying the pain in words, no matter how frugal the language, risked a diminishment of its caustic, dizzying, disorienting potency, his physical and mine emotional. Soon I would be speaking in rooms forever depleted of his voice, I would be breathing air that would no longer contain his breath. Even as I tried to control the pounding in my chest, my mind, hostage to surreptitious invasions of rationality, would coldly conduct a microscopic analysis of how to define my feelings precisely, to classify whether it was mourning for Harvey or anxiety for Sheherzad and myself having to live without him. Thoughts and emotions, conflicting and confusing, attacked simultaneously, smashing through any residual protective shield of hope, driving home the murky pathos of the coming emptiness in my life, the lonely days ahead, with a fierce, violent acuity that pierced with physical brutality, choking my parched throat, triggering waves of nausea.

Do other cancer patients experience variations on these themes, the vertigo of evanescent, soul-destroying, irreducible suffering? Do they run their weary fingers through serrated edges of anguish, say farewells in unspoken, unheard of languages in the silence of sleepless nights?

⚬⚭⚬

ONE OF THE saddest conversations I had with Per was several months after his bone marrow transplant. Just when everything appeared to be stabilizing, he developed one of the known and dreaded complications of the transplant procedure: severe pulmonary damage. After many rounds of therapies, some bordering on the heroic, Per finally knew that he was not going to make it.

⚬⚭⚬

BOTH HARVEY AND Per were dead within a few months of each other. Two lives lived with breakneck speed and intensity had abruptly exploded. They expanded, amplified, enlarged peculiarly in their stunning, outsized impact on those left behind precisely because they were snatched prematurely. I entered a fog-like space of my own, mechanically going through the motions, but all the time feeling riven, fragmented. Trying to be a reassuring mother, showing up at work, seeing patients, running a lab, winding up Harvey's scientific program, finding placements for a dozen scientists whose jobs ended unceremoniously. Dealing with estate issues, social security applications, hospital bills, insurance companies, grieving relatives, and well-meaning friends. Dealing at the same time with my own cosmic turbulence, the melancholic thoughts in my mind.

I felt a cleavage in my mind
As if my brain had split;
I tried to match it, seam by seam,
But could not make them fit.
The thought behind I strove to join
Unto the thought before,
But sequence raveled out of reach
Like balls upon a floor

—EMILY DICKINSON

THREE

LADY N.

A Loaded Gun

MARCEL PROUST SAID THAT THE REAL VOYAGE OF DISCOVERY IS not in seeking new landscapes but in having new eyes. I experience a slightly different version of this dictum practically on a daily basis, developing new insights through my patients' eyes. None could claim a vision more penetrating and acute than Lady N. She was high-spirited and boisterous, with a rowdy, uproarious personality that sparkled with wit and humor, possessing an uncanny habit of connecting seemingly unrelated things through common sense, extreme intelligence, inimitable humor, and pure and simple intuition. And most importantly, she had a blazing, sizzling passion for life writ large all over her massive five-foot, ten-inch frame.

Aged sixty-two, Lady N. swept into my clinic for her first visit in 2008 with this farcical, preposterous announcement: "FYI, I have been extremely anemic for at least twenty-five to thirty years, if not longer," she told me. "I also believe strongly that there *is* a genetic component to my MDS." She went on, "As you know, my father's sister's first child was born with no marrow in his bones." Although she had been anemic for a long time, her MDS had not been diagnosed until just before I met her. The first few years were not too hard, as her diseased cells were marked by a deletion in the long arm of chromosome 5. This special subtype of MDS is associated with slow progression, a longer survival, and an especially good response to Revlimid, a derivative of the once-infamous drug thalidomide.

❧

BACK IN 1999, I had personally prescribed thalidomide for Harvey, one of the first lymphoma patients ever to receive the drug on a compassionate basis.

When Harvey's cancer started manifesting a series of sudden, startling, painful paraneoplastic syndromes, we knew some form of therapy was now inevitable. Around this time, I heard data presented by an oncologist at a national meeting who had tried thalidomide in patients with lymphoma and had seen sporadic benefits. I immediately felt this could be a safer alternative for Harvey, who was still reluctant to start chemotherapy. I told Harvey I thought it was worth a try. What did we have to lose—a few weeks? Harvey listened to me and was willing to go along with my suggestion. Needing reinforcement for such an experimental use of the drug, we visited Harvey's primary oncologist in Chicago, Steve Rosen, a charismatic, deeply empathetic, kind, caring physician, a great friend, and the cancer center director at Northwestern. We reviewed Harvey's treatment options. Chemotherapy. A different kind of chemotherapy. Steve listened to my case for trying thalidomide. He agreed to prescribe the drug. Backed by Steve, as well as Owen O'Connor, chief of the lymphoma service at Memorial Sloan Kettering, I was able to get the drug on a compassionate, one-patient protocol basis for Harvey from Celgene, its manufacturer.

We started Harvey on thalidomide at 50 percent of the recommended dose because of the toxicity I had seen in MDS patients. The results even with this reduced dose were spectacular. Within forty-eight hours of starting, Harvey's facial edema started to melt visibly. By week's end, the pitting, uneven, grotesque puffiness had entirely disappeared, and his fine features reappeared.

LADY N.'S BLOOD counts eventually dropped, requiring intervention. As hoped, she responded well first to the red cell–stimulating hormone Procrit and then to Revlimid. The anemia improved beyond expectation, and she had an excellent quality of life, caring for her many cats, taking long drives visiting her numerous best friends, shopping and dining with her ninety-nine-year-old mother, and generally enjoying life to the full.

Lady N. would come to clinic for follow-ups regularly and endeared herself to everyone she encountered. Her openness, loud and hilarious remarks, self-deprecation, and a poignant concern for—and astonishing ability to recall—others' personal lives made her easy to like. Another unique quality was her matchless ability to communicate with the younger individuals who inevitably follow me in clinic. Whether they were high school students interning during summers, doctoral candidates writing dissertations on MDS, or fellows training in hematology, she would inquire about their backgrounds in a few sentences and then proceed to engage them through anecdotes and personal stories that were somehow tailored for their individual needs. I can recall numerous young fans, Matt Markham in particular, who kept in touch with her long after their rotations with me were done. Such was her attraction, such her charm.

She was a cat lady. Lady N. and her late husband toured with their beautiful feline army throughout America and Europe, earning admiration, winning awards, breeding and showing oriental shorthairs, amusing the clinic staff with endless, entertaining stories of her various award-winning trips. She created a memorial fund at Cornell University Feline Health Center dedicated to improving the care and well-being of cats in honor of her favorite cat, William. Lady N. was also an accomplished photographer of nature and of birds. She participated in research projects at the University of Vermont, including a study of the Indiana bats of East Dorset. She was a member of MENSA, played tournament bridge and chess, and was a natural with computers. She greatly enjoyed sharing her vast resources of knowledge in diverse fields and astonished her listeners by citing extraordinary facts during ordinary conversations. I adored her.

Lady N. was constantly examining her past to determine the root of her MDS—wondering if the kerosene heaters in a cabin where she spent holidays as a child might have contributed to her condition—and was always picking my brain for more satisfying answers than Google was able to provide about her future. She was especially eager to learn where the latest research on targeted therapy was heading. As I would describe some new drug we were testing in a phase 1 or phase 2 trial, she would become quite excited. "I am counting on you, my dear, dear friend, to make sure that I have at least another ten, if not twenty, years. Between the two of us and your colleagues, I am counting on it!" And she told me several times, "I want to be there when you make MDS a chronic disease like AIDS is now."

And then the inevitable happened, and she stopped responding to Revlimid. That left her transfusion dependent. Even as she was being pumped full of red blood cells from matched donors, her wicked sense of humor was ever present, and she would send me weekly cartoons that would make me smile or burst out laughing in the middle of clinic. Eventually, she was started on chemotherapy with Vidaza. It was not a pleasant experience. As the Vidaza continued into the fourth and then fifth month without any relief in the frequency of blood transfusions, an unexpected new symptom crept in. Lady N. began to experience inexplicable fatigue. She would wake up in the morning after an eight-hour sleep feeling like she had been pulling a cart all night. She was totally worn out by the simple act of brushing her teeth; washing and blow-drying her hair required at least three intervals of rest. Her arms felt like lead. She pumped herself full of coffee and took Excedrin and then Ritalin to shake herself out of the doldrums. Nothing worked. Week after week, she sat across from me in clinic and recounted the list of chores she had been unable to complete. We tried hyper-transfusing her with blood, maintaining her hemoglobin above 10 Gm at all times (the normal range is 12.5–16 Gm). Even she was perplexed by the profundity of exhaustion. She used to feel better when the hemoglobin was 7 Gm than she did now at 10 Gm. Ultimately, after ruling out all possible causes like nutritional deficiencies, thyroid dysfunction, drugs causing a side effect, we had to admit that she was suffering from a paraneoplastic syndrome.

We stopped the Vidaza, and that brought her temporary relief. She sent me the following note:

> Lately I've had so many transfusions I feel like changing my profession to "vampire" on hospital forms. . . . And as I like to tell people, I've done so much "blood doping" that I probably wouldn't be allowed to watch the Olympics on television. . . . Ok I jest, but I feel so much better. Gone is the peripheral neuropathy, the hot flash-like fevers at night, the dizziness and the mental foggies and a whole host of unpleasant side effects not the least of which is that when I'm on chemo I've felt like I've lost at least 50 IQ points. . . . It's nice to have them back.

We began to relax, celebrating her temporary deliverance from the deeply discomfiting symptoms, knowing full well that it would not last forever. She would storm into clinic, blowing kisses, handing out utterly unhealthy delights—cookies and doughnuts—high-fiving nurses and arguing with the receptionists, happy to be something of her usual unusual self once again. Everyone breathed a sigh of relief.

We continued to treat Lady N. symptomatically, but she was visibly getting worse, requiring more transfusions of blood and now occasional platelets as well. We became quite worried when Christmas 2014 rolled around and she told us that she was going to drive her mother to Vermont to visit family and friends. She tried to assuage our concerns about her "running around in these days of the new normal." "It just takes planning," she told us, "sort of like a military campaign." She insisted anything she could do sitting down, including driving a car, wasn't a problem—"that is, unless my hemoglobin is really tanking and my mind starts to get fuzzy." She did admit that "the vertical activities," like walking from her car to a shop's front door, do "have to be planned for rather carefully." And she had plans, including favoring stores where she could park near the entrance and lean on a shopping cart, but they were all clearly a willful denial of reality. Her absolute refusal to see what stared her in the eyes, her persistent demands for solutions from me, and her outrageous expressions of supreme confidence in my abilities in particular and of science in general to provide a cure for her left all of us involved in her care a little unsettled.

How someone with her level of high IQ, a member of MENSA, an extremely well-read and well-traveled woman of Lady N.'s extraordinary caliber managed to steadfastly, categorically, and decisively resist, ignore, and reject out of hand any acceptance of her looming mortality remains one of those perplexing things about humans that make us such complicated creatures. Since I had recently gone through the Omar debacle, it was only natural to compare Lady N.'s responses to her cancer with his. At thirty-eight, Omar, a brilliant young professor, distracted himself by obsessively researching treatment options and remaining hopeful until the end, yet at some intangible level, I sensed in him a silent, deeply melancholic prescience of impending doom. From the moment of diagnosis, he existed in a liminal space, suspended between life and death, waiting impotently, not knowing, perched on a threshold, unable to cross over or retreat, powerless to fully explain his own location. There was a delicate perishability about him, an unspoken despondency even as he ostensibly engaged in carefree celebrations of living. At other times, like the magician Prospero, reminding his daughter of the brevity of mortal life in *The Tempest,* Omar, too, seemed prepared to declare an end to the revels, *"We are such stuff as dreams are made on, and our little life is rounded with a sleep."* The aesthetic dignity of Omar's acceptance coming from inexplicable, peculiar, deep crevices of his psychic interior contrasted sharply with the flamboyant refutation of reality by Lady N., her obsessive postures of waiting, her perpetual expectancy, the flows and eddies of her piercing, scorching desire to live at all costs.

Celebrating her mother's hundredth birthday provided Lady N. with further reassurances of an inherited, robust, indestructible genetic makeup and presented her with a model to emulate: "The woman is a machine! She is also extremely stubborn! In many (but not all) ways, I'd love to grow up to be just like her. Especially to be one hundred years old, mentally together and well enough physically to be able to live by myself and do for myself the way she does. I mean, the woman is truly remarkable."

Around this time, Lady N. informed me that she had developed a whole new philosophy about her disease and how to cope with it. I asked her to write it down for my other MDS patients:

> *My mantra:*
> *I am NOT my cancer.*
> *I am not a "victim" because I have cancer.*
> *I am not a "hero" because I'm fighting cancer.*
> *I have no contract with life that will stand up in court. I could be crossing the street on my way to the garage to get my car and get nailed by a garbage truck.*
> *I will NOT allow people to marginalize me because I have cancer. (I find that people tend to marginalize you once they find out that you have cancer.)*

She also wrote down what the worst part of having MDS was, and how she responded. For her, cancer was like "climbing a mountain while wearing a knapsack and with every step it is as if someone is putting another brick or two in the knapsack. It is truly remarkable how much heavier and weaker I feel with each upward step. How do I deal with this? I try to get the same satisfaction from climbing a flight of stairs as I used to get from climbing a glacier, a mountain or the Alps as I did when I was a kid." And then she advised others about how to choose which mountains to climb:

> I have only a certain amount of energy each day and if I choose to expend that energy going out for a drive or for lunch in a restaurant or to the movies instead of making the bed or picking up or doing the laundry, that's fine. And if you come to visit me and disapprove of the mess or the unmade bed or unwashed dishes you have three choices: 1) you can ignore the mess, 2) you can clean it yourself if it really bothers you or, 3) you can leave.

෴

LADY N. RETURNED from Vermont and almost immediately afterward presented to the ER with a high fever, shaking chills, wild episodes of sweating, severe nausea, and uncontrolled vomiting. She was on the verge of septic shock. We admitted her to the hospital. The routine exhaustive workup for infections followed. Intravenous treatments to cover every possible pathogen were initiated. Again, as with the majority of such patients, no source for the fever was discovered. She began to deteriorate rapidly. Each morning, I stopped by to see her in the hospital. She looked at me wistfully from her bed, complaining about the shower and imparting acute asides. "The spaghetti they serve is so fake in this hospital," she said. "I call it *impasta*." As we tried to control the unidentified infection, presumably a fungal pneumonia, her white blood cells stopped maturing and started a steady, ominous climb in the blood. The MDS was transforming into acute leukemia in front of our eyes.

Talking to Lady N. as she fought the sepsis, I felt seriously deficient in my ability to explain the many paradoxes and uncertainties we were dealing with. In her case, the telltale signs of impending disaster had begun appearing a good six months before all hell would break loose. Back then, the leukemia cells brewing in her bone marrow were only just starting their hostile takeover and were still manageable in quantity. A new cytogenetic abnormality, along with a higher percentage of immature cells, was detected in the marrow. When I told her, she paled. "Okay. I guess this is not the news I was hoping for." But true to her motto—"Never give up—never give in!"—she said, "Why not treat me aggressively now? You always say, Dr. Raza, that the time to fix the roof is when the sun is shining. Not only is the sun going down rapidly for me, leaks are already appearing. How about doing something definitive now? Use me as your guinea pig. Try whatever you want. I trust you and will do exactly what you tell me." She was absolutely correct in demanding me to act then, a time when the leukemia was just starting to rear its ugly head. Isn't that why I had turned my attention to studying MDS in the first place—to find the leukemia early and treat it with a curative, preventive intent?

The problem for Lady N.—and for all cancer patients—is that unless the cancer presents early as a solid mass that can be surgically removed, there is no definitive, curative treatment that can be safely given to eliminate a small number of circulating cancer cells. All we have as treatment is chemotherapy that would end up destroying more normal cells than the few abnormal ones. In the presence of full-blown leukemia, chemotherapy is worth giving because the majority of cells in the bone marrow are leukemic. It is like saying we cannot treat your common cold, but if it develops into a pneumonia, we can.

In the background of MDS, a clonal cell had mutated in Lady N.'s marrow, losing any capability of differentiation, remaining an immature blast, a cell whose entire existence consisted of unceasing cycles of doubling its DNA followed by mitosis. The only potential cure for her would have been a bone marrow transplant. This involves killing every last cell in the patient's bone marrow, normal as well as malignant, and then trying to restart the empty marrow with fresh cells from a matched donor. Destroying the bone marrow carries with it so much toxicity and such a high risk of death that the procedure must remain limited to a select few, handpicked younger MDS patients. Lady N. was not a candidate for a bone marrow transplant due to her age and multiple co-morbidities with suboptimal function of heart, lungs, kidneys, and liver. At that point, almost six months since we first detected the earliest signs of transformation in her marrow, sepsis was complicating a rapidly advancing leukemic takeover in her body. Treat her for the infection alone, and the leukemia would get her. Treat the leukemia with the same old chemotherapy regimen and she would die faster from the suppressed, empty marrow, unable to hold the infection back. No matter what we did, her chances of survival would not improve. It was now a battle between the devil and the deep blue sea.

❦

THE STRATEGY FOR treating acute leukemia, followed for the past fifty years, is to kill as many abnormal cells as possible with a round of aggressive "induction" chemotherapy. This requires patients to be admitted to the hospital for several weeks, during which they receive what is known as the *7 + 3 protocol*: seven days of a drug called *cytosine arabinoside,* or *cytarabine* for short, and three days of the drug daunorubicin. These cytotoxic agents kill both the leukemia cells and all other rapidly dividing cells in the body, leading to the three most common side effects associated with chemotherapy—killing hair follicles, leading to baldness; killing cells in the gastrointestinal tract, leading to nausea and vomiting; and killing normal residual bone marrow cells, causing low blood counts and making patients susceptible to infections. Because those cell types proliferate at breakneck speeds, they are most sensitive to destruction by the chemotherapy. The bone marrow alone makes close to a trillion cells every twenty-four hours in a healthy adult. Once chemotherapy empties out the bone marrow, a period known as *aplasia,* it takes two to four weeks to recover. During this interval, patients end up with life-threatening infections requiring aggressive intravenous therapy with multiple antibacterial, antifungal, and antiviral drugs. If the marrow recovers with less than 5 percent leukemia cells, it is a complete remission, or CR. This is indeed cause for short-term celebration.

The problem is that a CR by itself is not sufficient. In a bit of mathematical medical jargon, one round of $7 + 3$ only destroys several "logs" of leukemia cells (where each log is a reduction by 1/10, so three logs would mean 1/1000 of the original leukemia cells). If the patient is left untreated after this, even when the bone marrow shows no microscopically recognizable leukemia, the disease relapses. In order to "consolidate" the CR, repeated rounds of $7 + 3$ or one of its variations must be administered in cycles. Because the human body can only tolerate a certain amount of cytotoxic assault at one time, a cycle is generally a month long with five to seven days of chemotherapy followed by a recovery period of two to four weeks. The patient is sent home briefly and readmitted for the next cycle within seven to ten days. When I started my training in oncology in the early '80s, we did some of the pioneering trials to determine the optimal number of "consolidations," comparing three, four, and eight follow-up, or postinduction, chemotherapy cycles. Eight was clearly too much; I recall only a handful of patients who completed this draconian prolonged torture. Today, two to four postinduction cycles are the standard.

The "hope" is to reduce the number to such a low level that the patient's own immune system can somehow deal with the "minimal residual disease," or MRD. Multiple technologies have evolved to detect one in a million or even one in a billion abnormal MRD cells. Even though we can detect those cells, we don't have anything more effective to offer than $7 + 3$ to kill them. Using the protocol again, however, would kill billions of normal cells while having a good chance of not killing those rare leukemic ones. The strategy fails in about one-third of patients, either from the beginning, because the dominant leukemic clone is entirely resistant to the $7 + 3$ and there is no complete remission to begin with, or because the MRD causes relapse of the disease.

It is hard to believe that since 1970, no better strategy has emerged. I remember hearing a talk in 1982 at Roswell Park when a visiting professor said, "We know very well that our children will look at us in disbelief and say, 'You gave *what* to your cancer patients? Chemotherapy? Were you out of your mind?'" Thirty years and many, many children, grandchildren, and great-grandchildren later, we are still doing the same. Just having to repeat the same conversation, the same statistics, and the same list of side effects to hundreds of patients a year for the past forty years is embarrassing and deeply depressing.

Had Lady N. lived to 2019, she might have responded to a new drug called *luspatercept.* Luspatercept was not developed to treat MDS patients. Like most successful cancer therapies, it arrived by their bedside purely by serendipity, developed for one indication, found to be useful for another. Luspatercept traps molecules that would otherwise bind to receptors on the surface of cells; when something is bound to those receptors, they initiate a signal that is important during the formation of bone. Overactivity of this pathway can lead to loss of bone. In patients with multiple myeloma, bone can be eaten away, resulting in creation of holes known as *lytic lesions.* This class of drugs was developed with the hope of blocking that signal and thereby reducing the number of lytic lesions in bones. When these were tried in healthy volunteers and in multiple myeloma patients, the researchers running the studies noted that the recipients' hemoglobin sharply increased, often to dangerous levels, ratcheting up so high in some cases that the patients had to undergo bloodletting. The researchers shifted course, and the focus was redirected to treating anemia instead. Enter MDS.

A phase 2 trial of luspatercept was conducted in Europe with encouraging results, particularly showing improvement in anemia of patients whose bone marrow contained *ring sideroblasts,* or early red blood cells where the nucleus gets surrounded by a ring of iron particles. It is an example of poverty in the midst of plenty. There is an abundance of iron (heme), but the red cell precursors are unable to

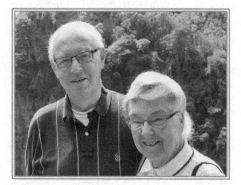

combine this heme with globin to make hemoglobin. The ring sidero-blasts cannot proceed without hemoglobin to become fully mature red blood cells. They drop dead, leading to anemia.

At Columbia University, we opened a multicenter phase 3 clinical trial of this agent in 2016 where 70 percent of patients would receive the drug and 30 percent would receive placebo. One such patient was Mrs. Fern Priestly; she had the ring sideroblastic anemia and was trans-fusion dependent, which were the two major eligibility criteria for the trial. Lady N.'s marrow also contained ring sideroblasts. The study was blinded, so we didn't know whether Fern was receiving placebo or the drug when we began, but the side effects she experienced, especially early on in the trial, helped her put two and two together fairly quickly. "I know I'm not on placebo," she told me, "because of how tired I feel after the shot every three weeks." You don't have to be a weatherman to know it's raining outside. "But it is slowly getting better each time. I think my body is finally getting adjusted to it." The study was for her, after nineteen years since being diagnosed with MDS, "the high point of the entire saga." She was so excited about the stabilization of her hemoglobin count with one shot of luspatercept every few weeks. "I have literally gotten my life back."

In one of the saddest, most tragic twists, dear Fern and her hus-band, Eldon Priestly, were involved in a deadly car accident. Fern died instantly on Sunday, August 12, 2018, and Eldon passed away from the mortal injuries he sustained, four months later.

How weary, stale, flat, and unprofitable seemed all the uses of this world.

—*HAMLET*, ACT 1, SCENE 2

೧৵৹

WHILE A PATIENT is participating in a study, every new complaint must be eyed suspiciously for possible relationship to the drug. Ultimately, the symptom may or may not be directly related, but extreme caution is necessary when new signs emerge under experimental therapies, as short- and long-term toxicities are inadequately known at the experimental stage. This is the price of novel drug trials. It became an issue with one of my patients on the luspatercept protocol.

In 2011, I met a patient who became my ideal within a few meetings. Gerson Lesser, a tall, handsome, fiercely intelligent, generous, well-read, thoughtful New Yorker of Jewish descent, is a fellow doctor, teacher, and researcher. He came to see me with his lovely, equally intelligent wife, Debbie. We became close as we settled into a routine of regular clinic visits. He had been politically active for most of his life, beginning with marching for the Spanish Republic during the Spanish Civil War. He spent hours at Zuccotti Park, the center of the Occupy Wall Street protests in 2011. A photo of Gerson at the protest went viral, "putting the lie," in Gerson's words, "to Rush Limbaugh's ugly remarks about the movement": "These protestors who are actually few in number, have contributed nothing. They are pure, genuine parasites. Many of them are bored, trust-fund kids, obsessed with being something, being somebody. Meaningless lives they want to matter." Gerson, at ninety-plus years of age, was out there with his walker every afternoon.

Once the medical part of his visits was over, we would spend twice that much time catching up on personal details, discussing politics and

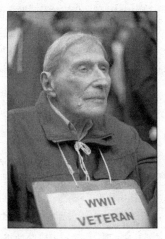

literature, science and music. He often brought me books he had just read or thought I would enjoy, I invited them to my apartment for book readings, and we went out to many dinners in lovely Manhattan restaurants. Gerson and Debbie have acquired a place in my heart reserved for only a special few. I feel incredibly fortunate every day for the opportunity my profession provides—bearing witness to some extraordinary lives, enjoying unparalleled, intimate glimpses into the most noble aspects of humanity. In the presence of such grace, all one can do is to be grateful.

By the time I first met him, he had been suffering from a chronic, slowly progressive anemia for eight years. Eventually, I put him on the luspatercept trial also. He, too, had a spectacular response, and his hemoglobin jumped by several grams to reach almost a normal level for the first time in over a decade, but he simultaneously developed shortness of breath on exertion. On the off chance that it was due to the medication, we withdrew Gerson from the trial. He promptly became transfusion dependent again and remains so to this day.

Even as both Fern and Gerson experienced dramatic responses to the trial drug, one died of a freak accident and the other could not continue, highlighting the uncertainties involved in the human condition. Nevertheless, luspatercept will be a welcome addition to the parched field of MDS therapeutics when it is approved by the FDA. The problem is that even when it is given to a hundred patients with ring sideroblast type of MDS, only thirty-eight will respond by becoming completely transfusion independent, while sixty-two will not, and based on experience so far, no one will be cured. It is discouraging to see that clinical trials today are designed in much the same way they were thirty to forty years ago. For example, it is clear that using ring sideroblasts as a marker to select patients for treatment was not good enough because not all patients responded. No serious attempt was made in the luspatercept phase 3 trial to understand why 62 percent of patients failed to respond and what is unique about those who did. We could have saved the pretherapy blood and marrow samples on the trial subjects and, once the outcome was known, compared the samples of responders and nonresponders by using the latest molecular tools. This comparison could have provided us with clues to preselect future potential responders. Equally disheartening is the attitude of the regulating agencies because they fail to demand more rigor from sponsors of the trial. What has the agency done to protect sixty-two of one hundred future patients who will have little response to luspatercept but will suffer the side effects of the drug and have to bear the exorbitant cost of therapy after the drug is approved? Nothing at all, unfortunately. The drug makers, on the other hand, expect a neat multibillion-dollar annual market for luspatercept between Europe and the United States once the agent is FDA approved. If I were younger, I would have concentrated more on the positive results for the 38 percent of patients on the trial rather than stress over the 62 percent of failures. Now that I am older, I cannot ignore the toxicities, nor the physical and financial tolls, that experimental medications take on patients. Even if Lady N. were alive today and tried luspatercept, there is no guarantee she would have responded and certainly no way of knowing for how long and at what cost of side effects. And once she stopped responding, her disease would still have progressed and killed her, either through transformation to acute leukemia or through increasing profundity of her cytopenias, causing the blood counts to plunge into irretrievable lows.

Such demoralizing news is not restricted to MDS and acute myeloid leukemia treatment. Vinay Prasad, a young hematologist-oncologist at Oregon Health & Sciences University, is a major critic of how the United States spends $700 billion on health care, identifying drug costs, conflicts of interest, poorly designed clinical trials for cancer drugs and diagnostics, and the fact that "more than half of all practiced medicine is based on scant evidence—and possibly ineffectual" as the major issues in the field. Prasad published an analysis of fifty-four cancer drugs approved by the FDA between 2008 and 2012. Of those fifty-four drugs, thirty-six, or 67 percent, were approved based on so-called surrogate end points—that is, on the basis of something other than a known effect on the tumor leading to improved survival. Indeed, follow-up over the next several years showed that thirty-one of those thirty-six approved drugs yielded no demonstrable gains in survival. What are we doing wrong? Perhaps the one-size-fits-all approach is the problem? Can we improve these grim numbers by custom-designing therapy to suit individual patient needs? Precision medicine.

◈

THE IDEA OF individualized therapy is attractive and logical on the surface. Take, for example, the drug Vidaza, which Lady N. received for six months to no avail. Other patients with MDS respond quite well to Vidaza, with the drug being effective enough that treatments—which can be debilitating—become less frequent with time. Mark De Noble, at eighty, was able to drive across the country with his wife after going on the drug in 2015: "It is February of 2019 now, and I continue to receive Vidaza for five days every six weeks and regularly visit Dr. Raza for my periodic bone marrow biopsies. My wife and I travel several

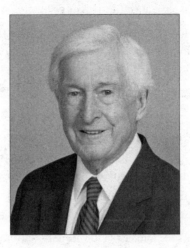

times a year, mostly by car, exploring new places and visiting family and friends. At home, we enjoy hosting friends and family. Now that we're retired, we volunteer once a month at a residential facility for fifteen troubled teenagers. As we all prepare a three-course dinner, we teach them how to prepare foods, handle kitchen tools, set a table, serve food, etc. Then we enjoy a delicious meal together."

Mr. De Noble had an extraordinary response to Vidaza while Lady N.'s counts did not budge on the same drug despite half a year's treatment. Under the microscope, their disease looked similar. In fact, Mr. De Noble experienced such complete and durable benefit from the drug that he earned a special moniker reserved for exceptional responders: *unicorn.* Traditionally, clinical trials of experimental agents are statistically powered to deliver response in a predetermined minimum percentage of patients. If the number fails to meet the end point, the drug is thrown out like the baby with the bathwater. This changed in 2012 as a result of a trial in which the drug everolimus given to patients with urothelial cancers produced overall dismal results in forty-four treated subjects but one of them showed a truly outstanding response. A deeper investigation into the reason for such exquisite sensitivity revealed the presence of unexpected mutations not previously associated with that type of bladder cancer, demonstrating once again the profound biologic variability within morphologically identical tumors. This one case led to the initiation of a pilot study, funded by the NCI, directed at identifying molecular features associated with exceptional responses. In the study referenced above, everolimus was the perfect drug for the exceptional responder, but was it worth having forty-four others suffer only the drug's toxicities without any appreciable benefits?

The ideal situation would be to administer the drug only to preselected potential responders. Identifying predictive markers that allow for individualizing therapy by matching drugs to patients remains the treasured yet elusive holy grail of oncology. To what extent is this strategy being pursued? More than 90 percent of trials ongoing around the country make almost zero attempt to save tumor samples for post hoc examination to identify predictive biomarkers. Even in the NCI-funded study of exceptional responders previously mentioned, only genetic mutations were investigated as the single potential predictive marker. What if the reason for response was not a mutated gene but abnormal expression of the gene at the RNA level, or that it resided entirely outside the tumor cell, related to the microenvironment of the tumor? Why are we not making the required efforts in as comprehensive a manner as needed? Who is pushing this short-term agenda driven by the singular goal of getting a drug approved with alacrity as long as it meets the bar of improving survival by mere weeks in a few patients?

A patient with MDS that I became extremely close to over the years was Barbara Freehill. She had a lower-risk MDS that evolved to an overlap myelodysplastic-myeloproliferative neoplasm (MDS/MPN). I saw her every two to three weeks as she was steadily transfusion dependent. Her poise, dignified personality, gorgeous looks, and her incredible wisdom combined to make her one of the most amazing people I have been fortunate to take care of. We could talk about anything under the sun. I treated her for a long time with Dacogen and then Revlimid. She was under my care, seeing me two to three times a month for several years

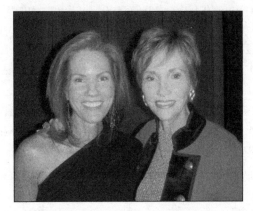

when one day she showed up without an appointment. My nurse came and told me Barbara wanted an urgent word with me. I went out to see her, and she could hardly breathe, so anxious was she. Her youngest daughter, thirty-nine-year-old Kendra Seth, was in the ICU. I will let Kendra tell you this shocking story:

I was admitted through the ER for a pain I was experiencing on my right side (I thought maybe I had pulled a muscle running). That pain quickly went from mild to excruciating. After a long night, a CAT scan revealed that I had a massive clot in my *portal vein.* The clot was virtually strangling all of the blood flow to my major organs. In order for me to *survive,* the clot had to be cleared as quickly as possible. After 3 failed surgeries & little hope for a plausible next step, my mom suggested that her doctor stop in for a "visit."

I begged my mom not to . . . after the failure of my "best chance" surgery I was at an all-time low both mentally & physically. My body seemed to go into complete revolt, although I hadn't eaten in weeks, I gained over 30 lbs in water weight virtually overnight. I couldn't bend my fingers or toes, or even roll over—I was literally a prisoner in my own bed.

Mentally I just could not wrap my head around how a year ago I had successfully climbed Mt Kilimanjaro—how my life had changed so dramatically in a number of months. The last thing I wanted was another team of doctors that only asked the same questions and provided no answers.

And then I met Dr. Raza . . . at the time she walked through the door we were discussing my "best" option which was a 5 organ transplant. All I could think about was getting home to my husband & 4 young children so I was all for it—shows you how desperate I felt. When Dr. Raza *quietly* came in, she didn't ask me all the usual questions, she spoke to me as a person, not a case—her humanity was immediately apparent. Dr. Raza suggested I be *tested** for a mutation in the gene Jak2 and when that came back positive about 10 days later it was our first *breadcrumb* to getting me healthy.

(*Note: My colleague Joe Jurcic, who had been consulted as the hematologist on service, had noticed the high platelet count also, and had preempted me in ordering the test.)

The most dramatic feature of Kendra's story is that she went from being considered for a five-organ transplant as she lay in the ICU, deathly ill, to being managed by aspirin alone. This happened because it was her underlying bone marrow overlap syndrome (MPN/MDS) causing her to have high platelets, which, in turn caused blood to form clots in large and small vessels. Aspirin reduces the clumping action of platelets, preventing clot formation. The life of a beautiful thirty-nine-year-old mother of four was saved because the right drug was matched to the right patient.

⚭

KENDRA'S CASE SUGGESTS a great plan: find a mutation by sequencing the DNA in the patient's cancer cells, match a drug with activity against the mutated protein, and administer it irrespective of which organ bears the tumor. This approach combines the best of available technology and preselection of patients likely to respond, resulting in therapy tailor-made to suit the need of an individual patient. Precision medicine. Customized health care. Targeted therapy. Predictive modeling. Optimized strategy.

All sound terrific. The wave of the future. The fashionable thing to do. Mostly, it does not work. Here is what happened. Two types of trials were conceived. In one, called *umbrella trials,* tumors affecting the same organ but presenting with different genetic mutations could be matched with targeted therapies. For example, one lung cancer has an EGFR mutation—and the best treatment for that patient would be an EGFR inhibitor like erlotinib—while another patient's lung cancer has a mutation in the HER2 gene, for whom Herceptin would be the right match. A second type of trials, called *basket trials,* pursues the same mutation as it appears in tumors in various organs; the idea is that the targeted therapy should work for all. For example, a mutation in the EGFR gene in a patient with pancreatic cancer should respond to erlotinib as well as a lung cancer patient with the same mutation. Many cancer programs have stepped forward to promote the idea of precision medicine because it seems the right thing to do.

There are several problems with the approach. First, it is extremely rare to have one gene driving one cancer. Second, even if such a mutation is identified, there aren't many effective, approved, targeted therapies with which to treat the patient. Third, when a genetic mutation is matched to a drug, response is not guaranteed; in fact, the response rate is 30 percent at best. And finally, if everything works as planned and the patient even responds to the targeted therapy, the response offers no more than six months of improvement in survival over unmatched therapies. And this is the fundamental problem with most of the approaches; cancer treatments either don't improve survival or the improvement is measurable in weeks or a few months, at tremendous physical, financial, and emotional burden.

How many thousands of tumors will need to be sequenced to find these rare patients, at what immense cost, and for what little benefit? Vinay Prasad argued in *Nature* in 2016 that the numbers will be very high; a sequencing program at MD Anderson Cancer Center was able to match only 6.4 percent of 2,600 patients with a targeted drug for identified mutations. A National Cancer Institute trial of 795 people who have relapsed solid tumors and lymphoma was only able (as of May 2016) to pair 2 percent of patients with a targeted therapy. Even then, Prasad reminds us, "being assigned such a therapy is not proof of benefit." Only a third of patients respond to drugs given based on biological markers, and median progression-free survival is less than six months. Prasad estimated that precision oncology would benefit only 1.5 percent of patients, such as those in the NCI trial.

At the 2018 meeting of the American Association of Cancer Research, David Hyman from Memorial Sloan Kettering Cancer Center presented data on tumors in more than 25,000 patients. Of them, 15 percent matched with an FDA-approved drug and 10 percent with a drug in clinical trials. Prasad found similar proportions in his latest analysis, where 15 percent of 610,000 US patients with metastatic cancer were eligible for an FDA-approved, genome-guided drug. But once matched, just 6.6 percent likely benefited. Similar finds emerge from a study in Europe. From 2009 to 2013, the European Medicines Agency approved the use of forty-eight cancer drugs for sixty-eight indications. Only for twenty-six, or 38 percent, of those indications was there an improvement in survival, with a median benefit of only 2.7 months.

When I have questioned the practical feasibility of conducting such trials at the cost of hundreds of millions of dollars, one answer I regularly receive is a rather self-righteous one: "Well, Azra, for those 6.6 percent of patients, the extra five to six months or more mattered." Of course the time mattered, although—since we're talking about medians—it's important to remember that half the patients would get less than the median benefit. And what about all the toxicity caused to the 93.4 percent who derived zero benefit from it? And all the wasted resources of sequencing thousands of tumors?

Take the example of the latest arrival in this area of precision oncology. In November 2018, the FDA approved the drug larotrectinib for the treatment of adult and pediatric solid tumors that express a neurotrophic receptor tyrosine kinase fusion gene (TRK). The trial of this small molecule, which led to approval of the drug, included a total of 55 patients, 22 percent showing complete and 53 percent a partial response. How long did the response last? Six months for two-thirds of the patients and a year for 40 percent. The test alone costs thousands of dollars per patient to find a very rare case. Treatment is likely to run in hundreds of thousands of dollars. For some two dozen patients who benefited for at least a year with this treatment, the approval of the drug is fantastic news. But bear in mind how small that number is in the face of the 1,735,350 new cases of cancer that will be diagnosed in the United States and the 609,640 who will die from the disease. This cannot be the most cost-effective way for us to move forward, yet such approvals are greeted as the new horizon, the game changer, the paradigm shift. It is my contention that these rare cases would be identified anyway through routine genetic profiling if we shift our focus to employing the genomic technology toward early detection. Instead of declaring victory, this approval by the FDA should serve as the impetus to envision better strategies for the future that can help a majority of cases.

Precision oncology ultimately fails because it ignores the evolutionary nature of cancer. As Theodosius Dobzhansky observed, "Nothing in biology makes sense except in the light of evolution." In 1837, Charles Darwin sketched a tree trunk in his notebook with radiating branches representing the evolution of species from a common ancestor. Today, a graphic representation of cancer with all its genetic diversity and presence of multiple competing subpopulations of cancer cells emanating from the primary tumor is superimposable on Darwin's tree of evolution. It has taken oncologists a long time to reach this understanding, thanks to a strange cleavage appearing among researchers early on. As molecular biology took off in earnest in the 1970s, investigators became convinced they would crack the cancer enigma. Reductionists, devoted to studying molecular genetic happenings in the cell, awash in overconfidence, drowned out the pluralists tracking the behavior of tumors as a whole. There was almost no cross talk between the two groups.

It is therefore no surprise that Peter Nowell's clairvoyance about cancer being an evolving entity, with all its attendant therapeutic implications, an idea hailed as truly revolutionary today, remained largely ignored when first published in 1976. Fortunately, my husband, Harvey, was an exception. He immediately saw the genius behind Nowell's paradigm, and he asked me to present the paper. Harvey was merciless in shredding one to pieces for the tiniest error during these weekly lab meetings. It was one's familiarity with details that impressed him; any misstep, no matter how small, would discredit the entire presentation. I had to study the paper very carefully and read up on all sorts of background material in order to present the ideas coherently. That single paper helped me develop a radically different view of cancer very early on in my career. At the risk of testing the patience of readers not initiated into the specialized, dense, telegraphic language of science, it is worthwhile reproducing Nowell's 138-word abstract from the classic paper "The Clonal Evolution of Tumor Cell Populations":

It is proposed that most neoplasms arise from a single cell of origin, and tumor progression results from acquired genetic variability within the original clone allowing sequential selection of more aggressive sublines. Tumor cell populations are apparently more genetically unstable than normal cells, perhaps from activation of specific gene loci in the neoplasm, continued presence of carcinogen, or even nutritional deficiencies within the tumor. The acquired genetic instability and associated selection process, most readily recognized cytogenetically, results in advanced human malignancies being highly individual karyotypically and biologically. Hence, each patient's cancer may require individual specific therapy, and even this may be thwarted by emergence of a genetically variant subline resistant to the treatment. More research should be directed toward understanding and controlling the evolutionary process in tumors before it reaches the late stage usually seen in clinical cancer.

That was more than forty years ago. Today, mapping mutational profiles in hundreds of individual tumors, combined with an astounding failure to develop any meaningful therapies for cancer in the interim, have confirmed the veracity of every word Nowell wrote. Simply stated, tumors also evolve by the Darwinian process of natural selection. Cancer begins in a single cell with one or more genetic mutations driving its release from growth-controlling signals. As the cell starts unchecked proliferation, its daughters pick up additional mutations, giving rise to multiple branches emanating from the tree. Each branch of cells carrying the driver mutation of the founder cell and the novel passenger mutations acquires novel metabolic and physiologic properties. Cells whose genotype matches the microenvironment develop a growth advantage, selectively expanding their population. Others wait their turn silently. No patient has one cancer.

There are countless cancers within each cancer. Since chemotherapy cannot kill every cancer cell, the surviving cells are selected to adapt and regrow. This is the reason why even the most successful targeted therapies fail; they only kill off the cells with peculiar characteristics susceptible to the treatment, selecting the outgrowth of others with biologic diversity.

Every cancer is unique, yet some common principles apply to all. First, the malignant process begins in a single cell for practically all known cancers. Mutations accumulate in key genes related to proliferation, cell growth, and cell death, eventually giving rise to a cell with a growth advantage. This cell divides rapidly to produce clones of itself. All the daughters will share the same foundational genetic mutations, but in addition, some of the daughters will sustain additional mutations that give them biologic characteristics that are distinct from the parent. Formation of such subclones happens constantly in a tumor, but usually, a few clones dominate at any given time while others remain on the sidelines, waiting for sequential recruitment. Of course, malignant cells also leave their natural habitats and wander off to form metastases.

The presence of innumerable, biologically distinct daughter cells with additional mutations, chromosomal changes, and altered nutritional and metabolic requirements is the reason why even the best of targeted therapies are of transient benefit. Treatment to which one clone is sensitive leads to the selection of refractory, resistant subclones and a more invasive disease. A biologically new cancer results with an entirely different natural history, novel rules of proliferation and differentiation, newfound invasive potential, unpredictable responsiveness to therapies. These frightening, abrupt transformations of the disease are a spectacle to watch through the clinical prism of changing blood counts, paraneoplastic syndromes, and immune reactions. As clinicians, we regularly witness this kaleidoscopic, repetitive dance of motley populations within populations of cancer cells unfolding in real time in vivo.

Competing groups of cells take turns expanding and shrinking; changing places, honeycombing, crumbling, only to be reignited into action by newly acquired copying errors in the reeling, replicating DNA strands, seeking comfort in uninhabited beds, forging alliances with cooperative bedfellows in marrow niches and safe havens of supportive organs. Occasionally, a leukemia arises in the background of MDS with such malignant ferocity that all we can do is watch the vertiginous descent into entropy, spellbound, helpless in front of so anarchic a rebellion.

The microenvironment of tumors plays a critical role in clonal selection and promotion. Properties of the soil vary in different areas of the body. When studying ovarian cancer, a tumor spreading by direct physical invasion in the abdominal cavity rather than traveling through blood or lymphatics, researchers found that subsets of cancer cells thrived in a site-specific manner. Characteristics of the microenvironment were differentially suited to promote the growth of one clone over another. One seed, one soil; change the properties of a seed through a mutation and it would have to find a new home. It is an important reason why preclinical cancer platforms employing cell lines and patient-derived xenografts are likely to remain wholly inadequate as models for drug development; they are devoid of the in vivo microenvironment.

∾

There is no sickness worse for me than
words that to be kind must lie.

—AESCHYLUS

The secret to success in life is relationships. The secret of relationships is trust. The secret of trust is acknowledgment of pure and simple truth. The problem in oncology, as in life, is that truth is rarely pure and never simple.

One historic incident that has stayed with me since I first read about it as a teenager growing up in Karachi involves Mr. M. A. Jinnah, the founder of Pakistan. He spoke to a crowd of approximately ten thousand at a public gathering in Agra, India, in the early 1940s, years before the partition of the subcontinent into India and Pakistan. Probably five hundred people in that crowd had a passing knowledge of English, and about fifty of the elite among them understood it well. Trained as a barrister at Lincoln's Inn in London, Mr. Jinnah spoke in chaste English with a British accent for forty minutes, and only in the last few did he address the commoners through a broken hybrid version of Urdu-Hindi-English. Shockingly enough, the crowd sat mesmerized throughout despite a complete lack of understanding. When asked afterward about what captivated them to such a degree, one man's answer was, "Look, it's true that I did not understand a word of what Mr. Jinnah said in English, but I have full trust that whatever he said was for my good and meant to protect me."

Was the man's blind trust justified? Trust is not just the sugarcoating glaze; it is indispensable, essential, vital. Too much willingness to trust is naive—a leap of faith that can earn deception. Yet a deeply meaningful blind trust is justified as long as the trustworthiness of the individual is already established. The man's trust was based on an intelligent and experiential assessment of Mr. Jinnah's previous actions, competence, reliability, integrity, and his demonstration of benevolence and empathy for the common man. Trust is not a static entity; it must be continually won.

Patients have the right to trust their physicians the same way Mr. Jinnah was trusted by his constituency. Do we deserve the trust?

In 1986, I had gone to Pakistan for a brief visit. One of the elderly female relatives at a family gathering, delighted to see me after several years, asked a curious question. "I don't care how many degrees a doctor has, even if they are known to cure cancer, if they don't have the reputation of *shifa* in their hands, I stay miles away from them. What I want to know is if you have been graced with *shifa* in your hands yet?" *Shifa* is an Urdu word loosely translated as "the healing power." It is the equivalent of blind trust in one's doctor—a powerful, intangible confidence that no matter how deadly their health challenges, and especially when medical knowledge is stumped, the physician alone possesses the wisdom to remain sensitive, to proceed in caring, empathic ways, always exclusively focused on the patient's interest.

Lady N. thought I possessed *shifa.* She expressed her confidence at least half a dozen times during every clinic visit. She trusted me with her life. I obsessively tally the number of ways in which I let her down, this terrified, trusting, vulnerable woman, sitting in the consultation room, her mind and body besieged from within and without, desperately seeking a lifeline I had no power to conjure. Lady N. and I both knew that she had a fatal illness, that it was simply a matter of time before she would enter the bedlam surrounding end-of-life issues. Obviously, I had no cure to offer, no magic bullet to eliminate the coming leukemia, and each time she expressed her implicit trust in my power of *shifa,* I reminded her gently of what was expected. She scoffed, she laughed it off, she changed the topic, sometimes she became agitated, abruptly walked out. I broached the subject of involving our palliative care team, which she dismissed out of hand. What about a psychiatrist? "I have been on antidepressants practically all my life. My mother thought I was hyper when I was two! I don't need more doping, thank you." Lady N. simply refused to accept that the end could come for her. She demanded therapy for her cancer, not her mind, willing to be a guinea pig for any experimental approach I could concoct.

Things spiraled out of control in her case with frightening speed. Within days, she was admitted to the hospital with a high fever. I sat on her bed early one morning as she struggled to breathe. We were, for once, without the usual team of nurses, oncology fellows, and medical students crowding the bed, craning their necks to catch snippets of our conversation. Strangely enough, the intimacy of solitude had a distancing effect, introducing a formality in our communication, an uncharacteristic courtesy with which to speak about unspeakable things.

"We have to intubate you now and place you on a respirator. You can refuse."

She caught her breath as the color drained from her face, then rallied and shot back, "Refuse and do what? Dr. Raza, I will *not* give up. Do whatever you can to keep me alive. For God's sake, my mother is alive at a hundred. I have good genes. Freeze my body if I die. I want you to clone me when you have the techniques worked out. I know you can. You are the only one I have full confidence in."

I kissed her and called the anesthesiology team. We wheeled her down to the MICU. Within minutes, she was intubated, placed on a respirator.

What followed was less about supporting life and more about prolonging death. There was zero chance that Lady N. would ever be able to breathe on her own again since her fundamental issue was not the rapidly progressive pneumonia but her untreatable, fatal cancer. Infections were flaring up precisely because all of a sudden, pathogens had a free pass in her leukemia-riddled body. The immune system was fast

approaching a state of total collapse as the bone marrow failed to produce the most critical first line of defense, white blood cells. I knew
precisely what frightful days lay ahead. She did not.

I am a clinician first, and my medical, moral, and ethical obligation
is to relieve distress and suffering caused by disease. I should enable
my patients to benefit from the best that science and technology has to
offer, not be hurt by it. Yet by offering to intubate her and connect her
to artificial life support, as if death were an option, did I fail to protect
Lady N.? What forces compelled me to offer her a choice of intubation,
inviting her to accept unspeakable horrors that she had no clue about?
The law, of course. What had I done to help Lady N. accept mortality?
Did I do enough to explain the hopeless nature of her leukemia, the
pointlessness of placing her on artificial life-support systems? Was it a
failure on my part as her treating oncologist that somehow I transmitted a false sense of hope to Lady N.? Did I use language that made sense
to Lady N. instead of confusing her? Or was it Lady N. whose nature
dictated revolt, who would never take things lying down, no matter
how much I tried to explain the hopelessness of her prognosis? What I
know beyond a shadow of doubt is that to intubate her and attach her
to a ventilator was the worst possible thing to do to her, and yet, against
my better judgment, I was forced to give her the choice. So was I morally wrong in knowingly letting her enter the hellish nightmare of the
next week? Where does medical and individual responsibility end and
societal responsibility take over?

Was Lady N. wrong to trust me? Where is my *shifa?*

⁍

TODAY, ANY TALK of death is considered morbid and unhealthy, but
in the mind-set a century ago—when war, disease, and famine raged
unchecked—it was an ever-present threat. Life expectancy was in mid-
forties at best. Rather than being a sad ending, often death was treated

as a new beginning. Emily Dickinson, imagining the scene of her final moments from beyond the grave, an unfathomable point of eternity, paints death arriving with the gallantry of a dignified escort:

> *Because I could not stop for Death—*
> *He kindly stopped for me—*
> *The Carriage held but just Ourselves—*
> *And Immortality.*

> *We slowly drove—He knew no haste*
> *And I had put away*
> *My labor and my leisure too,*
> *For His Civility—*

Not so, our Lady N. Drama queen that she was, she was not fading quietly into the twilight anytime soon, and no one was going to drive her carriage gently into the sunset.

Over the next week, an unrelenting chaos descended upon her unconscious body. She suffered every ignominy that a mechanical life-support system could possibly visit upon its subjects. Her body expanded grotesquely, unevenly, to accommodate six extra liters of fluid pumped in to combat hypotension, the fluid stagnating in strange crevices of her body because her failing kidneys were unable to expel most of it. Her eyes, circled by blue-black rings due to periorbital edema and bleeding, bulged from a shiny, swollen, unrecognizable, raccoon-like face. Her entire skin, forced to lodge pound upon pound of relentlessly multiplying, roving, vagrant leukemia cells, became studded with a smattering of rock-hard little mounds, referred to as *chloromas* because of their sickly green color, sprouting amid flowery patches of tiny red-and-purple petechial spots announcing shattered capillaries and profoundly low platelets. She had tubes coming out of every orifice, lines placed in multiple large veins from the jugular to the femoral. Monitors recorded everything from oxygen saturation and vital signs to the pulmonary arterial pressure and cardiac rhythm; colorful screens blinked from adjustable metal poles on wheels, beeping insistently, alarming visitors, alerting nurses, ignored, switched off, only to restart screeching in unison moments later.

Mortality steadily eroded the searing desire for eternity, piling a thousand humiliations at once on her decaying, battered, abused, assaulted, gigantic frame, shackled to the gadget-rich MICU bed with a hundred tubes and pipes. Lady N., suspended in a bizarre state between life and death, fought the funeral in her brain. Every groove, ridge, and fold in her cerebrum revolted. Every hair follicle on her skin, every cell in her organs, put up a fight. She refused to die. She pushed back, drawing upon astonishing psychological and physical reserves, producing a multifaceted tour de force of rebellion that challenged the limits of medical imagination and decorum. She managed to subvert the crippling blows of her fatal disease into an epistemology of endurance by her unyielding, uncanny, scandalously defiant posture of refusal.

Her 101-year-old mother finally stepped in. A devoted aide wheeled her into the MICU. Accompanied by friends of Lady N. and by her lawyer, she formally petitioned for her daughter to be taken off life support. An abrupt, eerie, unnerving silence replaced the racket of beeping and pinging alarms as machines switched off, IV lines were pulled, tubes yanked, monitors unplugged.

꩜

KEY OPINION LEADERS providing therapeutic algorithms rely on studies demonstrating success or failure of a strategy in the populations as a whole, but management of patients and the questions of existential challenges posed by each unique individual remain the responsibility of the treating oncologist. No degree of technologic improvement, national debates on "right to life" issues, or guidelines from evidence-based medicine can help in these deeply personal, intimate moments. Repetitive transmission of clinical trial results or regurgitation of statistical probabilities about chances of response and survival do not necessarily help patients. Devoid of emotions, recitation of facts is like a jockey without a horse. This moment calls for a serious reckoning. Patients disoriented and confused by the caprice of their rapidly evolving cancer and the absurdities of medical choices need more than medical advice from their oncologists. For their part, physicians must now harness all their own emotional, psychic, social, intellectual, philosophical, and even literary resources to engage with the patient and their families in repetitive, substantive conversations informed by empathy, kindness, and understanding. A more balanced, candid conversation about end-of-life issues, a frank explanation regarding the limits of medical and scientific knowledge should supplement the discussions of treatment options from the first meeting and continue as often as possible through subsequent encounters. Nowhere is the science of medicine replaced by the art of caring as in the final days of a terminal illness. Yet that is precisely where oncologists turn over the care of patients they have looked after for years to a new hospice team.

In addition to the end-of-life and do-not-resuscitate conversations, an equally important question is, why could I not offer Lady N. anything better than 7 + 3? Most large clinical trials conducted by cooperative groups of oncologists across the country in the past decades have concentrated on tweaking the doses, schedules, or formulation of the two drugs with minor improvements in the response rates. Harvey and I became so allergic to 7 + 3 discussions in every national meeting we attended that, following the formula of the great Paul Farmer, we also started using it to refer to individuals who use seven words when three would suffice. In the midst of a perfectly serious scientific session, or during a dinner conversation with guests, if anyone appeared to drone on tediously, Harvey would lean over and whisper, "Seven and three."

The latest entry into this arena, hailed as a paradigm shift by many reviewers and editorial contributors, is the lipid-encapsulated combined version of 7 + 3. In a large phase 3 clinical trial conducted at the cost of tens of millions of dollars, this new 7 + 3 version improved survival by 9.6 months compared to 5.9 months for the standard 7 + 3. Why is our bar for improving survival so low? Is 3.7 months the best we can offer our patients at almost ten times the cost of the previous regimen?

An improvement in the last fifty years in AML treatment has been that by using multiple parameters—including clinical presentation and biologic and genetic characteristics of leukemia cells—we can identify individuals likely to benefit from chemotherapy alone or those who are at high risk of relapse. Studies have shown that for the elderly (defined as anyone over sixty) or those with high-risk acute myeloid leukemia (that is, AML arising from MDS or after exposure to toxins like chemotherapy), even if a complete remission is produced in response to 7 + 3, the overall survival is not improved. The leukemia such as Lady N.'s that arises in the background of a myelodysplastic syndrome is notoriously resistant. In her case, 7 + 3 could be used to reduce the burden of leukemia in the bone marrow but would have to be followed by a stem cell transplant if the aim was to improve survival. Given her age and other comorbid conditions, a transplant was out of the question (it would kill her faster than anything else). Then what would be the point of torturing her in the hospital for weeks, treating her with agents that carry potentially lethal side effects? Why not simply provide the best supportive care available, with transfusions of platelets and blood, and treat infections as needed? Why not let them pass their last days at home with loved ones? Actually, oncologists do offer the choice of aggressive cytotoxic therapy versus supportive care with transfusions and antibiotics as needed. This is where we enter the strange circle where denial of the outcome of terminal illness, extreme fear of death, and the inextinguishable flame of hope merge together to cloud judgments. Almost all patients refuse supportive care and choose the aggressive approach. As did Lady N.

LADY N. PASSED away due to complications related to her MDS. Yet in a larger sense, MDS could not, and did not, defeat her. She defeated MDS by inspiring countless others she met because of her MDS. She dared to play Russian roulette with a loaded gun. She *was* the loaded gun possessing the power to die but without the agency to pull the trigger:

> *My Life had stood—a Loaded Gun—*
> *In Corners—till a Day*
> *The Owner passed—identified—*
> *And carried Me away—*
>
> —EMILY DICKINSON

I miss her greatly. At the oddest of moments—like when I see a cat, or an especially funny cartoon, or a scared young medical student, and most of all, because of a comment, a gesture, an expression, or a question from an MDS patient—her laughing face accosts me. I smile. I silently mouth the words . . .

Lady N., *Zindabad!* (Live long!)

| # KITTY C.

What Wound Did Ever Heal but by Degrees?

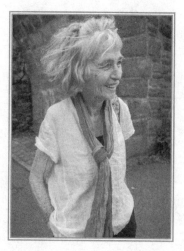

SUBWAY STATIONS IN MANHATTAN CAN TAKE YOU BY SURPRISE ON early Monday mornings before the rush-hour hullabaloo. One such morning, as I descended the steep stairs of the Fifty-Seventh Street and Eighth Avenue entrance to Columbus Circle for the A train to Columbia University Medical campus on 168th Street, I was struck by how pristine the place looked. Gone was the mess and mayhem of the weekend, the drunk, sweaty, overexerted, overpartied colliding bodies, rushing through stations, cramped into carriages. Every last discarded beer can and soda bottle, stray straw, soiled, drifting Kleenex, and plastic bag had been swept off the steps. Even the wet hobos had wandered off in flabbergasted weariness. Such moments are tender ones, with that unexpected morning neatness; the freshly swept floors exposing patterns of geometric formality, tiles radiating from a central pillar, stealing toward revolving horizontal arms of the entrance, almost nostalgic for the falls of boots and stilettos. The underground Turnstyle market was not humming yet, but the Bee Gees were:

> *Suddenly you're in my life*
> *A part of everything I do*
> *You got me workin' day and night*
> *Just tryin' to keep a hold on you*
>
> *… We can take forever just a minute at a time*
> *More than a woman*
> *More than a woman to me*

I was heading to a packed clinic where I would see anywhere from twenty to twenty-five patients and perform five to ten bone marrow biopsies on MDS and AML patients in the next twelve hours. From the car, I peered into the pitch black of the underground tunnel, overlaid with reflections of bodies bent on iPhones, half-asleep teenagers propped into upright postures by oversized backpacks, smartly dressed young professionals adjusting earphones. In the cool, quiet carriage, I opened the *New York Times* but was unable to concentrate, distracted by the mental cataloging of tasks ahead, matching actions to bodies, prescriptions to faces, wincing as I acknowledged the imperfection of my knowledge with each image. Still, some faces attached to precise clinic appointment times surfaced in my mind: *8:00 a.m. RG, 8:30 a.m. L. W., 9:00 a.m. Kitty C.*

I devised oblique methods for imparting bad news to one; to propose, with cheerful caution, a new experimental trial to another. I shored up the psychic reserves to negotiate impossible options with RG. I had become close to her through weekly encounters over years. I would be speaking on the phone to her scared and anxious daughter in Australia, who was unable to hop on the next plane because of her children. What were her worries and hopes? How could I help her take better care of her mother, living in the Bronx, who, with a hemoglobin of 7 g, practically fainted every time she climbed five flights of stairs yet who refused to take the elevator on the Sabbath? And that morning, as blasts were starting to show up in low numbers but with a disturbing consistency in her blood, I would be performing a bone marrow biopsy, checking for disease transformation from MDS to AML. Then what? In clinic with RG and her sweet, quiet, gentle husband, I would call her daughter in Australia and son in Boston, and when all of us had been connected, I'd discuss the next steps of treatment. They would all be tense, because last week, I had warned them of the coming bone marrow examination.

RG is seventy-one years old. She is an extremely loving and extremely anxious woman, and a frail one, weighing ninety-two pounds. She hugs me at least five times during every clinic visit. She reminds me how much trust she has in my ability to help her. Her children want her to move to be with one of them, but she refuses to go because she does not want to change hematologists. She cannot bear to see anyone else but me. It pained me deeply to think of how pathetic my abilities were (and are), how hopeless the treatments I would propose in case her MDS had turned to AML. After forty years, there was still only 7 + 3 to offer poor RG?

I suddenly felt a profound sense of grief. I felt lost. I thought of my friend Sara Suleri reading from her book *Meatless Days* when she came to speak at the University of Chicago: "For to be lost is just a minute's respite, after all, like a train that cannot help but stop between the stations of its proper destination in order to stage a pretend version of the end. Dying, we saw, was simply change taken to an extremity, and wasn't a thing to lose us but to find us out, to catch us where we least wanted to be caught."

The hurtling subway stopped at the 125th Street station in a fleeting impersonation of its grand finale, precisely matching the punctuated equilibrium of the clonal progression I was imagining for MDS cells in the marrow of another patient I would be seeing that morning, Kitty C. Her disease seemed to be stable for the moment, the dominant clone lying low, the smaller subclones coasting between spontaneous expansions and regressions. Nevertheless, she was harboring a time bomb in that marrow. *How long,* I wondered, *before the cells march to the next stop, acquire a new mutation, rest awhile, restart, and spin out of control? How long until the train wreck?*

⚮

KITTY C., IN her early seventies, had been diagnosed with MDS in June 2009 after her primary care physician noted that her hemoglobin was dropping. When it had fallen below 8 g/dl of blood, my hematology colleague David saw her and performed a bone marrow biopsy. The biopsy revealed that she had a lower-risk MDS with normal cytogenetics. In 2009, she became transfusion dependent, receiving blood every six to eight weeks or so. Initially, she was treated by David with erythropoietin, which stimulates the growth of red blood cells, and then with the FDA-approved chemotherapy Dacogen. After treatment, the intervals between transfusions increased, but not for long; within four months, she returned to her baseline frequency of blood transfusions.

David asked me to consider her for one of my clinical trials. When I first saw her in June 2010, she was profoundly anemic, receiving two units of blood every two weeks. Kitty and I instantly clicked. She was a quintessential New Yorker. Thin, scandalously liberal, single, given to long walks in Central Park and the New York Botanical Gardens in the Bronx, taking regular subway rides to attend lectures at the 92nd Street Y, art shows at MoMA, and classical music concerts at Lincoln Center. She was a voracious reader. We exchanged books and music, we talked about children and politics, Nora Ephron, dry skin, and *Moby Dick*. We laughed and we joked and we had serious discussions about every aspect of her profound anemia and the treatment options. We became friends.

I repeated a bone marrow biopsy and was pleased to see that the MDS was still of the low-risk variety, and the chromosomal test revealed a pleasant surprise. A small clone of cells in her bone marrow now showed a deletion of the long arm of chromosome 5, known as *del5q*. This is the same del5q abnormality that Lady N.'s diseased cells showed, associated with exquisite responsiveness to Revlimid. I gave Kitty the good news at our next meeting: almost 70 percent of MDS patients with del5q become transfusion independent for prolonged periods of time when treated with Revlimid. She looked surprised. "How come I was not treated with this before?" I explained that at diagnosis, her cytogenetics were normal, but with time, and following treatment with Dacogen, a subclone of cells emerged carrying this chromosomal damage. Clonal evolution in cancer is usually a sign of disease progression, but for once, chemotherapy had unraveled the presence of a "good" clone.

Kitty had a dramatic response to Revlimid. Within a month, her hemoglobin began to rise on its own, without transfusions. Week after week, we sat in clinic, gobsmacked as her blood counts steadily rose toward normal; high-fiving, we'd dance out of the consultation room into the hallway together, hugging, ready to declare victory from the citadel.

When she first hit the normal range of hemoglobin after several years of functioning with suboptimal oxygenation of the cells in her body, she sat in clinic, pensive, unusually quiet. "I feel so different suddenly. There is a new clarity. I can't explain what I am feeling. I need to sort things out." We talked for a long time about the toll anemia had exacted from her body. She remained thoughtful, trying to quantify, catalog, define her newfound old self. "Why don't you write about it?" I suggested.

"Not a bad idea," she said.

On her next visit, she brought me this:

I've been paying attention to my body as it responds to the new medication—as my hemoglobin ratchets up into the realms of the normal. I've been concentrating on the physical gains—being able, once again, to negotiate subway stairs, return to my daily walks around Fort Tryon Park, hills included, and in general, to just keep up. I've observed all this carefully and have been so grateful. But the big surprise came when I noticed something that I hadn't realized I had lost—my head. I have a sense of exhilaration as I find myself filled with ideas, making connections, feeling stimulated and finding it so much easier to express what's on my mind (nothing, mind you, brilliant or original, but still me). I'm thrilled with this recovery, doubly so because I hadn't realized how much I had lost and what a struggle it's been. I did not know how badly I felt all these years until I felt better.

Around that time, my colleague, fellow oncologist Siddhartha Mukherjee, and I were planning a fund-raiser for our laboratory research. With shrinking governmental support and increasing costs of cutting-edge technology, we desperately needed every extra dollar we could raise for our research program. Hugh Jackman, the great actor (of Wolverine fame), and his beautiful wife, Deborra-Lee, generously offered their home for the event, and a lineup from *Who's Who* was coming. Nobody wants to hear long, boring speeches at such events, yet we somehow needed to convey the gravity and urgency of the occasion. As we chatted one morning in clinic, I mentioned the fund-raiser to Kitty.

She exclaimed, "I worship Hugh Jackman! Wouldn't I love to be a fly on the wall at this function."

A light bulb blazed on in my head, and I asked her to be the featured speaker on the spot. At first, she demurred. She had never spoken in public before, let alone in front of so many famous people. I tried to reassure her. All she had to do was read the gorgeous note she had brought me. She finally agreed.

She arrived looking lovely on that evening in an off-white linen frock with her hair freshly styled, a string of pearls elegantly encircling her long, tanned neck. The quiet dignity she exuded that evening was captivating. We shared a glass of Prosecco, and she became engrossed in spotting the VIPs she could recognize. Standing around the cavernous Jackman living room was the top leadership of Columbia University, along with Wendy and Rupert Murdoch, Ivanka Trump, Donna Karan, and many other luminaries. Kitty C. did not show an iota of nervousness. She was deeply compelling in her honesty and sincerity. Her poignant story, a success story, told with heartfelt appeal to fund our program, was duly rewarded. We raised over a million dollars that evening. Money dedicated to cancer research. She was ecstatic. She posed for pictures with the Jackmans and sent them around to friends and family, reporting their delight during subsequent clinic visits. We were not just friends now, we were partners, sharing a passion to raise awareness and support for cancer research.

She remained in remission, taking Revlimid, seeing me once a month now instead of once a week. During these visits, we mostly talked about less pressing issues like how best to handle the diarrhea, a well-known side effect of the drug that came on with ferocious urgency, making her nervous about going out, reluctant to take longish subway rides across Manhattan. She tried many remedies over the next few months and eventually evolved a regimen combining Lomotil and altered timing of taking Revlimid to suit her individual needs. She found a modicum of relief. The couple of years that followed were remarkable in Kitty's enjoyment of the city; of her beloved sister and son, her friends; of her trips to see her brother, and a long-anticipated visit to China. Through it all, we met regularly, talking about everything under the sun, from Kafka to Stendhal, from the electrolyte imbalance and weight loss the diarrhea brought on, to her newfound love for ice cream and cookies. We recommended movies to each other, exchanged books and magazines, reviewed plays we had seen, trashed politicians we did not approve of, debated how to handle our adult children, and in particular, celebrated her marvelous response.

☙

THE LOWER-RISK TYPE of MDS, as a disease, does not progress in a linear manner but rather in fits and starts. I call it *punctuated equilibrium,* after Stephen Jay Gould's description of the process of evolution. Periods of stability are punctuated by a crisis, likely a genetic event leading to a new disease manifestation, followed by relative stability at the new normal. The stable period, during which a homeostasis of sorts is reached between the marrow's normal and abnormal cells, can last anywhere from months to years or even decades. During this state of relative quiescence, blood counts tend to remain unchanged. Then a subsequent event, probably another mutation, leads to the expansion of another clone with further deterioration in blood counts. Once again, a period of stability follows. And so on. Thus, lower-risk MDS tends to progress in more or less a stepwise fashion rather than following a pattern of gradual worsening.

The general rule is of course toward worsening blood counts, but applying it to patients is not always as neat. Occasionally, I have witnessed spontaneous intervals of improvements as well. The natural history of MDS can present with unexpected twists in individual cases.

For Curt Worden, another MDS patient, the question was whether the drug Revlimid that had produced a complete response could be stopped. In 2018, twenty years after his diagnosis in 1998, he reflected on what brought him to that point.

For me it came as a slow evolving surprise, seemingly out of nowhere. I realized there was something just not right—I was tired, and it was difficult to be active without shortness of breath. My skin was pale, colorless and sickly looking. I had never felt this way before. I was at the apex of my career, engaged as a news and documentary cameraman, travelling extensively, covering wars, conflicts and various assignments throughout the world. It was a physical job and now these symptoms created a significant obstacle to engaging my life's work. I distinctly remember working one day in Mexico City at a high eleva-

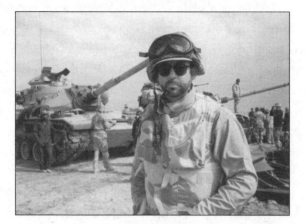

tion. To get the shots needed I had to climb a hill for the best view. I barely made it to the top and was exhausted and shaken from my inability to catch my breath. This was now very serious.

His case was indeed very serious. His hemoglobin had fallen to only 6.6 g, less than half of the normal value, and he was being transfused with three units of blood every three to four weeks. Blood transfusions are given most commonly in acute settings of trauma, gastrointestinal bleeding, during surgical procedures, and in cases of hemolysis. Although normal ranges of hemoglobin are between 12.5 and 15 g, getting a level past 8 g provides instant relief, and studies have shown that raising the hemoglobin to higher than 10 g provides no additional benefit than a level of 8 g. But the benefit is only short term, which explains the chronic, long-term transfusion dependency of individuals with congenital anemias like sickle-cell disease or thalassemia, or patients with bone marrow failure syndromes like aplastic anemia and MDS. Blood transfusions given in this setting improve the physical condition, but only transiently. Within days of experiencing relief, the symptoms creep back as the donor's blood cells start dying off in the recipient, until the low point of discomfort and weakness prompts the next transfusion.

Any stabilization of hemoglobin, even at lower levels, is a relief compared to this repetitive cycle, a jagged edge of ups and downs, improvement and deterioration coming with the precision of cardiac systole and diastole. Imagine the chaotic thunder of Mr. Worden's normal daily life spent on war fronts, dashing between enemy lines, dodging bullets, observing, recording, writing, filming stories of mayhem and massacre. The abrupt onset of anemia sapped his energy, muddled perceptive acuity, left him breathless and weak, unable to meet the demands of his high-pressure job.

Upon returning home, I went to my Internist and after a blood test was told that my Hemoglobin was 6.6 and I would need a blood transfusion. No diagnosis was available to me at that time—my age was 48, 20 years ago in 1998. Now, I found myself facing a very serious medical issue. I continued to have blood transfusions, taking in 3 units every 3 to 4 weeks. As this went on I still did not have a diagnosis, and I began receiving various treatments such as Aranesp with no valuable results But one thing was clear, my Ferritin (Iron) levels were climbing at a significant rate and had to be reduced. I continued to have chronic fatigue and to keep the iron levels in check I began chelating by injecting desferrioxamine subcutaneously, using a portable battery-operated infusion pump that was on my nightstand for 8 hours every night pumping fluid into my body that would bond with the iron and flush it from my system through urination. I was buying time.

Mr. Worden first came to me in 2005. I diagnosed him with MDS and asked if he would allow me to store a bone marrow sample in the tissue bank my lab maintained. He agreed, eager to participate in medical research. At the same time, I wanted to start him on Revlimid. He didn't have the del5q abnormality, but I was preparing to publish a large clinical trial in which a quarter of the patients who lacked del5q nevertheless became transfusion independent on Revlimid within three months. "I was ready to try anything to get out from under the cycle of transfusions and chelation," he wrote. In 2006, he started on a daily 10 mg dose of Revlimid. Within a few months, he was free of transfusions, although he needed the chelation therapy a bit longer.

> Remarkably, I was able to continue with my career and the physical demand it imposed on my body. I was strong again . . . I was happy to feel the way I did even with the knowledge there were no guarantees the future would be so bright as it was at that time.

Although Revlimid does sometimes work for patients without the chromosome 5 abnormality, the median duration of response is a mere ten months compared to two years for those who have it. Only a rare, anecdotal case is the exceptional responder, like Mr. De Noble is to Vidaza. Mr. Worden happily turned out to be another unicorn.

I moved to New York, and we lost touch. Ten years later, Mr. Worden abruptly returned to see me in New York with a curious question. He wanted, for financial reasons, to stop taking the Revlimid, as he was contemplating retirement. He was reluctant to do it on his own and wanted to know what I thought would happen if he stopped the Revlimid after all these years. I tried to go about it in a scientific, evidence-based manner and proceeded to compare genetic, cytogenetic, and clonal abnormalities between a fresh bone marrow sample and the old one that I retrieved from storage in my tissue repository. We found no new mutations, though he still had clear evidence of persistent lower-risk MDS by morphology. I agreed that it would be reasonable to stop the Revlimid. Surprisingly, his hemoglobin began to drop within two months of stopping. "Even after all those years, the MDS exploded into action without the brakes provided by Revlimid," he wrote. We resumed the drug as he became rapidly transfusion dependent, and fortunately, within a month of restarting at a lower dose of 5 mg, his hemoglobin returned to a steady 12.5 g.

Generally, if a patient is responding to any therapy, oncologists don't want to rock the boat and simply continue until it stops working.

The concern is that once we stop the drug, the abnormal clone of cells that had been held in check by the drug would start multiplying with a good likelihood that the predominant outgrowth of subclones would not be as sensitive to the previously administered drug. There are no guidelines about how to proceed when someone has been responding for a decade because unicorns like Mr. Worden are exceedingly rare. His case underlines the peculiar and patient-specific dynamics of MDS. He is responding thirteen years later to the same drug. This by itself is an anomaly. Additionally, he was able to resume taking the drug once again with a terrific response.

Beyond the rarity of his response, several additional peculiarities in this case were perplexing. The first was that the MDS clone of cells had been producing all the blood in his body for more than twenty years. This is not surprising in patients with lower-risk MDS who have not responded to any therapy. The proof that MDS cells are producing all the blood is evident from their transfusion dependency; they are requiring blood transfusions because their own bone marrow is not producing healthy enough cells. But Mr. Worden had become transfusion independent immediately after starting Revlimid and had remained that way over the course of twelve years of treatment, I had expected that the abnormal clone of cells in his marrow must have shrunk. Yet in his case, Revlimid had clearly done nothing to diminish the clone size. Second, the cells had remained exquisitely sensitive to Revlimid even after twelve years of treatment. He is presently leading a happy, retired life and comes to see me periodically. We have his bone marrow and blood samples saved in our tissue repository, and I am anxious to apply the latest technology to understand the biologic reasons for his exceptional responsiveness.

❧

IN 1975, MY brother Javed got married in Karachi. Among guests who came from America was Pam, a friend and pediatrician colleague of my sister Atiya. It was a hot July, and during many long, lazy afternoons, Pam and I bonded over books and mangoes as we sweated it out in hundred-degree temperatures, swooning over Bob Dylan, Shirley Bassey, and James Taylor. She was reading a book, the title of which fascinated me: *Zen and the Art of Motorcycle Maintenance* by Robert Pirsig. She left it for me, and over the next few months, I read the book several times. It left me profoundly moved and actually changed. Through this book, which I cannot claim to appreciate fully even now, I became interested in thinking more about issues of quality. To Pirsig, quality can be static or dynamic. Static quality represents everything definable. Then there is the dynamic type, driven by indefinable engines. Pirsig calls this the *metaphysics of quality*. Imagine being viscerally attracted to something before your intellect provides an objective reason for the appeal. This experiential, dynamic quality is beyond definition or expression in language. It is something that precedes intellectual comprehension, not something imposed but something deeply immanent within the realm of possible experiences.

Pirsig deconstructs both types of quality as he and his eleven-year-old son negotiate the mountains of Montana on a Honda 305 Superhawk, obsessed with the question of how to define, at an atomic level, that which makes a thing good. His meditations are a giddy tour de force consolidating physical, intellectual, and spiritual experiences, revealing glimpses of the essential, metaphysical mystery behind even the most rigid, stylized, and formal of scientific enterprises. Pirsig describes it all through the simple analogy of working on his motorbike; studying and exploring each aspect of the problem systematically, examining everything in the minutest detail, deconstructing endlessly, until finally discovering the root of the problem. The stringent, arduous labor alone, however, does not always lead to the moment of discovery. What drives his science, its crucial vitality that makes it come alive in all its throbbing, pulsating vibrancy is not the tedious planning but instinct, intuition—the metaphysics of quality. This impulse possesses the power to guide us as we negotiate our lives in the context of the larger universe around us, making the journey itself as important as arriving at the peak. "The only Zen you find on tops of mountains is the Zen you bring there."

Reading this book as a very young medical student, I felt as if Pirsig were speaking directly to me, providing me with a road map. There I was, a twenty-two-year-old with no experience but with lofty goals, embarking on a hybrid career that would combine an examination of the physical world through experiments and observations with the practice of medicine, the most humane, compassionate, empathic of sciences, where exceedingly intimate physical and psychological details are shared between two strangers within minutes of first contact. The answer I found in that book was how a dynamic, metaphysical quality could, and why it should, drive both my impulses of practicing medicine and science—why I should not recoil from but open myself wholeheartedly to feelings and emotions, to becoming deeply involved with patients, to exposing my own vulnerabilities without hesitation. At the same time, while designing exacting, methodical, rigorous basic science experiments, Pirsig taught me to welcome instinct, to examine its dictates, and to apply them fearlessly.

What I did not appreciate back in 1975 was how often during the most painful of journeys, as I witnessed dread and disease in others, I would experience sublime moments of grace. The Zen moments. Indeed, only the greatest of art can elevate without comforting. Pirsig freed me to partake of little pleasures while trapped and thrashed around in cyclones of sorrow.

> *I had no time to hate, because*
> *The grave would hinder me,*
> *And life was not so ample I*
> *Could finish enmity*
>
> *Nor had I time to love; but since*
> *Some industry must be,*

The little toil of love, I thought,
Was large enough for me

—EMILY DICKINSON

Kitty provided me with ample time for little toils of love, bring-ing moments of intense joy and satisfaction. The leisure of meeting regularly, every week or two, thirty or forty times a year, for years, allows discussions to continue in installments. Patients suffer much as a result of low blood counts; innumerable transfusions, recurrent infectious episodes land them in hospitals with life-threatening sep-sis. We live through the travails together. Kitty and I had such a rela-tionship. There was a Pandora's box of topics available to us when we met on a weekly basis; we opened it once and out came the practical implications of walking around the world deficient in hemoglobin; another time it yielded old age; another time sprang on us the issues of iron accumulation in the body from all the blood transfusions. We saw derangement and disorder arrive unexpectedly and often, after running a bruising painful course, settle down or vanish. We talked about the coming tornadoes about which we could do little. We pre-pared ourselves by dissecting with care and concern the finite disap-pointments in store. Kitty was always realistic and accepting of her disease. We took small pleasures in celebrating an unexpectedly high hemoglobin one week and Sheherzad's admission to Columbia Uni-versity next. We counted bruises; we marveled at hematomas forming at phlebotomy sites. Most days, we did not feel heroic, but we did our best to adjust to the ever-changing realities of her disease. We alter-nated between cringing and celebrating, but through it all, we stuck together as a team.

Then, as suddenly as they had improved, Kitty's blood counts tanked. After almost three years of a reasonable response, the benefits of Revlimid evaporated. I had anticipated this. She, too, knew what to expect because of our endless conversations, but even she was caught off guard when it actually happened. When I handed her the CBC report showing the return of her anemia, the blood drained from her face. She was genuinely taken by surprise. This issue of what the doctor says and what the patient hears remains baffling in general, but it is of special importance in oncology. Patients will concentrate on the positive, hopeful parts (some patients can respond to Revlimid for many years) and ignore the rest (others stop responding in months).

I was thinking about her disease, but Kitty was living through it. She was still feeling reasonably well; the worsening anemia was creeping so slowly that she had not felt any dramatic symptoms yet. Revlimid had stopped working, and we needed to come up with a new strategy to treat her worsening anemia. We repeated the blood counts weekly for the next month, and things continued to deteriorate. She started requiring blood transfusions once again. I decided to repeat the bone marrow biopsy and restage her disease. This came back showing evolution of her disease to a high-grade MDS with 13 percent blasts, or immature cells, in the marrow. A population of up to 5 percent falls within what's considered the normal range for MDS, while the presence of 20 percent blasts changes the diagnosis from MDS to acute myeloid leukemia, or AML. Kitty had had less than 5 percent blasts since 2009. This time, the cytogenetics were normal, but a genetic profile of her abnormal cells showed the appearance of the dreaded mutation in p53 associated with a poor prognosis and shorter survival.

The next choices were either an experimental trial or Vidaza, which she had not received so far. Because Vidaza is a hypomethylating agent similar to Dacogen, which Kitty had not responded to, it was possible that she would not respond to Vidaza either. However, I hoped that as she had not received any hypomethylating agent since 2009, four years earlier, that evolution under selection by Revlimid treatment could have rendered the dominant clone of cells sensitive to Vidaza. We discussed the pros and cons of this approach at length and finally started her on the abbreviated five-day course a month instead of the typical seven days. She was nervous:

Wed 7/10/2013 3:25 PM

Dear Dr. Raza,

I'm set to begin the Vidaza treatment on Monday

Since I'm to see you the morning before I begin, here are a few questions that have occurred to me—some just wishful thinking or delaying:

Anything to be gained by waiting a few weeks? Or lost?

Any relationship at all between Vidaza (Dacogen, also?) and reversing or slowing the increase of blasts in my marrow? I'm sure I know the answer but need to understand again that this kind of a reversal would be the very cure you're working for.

And is Vidaza my best chance (I understand 50 percent) to stave off dependence on transfusions and all that goes with that.

And (I know this is really magical thinking) would doing another bone marrow, biopsy possibly show a miraculous reversal in blasts?

I'll bring this with me on Monday.

Thanks
Kitty C.

Despite her concerns, she started treatment. I began to see her every week again. Our conversations resumed. On the whole, she tolerated Vidaza well but had moments of awful nausea, fatigue, and listlessness while being treated. A week after the five-day course, she would begin to feel human again, and by the third week, she was herself. However, she continued to receive blood transfusions at the same frequency. After three months of Vidaza, I did another bone marrow examination. The blasts had increased to 25 percent; she now had AML. That transition is what we had sought to avoid at all costs, because AML is a universally fatal illness.

One depressing morning, I sat her down in clinic to review all the options. It was a choice between a rock and a hard place. Elderly patients such as Kitty are not good candidates for either a bone marrow transplant or 7 + 3 chemotherapy. The alternative treatment, if there was one, was an experimental trial. "Well," said Kitty, "I am sure I don't want chemo." An experimental trial, with its possible toxicities and many more required bone marrow tests—"Ugh! I do hate them!" she said—held out only the possibility of questionable benefit. "To prolong my life by weeks? Maybe I will just get transfusions now and let nature take its course." I could not argue with her. Before she left the clinic that October morning, she gave me a long hug, said thanks, and walked out with her head held high.

We met in clinic the following week. The cytogenetic results from her most recent bone marrow exam were available. To my surprise, there were two out of twenty cells showing del5q. A small "good" subclone was rearing its head again. Given that she had already received several years of treatment with Revlimid, these emerging cells would seem likely to be resistant to therapy with the drug again, almost by definition. But then, she had not received Revlimid in almost six months. I suggested we try Vidaza and Revlimid together. In our relationship, I provided the expert "how" of medical treatment, but the informed decision had to be hers. She decided that she did not want to give up. "Dr. Raza, I trust you. If you think I should try this, write the orders."

∞

THE WAR ON CANCER

In the late '60s, chemotherapy was starting to produce remissions and even cures for some forms of childhood cancers. The picture for adults, however, still looked grim. President Nixon was ready to slash the budget for cancer research but for one woman, Mary Lasker.

Briefly, Mrs. Lasker, a wealthy businesswoman in her own right, married into more wealth, interested in the health care of Americans, was inspired and then obsessed with the problem of cancer. She consulted top oncologists and researchers about the best way to help. They unanimously agreed that meaningful impact on cancer would come through improved and expanded basic research. She decided to go after what she called "medicine for the people," stating on television how shameful it was that "less is spent on cancer research in America than on chewing gum." Mary recruited her friend Ann Landers to write a column appealing to the public to put pressure on President Nixon to increase funding for cancer research instead of cutting it. A quarter of a million devoted readers responded by contacting the White House, demanding the president's attention for this pressing need. What eventually followed is summarized in these now famous one hundred words from President Richard M. Nixon's 1971 State of the Union address.

> I will also ask for an appropriation of an extra $100 million to launch an intensive campaign to find a cure for cancer, and I will ask later for whatever additional funds can effectively be used. The time has come in America when the same kind of concentrated effort that split the atom and took man to the moon should be turned toward conquering this dread disease. Let us make a total national commitment to achieve this goal. America has long been the wealthiest nation in the world. Now it is time we became the healthiest nation in the world.

The media promptly dubbed it as Nixon's war on cancer. Following the stupendous infusion of money and resources into cancer, expectation for a cure swung high, many serious investigators declaring an end in sight by 1976. The great bicentennial came and went and there was no cure. Ten more years passed and still there was no light at the end of the tunnel. Slash, poison, and burn (surgery, chemo, and radiation therapies) continued to be the prevalent strategies. A few types of cancers did benefit (testicular cancer, childhood malignancies, lymphomas) but mostly because of more informed use of the existing strategies rather than any dramatic novel ones. Important biologic insights emerged thanks to basic research but failed spectacularly to improve the outcome for patients suffering from common cancers who continued to die painful deaths at practically the same rate.

A breakthrough seemed to have surfaced in 1998 when cancer mortality began to decline, but it turned out that instead of President Nixon's efforts to promote the war on cancer, credit for this long-awaited good news belonged to Dr. Terry Luther, the ninth surgeon general of the United States. Following the findings in the United Kingdom of a relationship between lung cancer and smoking, Luther had established the Surgeon General's Advisory Committee, which released its report on January 11, 1964, concluding that lung cancer and chronic bronchitis are causally related to cigarette smoking. Efforts directed at cessation of smoking that were started in 1960s were finally starting to show results in 1990s. Screening for colorectal cancers saved more than twenty thousand lives, and it was clear that cervical cancer could be 100 percent treatable if detected early through Pap smears.

Eleven years later, in 2009, Gina Kolata reported in her *New York Times* column the jaw-dropping statistics that despite the infusion of more than $100 billion into cancer research, death rates for cancer had dropped by only 5 percent between 1950 and 2005 when adjusted for size and age of the population. The war on cancer was not going well. The question was why not. Were we not spending the funds well, or was cancer simply an impossible problem? Since 1984, my answer has been a resounding yes on both counts. As someone who has been directly involved in cancer research since 1977, and obsessed with it for longer, I am a firsthand witness to the recurring cycles of high expectation and deflating disappointments in the last several decades. Because the stakes are so high, both in terms of life-death issues as well as the staggering amount of money involved, emotions tend to run high on all sides.

Even though President Nixon and subsequent administrations have continued to invest heavily in cancer research—the dedicated budget for the National Cancer Institute alone rocketing up to more than $5 billion, with additional funding, thanks to the "cancer moonshot" backed by President Obama and Vice President Biden—the monies are not being spent as wisely as they could be. For example, the funding agencies continue to reward basic research in petri dishes and mouse models that bear little relevance for humans, with the majority of investigators using xenografts. A review of where the research funds go reveals the inherent biases perpetuated by the peer-review process as detailed by Clifton Leaf in his eye-opening book, *The Truth in Small Doses: Why We're Losing the War on Cancer and How to Win It.* Enormous sums of money from the government continue to fund the same institutions and universities over and over. How seriously is one to take investigators from such institutions who author more than fifty abstracts for a single cancer meeting? Just look at the abstracts published by the American Society of Hematology meetings of the past couple of years and you will discover several such researchers, many authoring between fifty and more than one hundred abstracts each. If you consider the number of international meetings these researchers are rushing around to attend, I am confident you will find a minimum of 250 abstracts per year for each author. It is all a numbers game rather than thoughtful, quality research. The saddest part is that upon a serious examination of what is published, 70 percent of the basic research is not reproducible and 95 percent of clinical trials are unmitigated disasters.

Another problem in the funding crisis pointed out by Leaf, to which I am a witness, is that investigators are encouraged to ask small, highly esoteric, limited questions related to, say, a particular gene in a cancer cell. This results in thousands of publications on the same gene from multiple institutions involving a few dozen researchers without anyone examining the collective gain and making clinical sense of it all. Why?

Basic cancer research may one day be successful in identifying every signaling pathway that determines malignant transformation; however, it will be a long time before the entire process of cancer initiation, clonal expansion, invasion, and metastases is understood, especially in the context of the highly complex, poorly defined micro-environment in which the seed-soil interactions occur. Using this approach, an effective therapy for cancer can only be developed essentially after we understand how life works, how we age. Can our cancer patients afford to wait that long? Isn't the history of medicine replete with examples of cures obtained years, decades, and even centuries before the mechanism of action was fully understood (the most obvious being digitalis and aspirin)? The goal in cancer is not to understand it at its densest molecular level but to learn how to control it. Recognizing the complexity of cancer as a system, complete with emergent properties, isn't it better to turn to strategies that actually deal with complex systems?

The art of medicine, once based purely on experience and observation, a hostage to tradition, gradually evolved into a practice increasingly driven by scientific evidence. More recently, it has undergone an unexpected transition by morphing into a monstrous business enterprise. For oncology, this milestone was reached in the 1990s when the pharmaceutical industry suddenly woke up to the realization that developing cancer treatments offers an untapped market of infinite monetary gains. The last thirty-five years saw a sweeping, radical change in oncology as drug development responsibilities shifted from academic and government-sponsored institutions to industry. Of course the ultimate aim for both is to bring relief to the cancer patient, but the latter added a profit motive as an attractive by-product. Under the control of companies whose investments easily reach into billions, far outweighing the paltry sums available before, each new drug was presented for clinical trials as the great, long-awaited panacea. Sadly, in a tragic anticlimax, the vast majority proved to be useless at the bedside, the remaining few painfully limping to meet the primary end point by improving survival measurable in weeks. Whose responsibility is it to reject such derisory, absurd end points? The FDA, the NCI, the institutional review boards, the patients, their advocacy groups, or the oncologists?

The problem is that we have all bought into this grotesque enterprise, cornering ourselves into an untenable situation, carelessly squandering precious resources and unwittingly harming lives, damaging the overall well-being of the community. A recent study titled, "Death or Debt? National Estimates of Financial Toxicity in Persons with Newly-Diagnosed Cancer," published in the October 2018 issue of the *American Journal of Medicine,* tabulates the chilling economic burden borne by patients with newly diagnosed cancer. Using the Health and Retirement Study Data, this longitudinal study identified 9.5 million estimated new cases of cancer between 1998 and 2012 in the United States. Two years from diagnosis, 42.4 percent of individuals had depleted their entire life's assets, and 38.2 percent incurred longer-term insolvency, cancer costs being highest during treatment and in the final months of life. The most vulnerable groups were those with worsening cancer, older age, females, retired individuals, and those suffering from comorbidities like diabetes, hypertension, lung and heart diseases, belonging to a lower socioeconomic group, or on Medicaid. Given the sensitive nature of discussions involving life-and-death issues, both oncologists and patients shy away from engaging in cost-related issues—oncologists for fear of introducing even the appearance of a bias in therapeutic choices.

Emotional and economic issues notwithstanding, yet another problem of handing over the task of drug development to industry is an indirect dampening of innovation and creativity. Pharmaceutical industry leaders anxious to maximize shareholder values see that the fastest route to making a buck in this rush-to-riches approach is one that builds on the success of others by producing biosimilar agents instead of investing in their own research and development efforts to identify radically different solutions. A glaring example of this approach is paclitaxel (Taxol), a drug that kills cells by inhibiting mitotic activity. Following its success, twenty-five drugs were developed by various companies aimed at the same target. Several billion dollars later, a response rate of 1 percent was seen in more than two thousand patients treated for a variety of solid tumors, establishing beyond a shadow of a doubt that mitosis is not the ideal target in cancer cells.

In an exceptionally candid, courageous summation of the John Conley Lecture, T. Fojo and colleagues come to several sobering conclusions:

The rapidly rising cost of cancer therapies, the regulations governing their adoption by public and private insurers, and the increasing economic risk of drug development have had the unintended consequence of stifling progress by diverting enormous amounts of time, money, and other resources toward therapeutic indications that are arguably marginal. Why else would we pursue gains of a few weeks to a few months with a new drug or as an expanded indication? And rapidly rising costs have also stifled innovation and creativity by promoting a me-too mentality. Why else would the portfolios of companies overlap so greatly with drugs so similar and with differences that either do not exist or that will only be discernible with trials that enroll hundreds if not thousands of patients, the numbers needed to establish statistical significance for nearly imperceptible differences?

A curious love-hate relationship has developed between academia and the pharmaceutical industry. On the one hand, major research findings in academia developed through NCI funds or the research and development efforts by industry, conducted under great secrecy, result in the identification of potentially useful novel strategies. To bring the discoveries to the bedside, clinical trials are conducted by academic oncologists but sponsored and funded by industry. This forces the industry and academia to become reluctant bedfellows. In order for a drug to show efficacy, the FDA demands that it be tested first in animal models. By now, every reader knows that such models are not relevant to humans. To make matters worse, when the drugs are approved for human trials, they can only be tested in patients who have been previously treated with some other established medication. Many agents that might have proved effective in earlier stages of the disease are therefore missed.

Finally, very few, if any, surrogate markers are used to gauge the biologic effects of drugs used in clinical trials. The surrogate or biomarkers include proteins produced by abnormal genes as well as processes that distinguish cancer cells from normal cells, such as formation of new blood vessels or angiogenesis. If a drug does not produce the desired clinical end point, it is then likely to be abandoned completely, even though its biologic activity could be harnessed for more effective use in combination with other agents.

As the internet dot-com bubble burst in the '90s, the biotechnology industry was the big winner since some of the best minds in the country made lateral moves and began to invest their talents in this area. The striking changeabout since 2010 in the pharmaceutical industry has been its ability to attract and retain high-caliber academic scientists and clinical investigators. Even with this vital infusion, it takes a decade and a prohibitive billion dollars for a pharmaceutical company to get a new drug approved, most of the money having been raised from the private sector, which is clamoring all the while for a profit. Following the arduous R&D process and the tedious, time-consuming, and labor-intensive animal studies, by the time a clinical trial is undertaken in human subjects, the stakes are already too high and companies are struggling to demonstrate the tiniest statistical benefits over each other's products.

Where drug development research is concerned, humans must remain the measure of all things. No model, whether it is in vitro cell lines or in vivo animal models or even freshly obtained cancer cells from patients, accurately predicts what will happen when a drug is actually administered to humans. So why not start with giving the agent of interest to humans directly, bypassing the misleading model systems altogether? It is possible to do this through the mechanism of phase 0 trials. The ideal manner to conduct clinical trials would be to take them through the traditional four phases as prescribed by the FDA but at each phase to examine as many biologic and clinical markers as possible in the subjects using the latest technology. If thirty participants in a phase 1 trial have their blood, bone marrow, microbiome, serum analytes, and all available tumor cells studied thoroughly using panomics, AI, imaging, and nanotechnology, then chances are high for identifying surrogate markers for positive and negative effects of the trial agent that may not yet translate into an actual clinical response. This information could help enrich recruitment of potential responders into the next phase of the trial by preselecting only those who show positive biomarkers of response. It is the best and only way to identify possible responders to a given strategy. It is so logical that you would be justified in wondering why this is not already happening.

The unfortunate reality is that not a single marker for response is examined in the majority of clinical trials being conducted even today. Why? Because this is how the system has evolved. The pharmaceutical industry sponsoring the trials is only interested in reaching a statistical end point to get their agent approved. The companies have usually invested almost a billion dollars already to bring an agent to the point of a phase 3 trial. It would add a staggering amount of money to their stretched budgets to perform such detailed biomarker analysis. I suggest saving all the money being squandered on testing the agents in pretherapy, preclinical models of cell lines, and mouse models and instead investing the resources in biomarker analysis. Some bold changes are needed at every level. To harness rapidly evolving fields like imaging, nanotechnology, proteomics, immunology, artificial intelligence, and bioinformatics, and focus them on serving the cause of the cancer patient, we must insist on collaboration between government institutions (NCI, FDA, CDC, DOD), American Society of Clinical Oncology, American Society of Hematology, funding agencies, academia, philanthropy, and industry. The success of many landmark projects of our time, such as the Human Genome Project, the Human Microbiome Project, and the Cancer Genome Atlas, are examples of collaboration between scientists around the world and can serve as a model for the First Cell Project aimed at developing the technology needed for early detection and prevention of cancer.

◊

KITTY STARTED WITH the combination therapy, and once again, we fell into our weekly routine. She would come in and get the CBC done. We would meet and look at the hemoglobin level, white blood cells, and platelets together before I sent her to the infusion center for eight hours if she needed a blood transfusion, or she would make a return appointment for next week if the hemoglobin was acceptable. With Revlimid, her diarrhea returned. She restarted her old regimen of Lomotil and dietary restrictions. Six weeks into the combination therapy, her hemoglobin, instead of falling, had jumped up by a whole gram in one week. We thought there was a mistake and repeated the count. No mistake. Amazed, we did not want to overinterpret the results and decided to wait another week before opening champagne. The following week, her hemoglobin was even better. With this combination, Kitty did unexpectedly well. She required an occasional transfusion, the blasts did not decrease by much, a March 2014 bone marrow biopsy showed 22 percent, but at least they were not galloping out of control. We became cautiously optimistic. She continued this treatment with minor tweaking of Revlimid doses and varying intervals between Vidaza cycles.

Another year went by. Her nagging anxieties relieved, she resumed her activities. No, she did more—she extracted life out of life.

Thu 1/1/2015 3:20 PM

Dear Dr. Raza,

Well enough and happy enough, I got down to Lincoln Center on the A train last night to sing in the New Year, joining with a friend and few thousand other people in the audience as we sang "Auld Lang Syne" accompanied by the NY Philharmonic. Can't think of a better way to celebrate and keep moving on. I never thought, expected to greet 2015!

Thanks. And my best wishes to you for all good things in 2015—love and health and delightful surprises.

A friend who lives in North Carolina called me to tell me that she had just received her invitation to the January 20 EVENT (She was a donor at the last fund raiser). Since I haven't heard anything I thought I better say something. Should I contact someone?

All my best,
Kitty C.

The "event" was our next fund-raiser. This time, we had Paul Simon, James Taylor, Diana Reeves, and many other greats performing at Lincoln Center to benefit our research program. Kitty was excited to attend and to bring us sponsorship from friends. This interlude turned out to be full of enchanting activities for Kitty. She had learned to value each good day, and she was determined to make the most of it. She traveled, socialized with friends and family, attended performances at Lincoln Center, enjoyed her walks in the park and trips into the city to visit museums, attended lectures, saw movies, ate in Chinatown. And we talked. We talked all the time. We had our weekly routine in clinic, where we would dispense with the medical issues with alacrity and then relax and start comparing notes on our weekly activities. How privileged I have felt, meeting and befriending such remarkable souls. Work can really be more fun than fun.

Sat 2/21/2015 12:57 PM

Dear Dr. Raza,

Michelle Tapar interviewed me at home by telephone on Thursday. I told her "my story" including the significance of a center devoted to research and treatment of MDS and the depth and extent of the expertise brought to bear on each step of my treatment over the years.

She recorded my story but did explain that they have no plans to make any more films for the time being (They've completed the set that is currently being shown) and are now collecting stories for future filming. When and whether they do more will depend on a "number of factors." In the event they resume filming, she said that they will contact me. And in that event, I'll be ready and willing.

All my best,
Kitty C.

I repeated a bone marrow biopsy in August 2015. The aspirate was inadequate and blast percentage could not be accurately assessed. In fact, compared to the previous marrow test of March 2015, these results were no different. She had a 17 percent blast count in the aspirate and 15 percent in the biopsy back then. In addition, both marrows continued to show a small clone of del5q cells. My conclusion was that at least her disease was no worse.

Kitty's blood counts slowly stabilized; the platelets were back in the 100,000 range, but it was clear that the treatment was proving to be too toxic to the bone marrow. I needed to do something different now. I suggested a short cycle of two to three days of Dacogen instead of Vidaza along with the Revlimid. She had not received Dacogen for more than five years by that point. She had several cycles of this, and a repeat marrow check showed continued disease stabilization.

But right after the fifth cycle, she developed a high fever and was admitted to the hospital. She had a prolonged admission, diagnosed with pneumonia that did not respond to antibiotics but that eventually responded to antifungals. She had more than a liter of fluid removed from the lungs. Slowly, she improved and was discharged home after several weeks in the hospital.

In February and March of 2016, she only had 1 percent blasts circulating in the blood. By May, they were up to 10 percent. In June, they were in the 40 percent range. The increase could partly have been because of her infections. She had also received the white blood cell–stimulating growth factor Neupogen. We decided to wait it out. Leukemia has other ways of declaring itself. After she recovered from the pneumonia and was off both the growth factor and antifungal agents, her circulating blasts still continued to rise. She refused another bone marrow test.

In July 2016, Kitty turned eighty. She had not expected it. She was pleased. Although she didn't want another bone marrow screening, she was still ready for more treatment. I started her now on a combination of Dacogen and another chemotherapy called *6-thioguanine* (6-TG), using doses so small they were practically homeopathic because the treatment itself posed a serious risk of dangerously lowering the white blood cell count and suppressing the immune system further. It is a fine line between killing the leukemia cells and hurting the patient with aggressive, cytotoxic therapy. After this first course, in the third week of August 2016, she again presented with fever and a worsening pneumonia. She was hospitalized for three weeks that time, released on September 14, taking antifungals, antibiotics, antivirals, and Flagyl as an outpatient. They were brutal, wreaking havoc on every organ in her much-assaulted, enfeebled body. Suddenly, her sense of taste was gone. She said to me with wonder, "I had no idea until now how much of appetite is tied to taste." She stopped eating, forcing down a few sips of those dreaded Ensure Plus shakes. She continued losing weight.

We repeated a bone marrow biopsy on October 12, 2016, and this showed 78 percent blasts. I treated her with Dacogen and 6-TG for three days from October 19 to 21. She tolerated the treatment well. Unfortunately, it wasn't effective. The blood counts dropped dramatically. Time went on, and the counts failed to improve. Then, slowly, menacingly, the blast count started rising in her blood. When her white blood count started to increase rapidly, she was too frail for high-dose chemotherapy; I started her on oral hydroxyurea, another chemo, instead.

She refused admission to the hospital. Ever.

❧

NOWHERE IS THE mind-body dualism more acute than in these final stages when the footsteps of approaching death become louder by the day. The protracted, harrowing, exhausting, tormented battle with MDS, and then AML, was finally coming to an excruciating finale. A part of Kitty had quietly gone missing. She was drained. She brought her sister and son for a valedictory meeting. We crowded into the little consultation room for one final meeting. Her beloved son sat silently, choking back tears. The scene seemed staged, contrived, our postures oddly stylized, as if we were all playing rehearsed parts in a play. She looked frail and emaciated. The chic outfit hung on her like a shroud, exaggerating her skeletal contours. She sat across from me, rallying whatever residual psychic resources she could from crevices unbeknownst even to her until just that moment, speaking slowly and deliberately, with an impossible dignity. She said, "I can't eat, I can't walk, I can't read. I don't *want* to. I have no desire to do anything anymore. All I feel like doing all day is sleep." She took a deep breath. "I am dying."

She requested hospice care.

Kitty died in the spring of 2017.

Death came by a thousand cuts.

In those twilight days, her son took tender care of her. In the beginning, we spoke on the phone every day. Then she became too weak to talk, and our long-distance conversations dwindled, became forced. Eventually, we ran out of things to say. One evening, I was in an Uber, caught in traffic on Fifth Avenue, late for a meeting on the Upper East Side, when my cell phone rang. It was her son. He swallowed before he could speak. "Dr. Raza, thank you for all you did." He did not have to say more. I stared at the rushing pedestrians, the throng of cars, yellow cabs, buses, a lone policeman thrashing his arms, guiding the mad traffic. Everything around me was the same. My eyes had changed. A tristesse enveloped the tapestry of midtown Manhattan. I heard her voice from our first meeting eight years earlier.

We had met in a stuffy, airless, aseptic consultation room on the ninth floor of the Herbert Irving Pavilion. Kitty, with her dazzling smile, her fine features, clear blue eyes, her gorgeous halo of startling, salt-and-pepper curly hair, her slight frame, her stylish, loose linen top and baggy pants, book in hand. I noticed her unusual shoes with straps climbing up to mid-calf, brown leather, with comfortable-looking round toes punched with holes for air. "You like walking?" I asked.

"Love it," she said. "And you?"

"I am a runner," I said. "Three to five miles a day."

She smiled. "Figures. You are just what I imagined. Someone who starts by racing the day. Exerting yourself to the full in whatever you do."

༄

A COUPLE OF months after Harvey died, little eight-year-old Sheherzad developed the flu. Any respiratory illness aggravated her chronic asthma, and for the next forty-eight hours, she struggled to breathe through nebulizers and inhalers, running high fevers and staying up nights with a hacking cough. It took a week for her to experience any relief. One early morning, I was working in the family room when she came out of her room crying inconsolably. I assumed she had a relapse and was worse. She was unable to answer for a few minutes as her little body shook with sobs. Finally, she was calm enough to explain. "Actually, Mom, I feel fine. But now I know how horrible it is to be sick and how good it feels to get better. My dad never got better," she said, bursting into a fresh cycle of crying.

After Harvey died, I found myself feeling disconnected from the world, distanced, alienated almost. For almost five years, the focus had been entirely on his illness, every action, every thought related somehow to the lymphoma. Now, I suddenly had nothing to do, no frantic doctors' appointments to keep, no overnight hospital stays, no need to coordinate consultations with ten experts, no anxiety to scan fifteen test results, make complicated decisions, face impossible choices, all the while arranging babysitters for Sheherzad, seeing my own patients in packed clinics, running a research lab. No more soul-wrenching pillow talks. More than the physical issues, it was the intellectual sterility I experienced that was entirely new and profoundly unsettling, a deep desolation oozing out of every sulcus and gyrus in my cerebrum, preventing me from thinking properly, making me unable to concentrate. I felt an indescribable hollowness. Like a dreamer who woke up, could not remember the dream, but remained stirred by the feelings, I drifted through the days listlessly, missing Harvey, and curiously enough, missing what I used to be like when I was with him. It was as if I had to reacquaint myself with a new post-Harvey me. I could not listen to music. Work remained the only distraction. Several months passed. I decided to do something about it. I ordered the hundred great books of the Western literary tradition (there are many such lists; I went for the fancy Easton Press ones, gorgeously bound, a delight to stare at, hold). For the next three years, I immersed myself in reading, starting with Euripides, Aeschylus, Homer, Plato, Augustine, all the way to Cervantes, Dostoevsky, and Rousseau to Elliott and Thackeray, Dickens and James, Wharton and Melville. It helped me orient myself back to being me, back to life, to grieve, to accept and eventually to move on. Fiction helped me mend, saved my sanity. Books seemed to bring time to a halt, the stories forcing me to pause and take stock of my own surroundings in the context of the unfolding fictitious dramas.

How do oncologists deal with dying patients day in and day out, caught in the amber of soul-destroying moments when people running out of time catalog their swelling regrets, their vanishing options, in a maelstrom of disorder and disease? And how do we deal with the grief once we lose them? Reading fiction, especially the classics of both Urdu and English, has helped me do both in a way that I could not have managed otherwise. By blurring the us-versus-them margins as I stood in the shoes of various characters and felt their joys and sorrows, fear and pain, it helped me appreciate the complexity of lives beyond the complacent, self-satisfied, simplistic Manichean duality of good and evil. My empathy for characters surged in direct proportion to the level of emotional engagement I experienced in a story. Fiction polished my cognitive and intellectual skills to read emotions in others, gauge anxiety levels, diagnose psychosocial fragility. Fiction gave me the equanimity and self-control to follow the advice of Emory Austin: "Some days there won't be a song in your heart. Sing anyway."

Obviously, no two patients are alike in how they face the end, and each one has individual needs. There is no algorithm to follow. The only practical approach is to let patients teach us what they need at any given moment, one at a time. The key is to listen when patients talk. To listen seriously. Listen more "hearingly," the kind of listening that the blind develop naturally; listening for what is not said, listening to understand. Patients tend to hold back their tormenting concerns, the worries keeping them up at night. These require concentrated listening. Doctors are known to interrupt patients every eighteen seconds on an average.

Ultimately, nearer the end, nature itself quietly takes over, becomes the guide for patients, and patients in turn teach us what to do and how.

Kitty was one of my best teachers. She took me from crayons to perfumes.

| # JC

One Touch of Nature
Makes the Whole World Kin

JC WAS VERY SICK WHEN I FIRST MET HER. SHE WAS DIAGNOSED with acute myeloid leukemia days before our first encounter in clinic at Roswell Park Memorial Institute in the early 1980s. She would make me acutely aware of the inadequacy and dismal failings of the cancer paradigm, the ghoulish therapies, their macabre side effects. It was the first time I felt like a fraud, having only the same old dreadful drug combinations to offer her, knowing that since she had a particularly virulent form of secondary AML, her chances of surviving two years were essentially zero point zero zero. After meeting her, I desperately yearned to be a more effective healer, a smarter scientist, a better person. I was thirty-two years old at the time, having just completed my fellowship in medical oncology. Most of the AML patients I had seen until then had been older, sixty and above. JC was someone I could picture myself having a drink with, hanging out, having fun. She was thirty-four.

She was dazzling—tall, with gorgeous blue-black skin, astonishingly graceful, hysterically funny, with an infectious laugh. "Artificial intelligence is no match for natural stupidity. If a girl is smart, Dr. Raza, she does not need brains!" JC was both smart and had brains. She was admitted for weeks on end to receive aggressive courses of 7 + 3 or one of its variations. As the chaos of a day in a busy leukemia service subsided, my long list of must-do things mostly checked off, I would invariably find my way around dinnertime into her room.

Weary, exhausted, like an addict, I sought her grace. She would be waiting. We were like vitamins, supplementing each other's minimum daily requirements. One evening, as I arrived in her room around 9:00 p.m., she handed me the Jell-O she had saved from the dinner tray, asking, "Are you always on call?" Before I could say anything, she roared with laughter, infinitely pleased to provide the answer herself. "Of course you are! You are an on-call-ogist!" Death-bound, she remained irrepressible.

She gagged, puked, retched, and carried on with rampant good cheer. "They are looking for pneumonia in my lungs like its buried treasure!" She laughed with an unbearable lightness. "I had a lot of notions today, but no motions," she would seriously report. Instead of recounting some fresh horror that life in a cancer ward, with its indifferent, bizarre twists, had dumped her way, JC would recount mother-in-law jokes ("Dr. Raza, my mother-in-law has only one problem. Breathing. She also has a strange growth on her neck. Her head."), or report upon the harried young intern who had seen her earlier ("He is so green, he thinks I left my white cells and platelets at home!"). She would complain about the blood transfusion ("I feel woozy. My donor had so much alcohol in his blood, you should be cleaning OR instruments with it!") or how hard it was to eat ("This morning when the food cart came by and the lady asked me if I wanted my eggs fried or scrambled, all I could say was, 'Intravenous, please.'"). In those days, I was obsessed with Louis Safian's *2000 More Insults,* which my sister Atiya, in her infinite wisdom and consummate familial insight, had sent to Karachi in 1973, knowing how her siblings would shriek maniacally with delight, trading caustic one-liners from the book. The only person I ever met outside of the Raza family who shared our corny sense of humor and kept a copy of the book by her side was JC. "Your favorite pulmonologist came to see me today," she would deadpan. "I wish I used a hearing aid so I could shut him off."

I would shoot right back, "Agreed. He is a constant source of ear-itation!"

We would high-five and dissolve into hysterics.

She also arrived with a fantastic story. While pregnant two years earlier, she had developed an inexplicable fetish for the smell of gasoline. Against her better judgment, this led her to the corner gas station, where she'd regularly purchase a dime's worth that she kept in a little bottle, tucked away in her bag. JC was no fool. She knew it was wrong. She knew it could harm not just her but the precious cargo on board. With the compulsion of a doper, she stole moments throughout her crazy-busy working day to unscrew the tiny bottle, inhale the toxic fumes deeply as if they were specially concocted fragrances sent from high heavens for her private consumption. After nine months, she delivered a healthy set of twin girls. Shortly thereafter, a profound drop in her blood counts appeared on a routine postpartum check.

She had been unconsciously expecting it and was prepared for the worst. The obstetrician referred her to a hematologist. A bone marrow study showed myelodysplastic syndrome. Cytogenetic analysis revealed a total mess. Multiple chromosomes were randomly broken up, damaged, duplicated. Some were missing whole arms, others had additional material piled on, still others had translocated and exchanged reams of DNA with fellow chromosomes. Practically none was entirely normal. A textbook case of aneuploidy. Such a complex picture is most commonly associated with a secondary type of MDS, one with a traceable primary cause such as exposure to DNA-damaging agents. Almost certainly, she had brought this upon herself with the gasoline fixation during pregnancy.

Her only chance of any reasonable long-term survival was an allogeneic bone marrow transplant. She had no siblings, which, especially in those early days, meant finding an unrelated donor for her was next to impossible. Even today, the national bone marrow registry shows that only 25 percent of African Americans find an unrelated donor, versus 75 percent for Caucasians, 45 percent for Hispanics, and 40 percent for Asians. If an African American does match to a donor, 80 percent of the time, it is the *only* potential match in the registry. One of the biggest problems for all races is that only 2 percent of the population is on the donor list. An incredibly brave woman, Susan Brecker, set out to change this bleak outlook.

In 2013, I was seeing an MDS patient in clinic when her daughter asked me if I knew Susan Brecker. I did not. It turned out that Susan's husband, the great jazz saxophonist Michael Brecker, was diagnosed with high-risk MDS, and his only chance was a stem cell transplant. No match could be found for him in time. Susan had made a film, recounting the story of three cancer patients, two of whom received matched unrelated transplants, survived, and are leading normal lives, while her husband died for lack of a donor at fifty-seven years of age. My patient's daughter had seen the film and sent it to me. *More to Live For* tells deeply moving stories. I immediately started searching the internet for Susan's contact information and eventually found her. My colleague Siddhartha Mukherjee and I met her together for lunch at the Columbia University Faculty Club. It was the start of a wonderful partnership.

More to Live For was successfully screened at dozens of schools, college campuses, churches, and social events. After the film, drives recruited potential donors for the national bone marrow transplant registry. All it requires is a cheek swab, not even blood, to be registered as a potential donor on the list, and if called upon to donate, stem cells are recovered from the blood in 70 percent of the cases. It is that easy. Susan's efforts have saved more than a hundred lives already. She said she was ready to do more for MDS patients now that the film project was over and the awareness campaign for increasing donor registry was well on its way independently. Siddhartha and I jumped at her offer, as we were planning our next fund-raiser to support research efforts in MDS.

Susan is a rare combination of high intelligence, total commitment, deep empathy, and a one-woman powerhouse of infinite, indomitable energy. Within weeks, she had recruited big-name artists like Paul

Simon, James Taylor, Diana Reeves, and a host of others, along with an incredible emcee for the evening titled, "The Nearness of You Concert," held on January 20, 2015, in the Appel Room of Jazz at Lincoln Center. The artists volunteered their time because of their deep love for Michael, and Susan added to their commitment to cancer research. The elegant and articulate ABC anchor of *Good Morning America,* Ms. Robin Roberts, an exceptionally courageous woman who agreed to serve as the welcoming host for the evening and who has talked about her MDS diagnosis and subsequent stem cell transplant publicly, was an honored guest for the evening. I felt oddly drawn to her, following her with my eyes as she mingled with the guests—many of them my MDS patients—exchanged stories with them, and posed for photographs, and I suddenly realized the source of that inexplicable connection. She reminded me very much of JC. The same body language, easy laugh, extraordinarily charming personality, empathy oozing out of every pore in her body.

JC was not fortunate enough to find a matched unrelated donor, which meant that, until her MDS developed into acute myeloid leukemia, there was not much that could be done. Once she had AML, her doctor told her, they would use "the big guns." She began seeing the hematologist every few weeks, until her anemia became profound and she required regular blood transfusions. This continued for another few months. It was a few months after that when she had developed acute leukemia in 1984 that she came to see me. I treated her, attempting to improve her chances of survival, but it was JC who ended up improving my life.

⬙

JC WENT THROUGH the painful phases of induction and consolidation chemotherapies under my direct care. Once, during a particularly savage cycle, I sat on the edge of her bed, and, in a feeble attempt to distract her, instead of telling her a joke, I recited a poem I love:

This condition of life
is not for the whole year
only the few months when it rains.
The blazing fire of the drywood
will cook rice in no time.
And
whatever is there
will come back into view
sharp and clear.
When the rains depart
we will put out in the sun
everything that is wet
woodchips and all.
Put out in the sun
we shall
even our hearts.

—SUBHASH MUKHOPADHYAY

She burst out crying. So did I. It was unreal. I was thirty-two, starting my career. She was thirty-four, dying.

❧

JC SURVIVED THE sickening rounds of chemotherapies and did get better. There was nothing more to do but wait and hope that she did not have a relapse. I began to follow her in my outpatient clinic once every two to three weeks, and then once every four to six. She and I started talking more about nonmedical issues, and as we learned about each other's lives, we became closer and closer. Both of us knew that her chances of a durable remission were not great, given the high-risk nature of secondary leukemia like hers. I can still feel the anxiety we tried to hide from each other as we waited for the results of her blood tests in clinic, distracting ourselves with small talk.

The leukemia relapsed a year and a half after her initial diagnosis. Most of this time had been spent in the hospital, her gorgeous body racked with fevers, her insides eviscerated as the gut revolted against the cytotoxic drugs that did little good and much harm. The end came faster than either of us suspected. Her disease spun out of control in a matter of days as the malignant cells started doubling exponentially. When she realized that we had emptied our arsenal, JC requested admission to the hospital for her terminal illness. I admitted her and started low doses of chemotherapy to control the rapidly increasing blasts in the blood, knowing perfectly well that it would do nothing for the underlying bone marrow disease.

As I rounded each morning, making believe with all sincerity that balancing her intake and output of fluids was the crucial order of the day, the inadequacy of my pathetic nontreatment plan slapped me in the face. JC was dejected, withdrawn. I longed for the days when she teased me, but a wan smile would be all she could muster, gently, almost tenderly, acknowledging my feeble attempts at lightheartedness, successfully aborted before they began. I listened to her heart and lungs, palpated her abdomen, examined the swollen ankles, shiny now with skin stretched tautly, nauseated by my own bogus good cheer. Young bodies are not made for dying. They are hard to demolish even for so malignant a disease: two steps forward for cancer, one back toward life, as the body staged astonishing comebacks, rallying organs in a confounding, irregular sequence. One day, the lungs look clearer on x-ray; the next, the creatinine levels tank, then the pneumonia improves only to be followed by the liver starting to shut down. She lost weight and hope, she stopped eating, forgot how to laugh, quit the morning and evening walks around the ward. She hardly left the room anymore.

And then, suddenly, something snapped in her. An unexpected vehemence resurrected her withering, skeletal frame, imbuing her with a newfound palpable energy. JC asked for pen and paper, and she started writing. Furiously. Gone was the exhaustion and lassitude, gone the dozing stupor; the internal dismantling was abruptly suspended by the force of her intellectual zeal. She was a woman possessed. She filled legal-sized notepads, emptied pens, demanded more paper and extra ballpoints at odd hours of the night and day. There were few tomorrows remaining, and she was not wasting a single one of them. Her mind composed feverishly as the body decomposed. Over the course of a long career spent taking care of countless terminally ill patients, I have witnessed this sporadic burst of end-of-life force enough times to know it is real; dishevelment of a body being gradually laid to waste, reassured sweetly through a cleansing, terminal lucidity. How this happens—how she got enough strength in those emaciated carpals and metacarpals to balance pen on paper for hours on end, how she reassembled her dwindling psychic resources, how she filled page after page as her head pounded from profound hypoxia—remains a mystery.

She did not volunteer information about what she was writing. I was too afraid to ask. Until one evening, when we were alone, I did. "Sit down," she said. For a while, she remained silent, looking out the window. In that moment, as the fading sunlight cast oblique shadows on the pale walls of her hospital room in the newly renovated Carlton House, I became acutely aware of the glaring disparity—the fragile, crumbling state of her body, a sorry vessel to house so capacious a soul. She, of the *2000 More Insults* camaraderie, seemed ready to put the body away for good. It was humbling to imagine the gravity of her task. In telling me what she wrote, she was acknowledging the end. *Khattam-Shud.* She turned her face and looked at me with a shadow of the old smile. "Even the germs can't stand me anymore. I guess it's time to go." She swallowed hard and blurted out, "I am writing letters I want my two-and-a-half-year-old twin daughters to open on each of their birthdays." She hesitated, looked askance at me, almost bashful. "Keep me alive until I reach their twenty-first?"

By the time JC died two days later, she had barely completed the letter for their twelfth.

I HAD MY eureka moment as I signed her death certificate. JC died because her leukemia was too advanced by the time I saw her. It had taken her a year to cross over from preleukemia to leukemia. I should have treated her at the earliest, preleukemic stage of the disease. Surely, it would be easier to control MDS rather than AML. From that day on, I announced to Harvey that evening, because of JC, I was going to concentrate on studying and treating MDS. Even at the ripe old age of thirty-two, it was clear to me that the animal models were far too simplistic and artificial, utterly incapable of recapitulating a fraction of the complex disease I had seen evolve in JC's case. The only hope of dealing with so deadly a foe was to detect it at its earliest stage and apply the best available scientific technology to find ways to arrest it before all hell broke loose. If I studied both MDS and AML stages of the disease, I thought, I could define the biologic milestones that mark how preleukemia cells cross over to the frankly leukemic stage. From that, a better understanding of the natural history of the malignant process would emerge, hopefully, yielding novel potential therapeutic targets on the way.

Harvey's response was, "Az, your idea is spot-on, but I can warn you right now, you will never get a grant funded. MDS is too rare a disease. No one can even pronounce it properly, let alone support your work." Of course, I did it anyway. And also got grants funded. Had I gone to school in this country, my research would have involved attempts to reproduce the disease in mouse models or to create tissue-culture cell lines from patients' malignant cells. Being an outsider, I had the audacity to follow instinct rather than custom. I would save every cell I could from every future patient I saw and study them thoroughly. It never occurred to me to do otherwise. While Harvey always provided his intellectual and moral support for my work, he never got interested in MDS and continued his AML work as before. Ours proved to be a great complementary partnership as the two of us were studying different stages of the same disease and compared notes constantly, learning from each other, providing unique new insights for experiments we designed independently and jointly.

To that end, I began my tissue repository, collecting sequential samples from each of my patients throughout the evolution of each patient's disease. The repository was and is backed by a computerized data bank containing detailed clinical and pathologic information on each patient. The repository is unique in that it provides the ability to look back on survival data spanning three decades. Such a retrospective view of the disease is critical to understanding what makes some MDS patients develop AML or why some succumb to MDS within two years while others survive five, ten, or even twenty years. The serial samples can be interrogated using the latest technologies encompassing genomics, transcriptomics, proteomics, metabolomics, and even panomics. The resulting biologic insights will be invaluable. It is the only way to understand the initiation, progression, invasion, and lethality of the disease, responsiveness to given treatments, the natural history. Once important biomarkers of leukemia cells emerge through this high-throughput technology, identifying and targeting the first leukemia cell will be possible. It is because of the repository that I was able to define detailed cell cycle kinetics of both MDS and the leukemia that subsequently develops, giving patients infusions of the thymidine analogs bromo- and iododeoxyuridine in those early days, so the dividing cells could be labeled in vivo. We showed that, contrary to previous assumptions, the bone marrow cells in MDS patients are hyperproliferative. I also used the precious samples from hundreds of MDS patients to figure out that the low blood counts—despite a proliferative marrow—result from premature death of the clonal cells by a peculiar mode of suicide called *apoptosis.* Finally, we showed that this cell death is, at least in part, mediated and accelerated by pro-inflammatory proteins, tumor necrosis factor (TNF), and transforming growth factor beta (TGFb). It naturally followed that blocking TNF and TGF would lead to less cell death, more mature cells entering the bloodstream, and improved counts. The first such drug with anti-TNF effects was thalidomide, and when I gave it to MDS patients, it produced complete responses in 20 percent of the cases. This led to the development of

Revlimid, the drug from which Lady N., Kitty C., and Harvey benefited. More recently, the drug luspatercept has shown activity in MDS.
It acts by inhibiting the TGF family of proteins.

All these advances occurred because patients agreed to donate their
blood and marrow cells to the repository. In these thirty years, I have
met maybe a handful of patients at most who refused. The rest, 99.99
percent, instantly agreed. Of course, pulling extra marrow causes some
extra pain. Introducing the large needle through an electric drill or brute
physical force is not too uncomfortable because we numb the entry site
thoroughly, but once we start pulling through a syringe, marrow starts
moving inside the bone, waking up thousands of nerves per millimeter,
causing a profoundly uncomfortable sensation. It is not exactly pain,
but unpleasant. I have performed thousands of bone marrow biopsies
on patients and continue to perform a dozen or so every week even today. Yet I am humbled each time a patient acquiesces. "Dr. Raza, even
if it does not help me, it could help someone else. I trust you. Do what
you have to do." Some patients have donated samples dozens of times;
they know what's in store for them. They do it so it may help us find
better solutions for future patients. How is it possible not to hang our
heads in deep gratitude in front of such unparalleled grace?

How, too, is it possible to not try to do more? The repository constitutes an invaluable resource, holding the key to addressing fundamental questions, some common to all cancers, not just MDS and
AML. Over the past several decades, in every instance that we have
studied samples from the repository for research purposes, we have
uncovered exciting biologic information and published our results in
the highest-profile peer-reviewed scientific journals. However, these
small-scale research projects, many in collaboration with scientists
around the country, are limited in scope. They have answered important, but specific, basic questions about one or another aspect of the
disease. These have been performed on a limited number of samples,
a few hundred at best. Once the human genome was sequenced and
technologies were brought up to economies of scale, I was anxious to

undertake a careful, systematic study of thousands of samples sequentially obtained on patients as their diseases evolved. Grants I applied for received regular rejections. I was faulted for not using a system that could be manipulated, such as animal models.

While in vitro testing and animal models are good for studying basic aspects of understanding gene functions and interactions, defining signaling pathways, and observing effects of knocking genes out in controllable, well-defined, simplified systems, I am interested in therapy-driven research. How can I develop better treatment options for my patients? Mouse models are practically worthless for cancer drug development, but funding agencies and the current scientific culture are so heavily invested in the system that nothing can make them accept the folly of their failing models. Hundreds of scientific studies have already shown that there is close to zero relationship between efficacy in animals and what happens in humans. What more evidence is needed than a greater than 90 percent failure rate of drugs brought to the bedside through such inappropriate, irrelevant preclinical platforms? Yet grants are not funded in general without animal models. What accounts for this deliberate blindness? The only reasonable explanation is that the survival of these grants depends upon remaining blind. The oncologist equivalent of this insanity is on daily display when hours are spent upon obsessively balancing electrolytes while the entire body succumbs to cancer.

No grants are available even to support the maintenance of the tissue repository. What has allowed my biobanking attempts to continue are philanthropy and generous patients. If it were not for fund-raisers to which our benefactors, friends, patients, and their families contribute wholeheartedly, I would have to pour the samples down lab sinks and call it a day. I have seen this happen once. As a well-known cardiologist shifted her laboratory program to a new hospital, her old employers refused to let her move her repository, and out of spite, the institution trashed each one of her samples with glee.

FRUSTRATED BY THE limited availability of resources, I had to become more creative. Why should my patients and I be hostage to rules devised by a few individuals who have little idea about what cancer is in real humans? For God's sake, we are living in the most affluent country in the world in the most affluent time in the history of mankind. Surely, there are other resources to be tapped, alternate ways of funding the tissue repository project. I decided to go public. I spoke out at every opportunity I had, in grand rounds and tumor boards, dinner lectures and national meetings; I wrote opinion pieces, gave interviews, harassed private foundations and industry moguls to do the right thing. Everyone politely listened, agreed, and went home to continue doing whatever they were doing. Nothing happened.

During the Christmas break of 2014, I woke up one morning, particularly distressed. Lady N. had died. I was struggling to find a new option for Kitty C. I would see twice the usual number of patients in clinic the week following Christmas because of the holidays. The jolly good cheer of the season brings impractical hopefulness to patients. They yearn for better solutions. I wanted to offer them better solutions. I was feeling the pressure. I was feeling even more frustrated by my helplessness. I was confident I could find many answers if only I was able to conduct a thorough, systematic study of samples stored in the tissue repository.

Half-heartedly, I opened a stray magazine and read that a sportsman was rewarded with a record seven-year, $126 million contract.

That did it.

What kind of a society are we living in where a sportsman is compensated with hundreds of millions of dollars for ball games, and I have to beg and borrow, grovel and plead, for paltry sums of money to find better treatments for *cancer?* Cancer is no longer a disease that happens to others. Most of us have one degree of separation from it at best. So why such grotesque disparity? Such heartless indifference? Samples of bone marrow and blood obtained over three decades from thousands of patients through unbearably painful procedures, drilling into bones, stabbing at collapsing veins, remained frozen, languishing in liquid nitrogen, for lack of funds. The entire budget for cancer research through the National Cancer Institute is $5 billion, accounting for less than 0.1 percent of US federal spending. What I needed for my work would constitute a fraction of that athlete's obscene compensation package. It was and is unconscionable.

Extreme ailments require extreme cures. Desperate times call for desperate measures. Wrapped in water-resistant layers of stretchy, moisture-wicking fabric, gloved, monkey-capped, goggled, booted with thermal socks and light sneakers, I went for a long run along the Hudson in twenty-two-degree weather to clear my head. It was apparent that the strategies I had tried were not working. I obtained enough money every year to continue to fund the repository and my dedicated group of lab scientists and researchers, publishing important enough clinical and basic biologic studies to remain a credible voice in the field. But I needed a more serious investment in my research plans now. Who could help? This kind of support was beyond the scope of the usual suspects entrusted to fund scientific research, such as the NCI. The only option would be to somehow interest individuals with the bandwidth to undertake such a vital project. What I needed was an old-fashioned patron.

To begin, I pictured myself as a socially conscious, good-hearted, compassionate, and exceedingly rich person wanting to do something to help humanity. If I wanted to identify an authentic cause to support—preferably, one free of countless intermediaries, tax-exempt organizations, and professional fund-raising agencies—I would have to undertake a lot of research. It could be challenging. Maybe there is someone out there waiting to hear of so deserving a cause as accelerating cancer cure? Fueled by the ever-present faces of frantic patients desperate for respite, I decided to approach the rich of the land directly. I sincerely believed that if only they could see what a fantastic opportunity it was to help cancer research in a meaningful way, they would be falling over each other to come to my rescue. Only one problem remained: How do I reach them?

A light bulb flashed on in my brain. In the middle of my jog on that freezing morning, I made a sharp right onto West Eighty-Sixth Street toward Barnes & Noble on the corner of Broadway. I purchased a copy of the latest *Forbes* magazine with its list of the one hundred richest people and spent the entire day chasing down their mailing addresses. Most could only be reached through the respective philanthropic arms of their companies. Nonetheless, I addressed the actual billionaire by name and wrote a brief, personal letter to each. I described the miracle of the unique tissue repository. I explained the evolving panomics technology available to study these samples. I expressed high hopes of finding novel targets of early detection and therapy that could be identified through such studies, targets that would allow us to arrest the disease at its inception. I made the case that defining the molecular, genetic events as MDS progresses to AML could possibly help us understand a universal set of principles, algorithms all cells follow in the process of acquiring immortality: the genes activated, the pathways ignited, the proteins shut down, the immune checkpoints silenced as a premalignant cell becomes autonomous and frankly malignant. The studies on the MDS-AML tissue repository samples could help us understand prostate and breast cancers, lung and GI tumors. I told them that the implications were infinite and exciting. I requested their support to provide the resources to do it. On December 31, I carried a large cardboard box of envelopes, addressed by hand, and stuffed them into the corner mailbox.

Over the next few weeks, I waited with bated breath. I received ten responses. All were form letters, obviously, regularly mailed to supplicants like me by clerical staff. No billionaire had actually read my letter. I was sure of it, because if they had, why would they not have responded positively? Three months went by. I busied myself again with writing endless grant applications. I forgot all about the Billionaire Project. One March afternoon, I was working in my office when the phone rang. "Hello, Dr. Raza, this is Patrick Soon-Shiong. You wrote to me some time ago. Sorry, I am just physically opening my snail mail.

Needless to say, I am calling you because I am very impressed by what you have done with banking the tissue samples for three decades. Congratulations. I think we should meet."

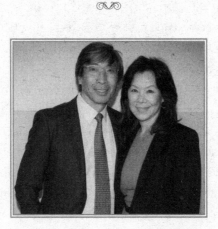

HE WAS DIFFERENT from how I had imagined him to be. For one thing, Patrick has the softest voice. After knowing him for these past few years, I still cannot imagine him ever raising it; in fact, when he wants to make a point, he lowers it even more. For another, he has the sweetest relationship with Michele, his beautiful wife. Their comfortable, carefree exchanges are hugely reassuring, grounding them in a deeply human way. The day of our first meeting, Dr. Abdullah Ali, the brilliant director of our MDS Research Program at Columbia University, and I had arrived at their sprawling Bel Air mansion a half hour ahead of our appointment. The guard on duty refused to open the heavy iron gates and instructed us rudely through a slit to wait outside. We had crossed the street and were standing under a tree to avoid the blazing California sun when an SUV drove up. The young driver scrutinized us as the gates opened and the car slid in. Minutes later, the driver emerged from a side gate, introduced himself as Phil Yang, Patrick's assistant, and apologized for the guard's treatment of us. He escorted us in and invited us to make ourselves comfortable in the beautiful conference room, equipped with the latest audiovisual equipment with an open patio surrounded by gorgeously manicured plants and hedges. The warmth of Phil's welcome relaxed us, and soon Shahrooz Rabizadeh, the director of Patrick's scientific enterprise, arrived with laptop in hand. With Phil's and Shahrooz's assistance, we loaded my slides and waited for Patrick.

He appeared on the dot. He had just finished his morning exercise routine and was freshly showered and shaved, ready for another action-packed day. He greeted us with a kind smile and much curiosity. Soon after the pleasantries were over, we got down to business. I began my formal presentation. It was a marvelous experience. That Patrick is exceptionally intelligent goes without saying. The astonishing part was the lightning speed with which he grasped the import of what I was presenting. Despite being a surgeon who had probably not encountered the acronym *MDS* since his medical school days, Patrick instantly understood the underlying complexity involved in defining the natural history of this heterogeneous disease. He asked many relevant questions, summarized the issues at various points in my talk, debated intricate technical details with Abdullah, and directed thoughtful clinical, patient-related queries at me.

There was to be a big omics meeting the next day at his home-office complex to which cancer center directors and reputed scientists from around the country were invited. Patrick asked me to present my ideas, helped me choose the slides, framed the critical questions, and ended up with a series of proposed studies for collaborative work. I was really impressed by the breadth and depth of his knowledge. Michele floated in lightly, looking beautiful in a summer dress, trailed by assistants, to whom she was imparting instructions on placement of chairs, directing where lunch tables were to be laid, setting the agenda for the day, planning an evening excursion for the entire group. She came over to where we sat and gently inquired if we were ready for lunch. Patrick took me on a walk around the impeccably landscaped garden, showed me around, pointing out favorite trees and plants, eventually arriving at a gazebo with a breathtaking view of the picturesque lands around. We ate a light salad and talked. We took another walk, enjoying the pastoral splendor in the middle of a buzzing, hyperactive city, and continued our scientific discussion. By the end of five hours, we had developed an exceptional understanding of each other's missions. The friendship with Patrick and Michele, started on that sunny morning in 2015, has only deepened with time.

What bonded the three of us inseparably was our shared mutual concern for patients. In one meeting, I sensed the profound empathy this couple has for human suffering and for their relentless, insistent, fearless commitment to alleviate it. It is Patrick's and Michele's respect for others that marks all their manners; one way in which they best show it is by thoughtfully listening to what others have to say. A scientist can become consumed by devotion to facts without caring about what their value is to humanity. Patrick and Michele have avoided that suffocating trap.

They were born in South Africa, where they were no strangers to prejudice and discrimination, but they never let it defeat them. Their journey from Port Elizabeth and Johannesburg through Patrick's residency in Canada, to a UCLA professorship, performing the world's first encapsulated human-to-human transplants of islet cells from the pancreas and the first full pancreas transplant on the West Coast, then as a NASA researcher, developer of Abraxane (a form of chemotherapy for breast, lung, and pancreatic cancer), and corporate CEO is the stuff of legend by now. But the man's story is perhaps more worthy than the legend of it.

The first two pancreas transplant patients at UCLA did fabulously, except they both rejected their transplant. Pancreas transplant rejections are the most frightening thing, because you've hooked the pancreas to the bladder. When the organ rejects, port-wine blood pours out the ureteral catheter. I said to myself, "Wow, do I really believe this is the right thing to do to a patient?" Which led me to tell my chairman that I'm going to shut down the program of which I'm the director. I decided that I needed to understand regenerative medicine. I got interested in the immune system because I was trying to induce tolerance, and that is when I learnt that cancer cells have figured out how to induce tolerance, to tell your body "don't eat me because I'm actually you." So the irony is that the first part of my career was to induce tolerance for transplants, and the second part was to break tolerance to actually tell the body to kill cancer cells.

As physicians we're trained to be reductionists. We rigidly follow protocol. But life is not that way. Cancer is not linear—it is completely non-linear. It lives in the science of chaos. There's no single point of control. You need to attack it in a non-linear fashion across time and space, monitoring it and truly dancing with it. If you biopsy a patient with breast cancer twice in the same day, once in the breast and once in the lymph node, you can get cancer cells with different sequences. This heterogeneity breaks all these reductionist assumptions, because which target are you hitting and what made you choose it? The only chance we have, in my opinion, is to do what I call micro killing and macro killing at the same time. Micro killing meaning you go after these little targets, maybe even using a little chemotherapy. And macro killing meaning either surgery, radiation, or immunotherapy.

Patrick is particularly allergic to the widely held dogma that DNA alone holds the key to a cancer cure. He has been advancing a more comprehensive study of cancer and its microenvironment that includes detailed DNA, RNA, and protein measurements. Patrick has also consistently pointed out the damage inflicted by the traditional high-dose chemotherapy regimens to the immune system, the very system we need most in the fight against cancer. He has initiated multiple, very exciting clinical protocols employing cellular therapies and vaccines combined with more conventional approaches of chemo and targeted therapies in cases of advanced cancers.

Around 2015 Vice President Biden called me about his son's brain cancer, and I got involved with some of the diagnostics. His son passed away in May of 2015. By October I had written a two-page white paper talking about accelerating cancer immunotherapy using genomic sequencing and big data. My job as a physician, a surgeon, a cancer oncologist, immunologist, NASA ex-scientist, and former CEO is to orchestrate all of this. We are pursuing a very, very ambitious program. I'm not saying we're going to cure cancer by 2020, but maybe we'll be able to activate the body's T cells to fight it.

Michele and Patrick helped me in one unexpected but highly desirable way. They gifted Columbia University with an endowed chair, the Chan Soon-Shiong Professorship, which I was named to receive and which has provided me with protected time to devote to clinical and basic research. In a long-running interview, Patrick shared with me his strong belief that the cancer cell creates an evolving, changing environment in response to the treatment we impose on the patient. Hence, he believes that basic research needs to be performed within the dynamics of a clinical treatment, rather than at a static point in time. As a consequence, he has devoted his resources in developing a cancer vaccine by activating the patient's own immune system and wishes to support basic research in the characterization of the cells surrounding the tumor in real time. Patrick and I remain in touch constantly and debate cancer therapy questions regularly.

As for finding patronage for my tissue repository, I remain at square one.

For Patrick and Michele, the goal has never been just about following their passion for self-satisfaction. Their goal is to unite their passion with compassion in the service of humanity. Such a quest is led less by eyesight and more by insight. They have aimed high, they made big plans, and they work relentlessly toward their goals. It will be a lifelong journey, because in the words of Charles Evans Hughes, "medicine is testing us every day as is life itself. Success must continuously be won and is never finally achieved. Every day puts at risk all that has been gained. The greater is the gain, the greater is your risk of loss. One must never look at the end of the road, as one is always at the beginning of a new one."

⚮

I REMEMBER A day, earlier on in her disease, when JC was in an uncharacteristically somber and reflective mood. She sighed and confessed that she regretted not having valued her family more when she was well; she especially mentioned the pointless, inane arguments with her live-in mother-in-law over trivial issues, leading to days of unpleasantness. Facing a lethal illness at the age of thirty-four, JC wished for a second chance so she could show everyone the better angels of her nature. Confinement by disease allowed her to free her spirit, made her more generous. After being in remission for a year, one day she was in clinic for a visit and mischievously confessed that in the middle of a recent jaw-jaw with her mother-in-law, she had suddenly stopped in her tracks as she realized how "normal" she must be feeling. She had reverted to her whining, entitled, temperamental, vacuous predisease self. "And those are some of my good points!" she groaned. "I tried to emerge a pearl out of the oyster of my illness. Instead, I have ended up impersonating the old crab. Warning, Dr. Raza! When you find me being nice, suspect relapse."

Maybe it was because those were my salad days. Maybe it was JC's ravishing personality. Her youthful, stunning good looks, her vulnerability as a new mother, her wicked sense of humor, her poise, her willingness to befriend and school a fresh, insecure, junior attending physician in ways of knowing cancer, ways of knowing life. Aristotle defined tragedy as a moment of discovery. The discovery has to be, somehow, purged. When Oedipus found out that he had killed his father and married his mother, he had to blind himself, wandering off as some kind of a prophet. The years with JC shattered me in ways I was not aware of until I tried to put myself back together. The destruction and reconstruction process, painful, stepwise rehabilitation of my soul, marked by many false starts and regressions, was my equivalent of blinding and un-blinding myself. I stopped being the newly minted warrior oncologist. I emerged as someone who was no longer startled by cancer's infinitely unpredictable, testy tolls, its gruesome cruelties; rather, I became an adult who had learned to stop twinning the suffering of individual patients. The mystery of the world is the visible, as Oscar Wilde pointed out, not the invisible. JC helped me make that leap from dallying in the abyss of cancer's ruthless nihilism to consideration of more humanistic, humanitarian issues of life and death. JC gave no lectures; she wrote no books. It was her sober acceptance of the unspeakable tragedy in a thousand little gestures that slowly but surely parted the curtain, allowing me to witness grace in all its heroic splendor. She gave my eyesight the insight it needed. JC made the invisible visible and opened entire new mysterious worlds for me to wander in as I negotiated each new patient who came with their own unique set of cryptic and mysterious challenges.

The best tribute I could pay her when she died was to pledge my life to study and cure the disease that took hers. If I have seventy-two more lives, I would pledge myself seventy-two more times to JC.

If equal affection cannot be, let the more loving one be me.

—W. H. AUDEN, "THE MORE LOVING ONE"

| # ANDREW

Was Honesty a Choice?

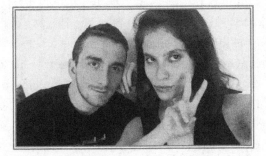

MY DAUGHTER, SHEHERZAD, BROUGHT HIM OVER ONE EVENING after school in 2009 when they were fifteen. "Meet my new GBF [gay best friend], Mom." And before I had time to look up, "*Khuda hafiz,* we are going to play video games in my room. Oh, and we are starving." As they flew into her room, Andrew doubled back. "Hi, Azra," he said. "Thanks for having me. I am excited to try the famous Pakistani food everyone talks about." He was the polite one, always. I will let Sheher and Andrew's sister Kat, older than him by two years, tell his story in their words.

∞ KAT ∞

In April 2016, Andrew started getting weak in his right arm. Couldn't do push-ups suddenly. Dad recommended a chiropractor, who told Andrew it was a pinched nerve. He advised various exercises. No benefit. In the last week of April, we went upstate for a family friend's birthday. Andrew was self-medicating with old opioids. He took Percocet, which did not help. We finally decided to go to the local ER. He was thoroughly examined, told once again that he had a pinched nerve, given stronger pain meds. The next morning, back home in Brooklyn, he was dizzy and could not get out of bed. Our mom and grandma were returning from vacation in Europe. I called my uncle, who is a pediatrician. He asked us to take him to the ER. My dad drove him. He was in the ER all day.

It was a Sunday, and the MRI machine was backed up. By 8:00 p.m., I was informed that the technician had left for the day and it would have to wait 'til morning, so they admitted him. He developed urinary retention. A catheter was inserted. I was on my way to the hospital the next morning and called him once I got off the train. I still remember that moment. I was on Thirty-Fourth Street. The doctors had just come in. Andrew put me on the speaker. The doctors said they were not specialists, but there was a large tumor in his spinal cord and he would be sent to the specialists, who would decide what to do. This was now Monday morning. They transferred him to the neurosurgical team. The tumor board apparently met and decided to take the tumor out. We called Mom, who was getting on a flight back home from a cruise in the Baltics. It was just Andrew and me. Mom was in hysterics the whole flight home, with Grandma trying to calm her down. They came straight from the airport to the hospital. He was operated on Wednesday, a seven-hour surgery. It was a nine-centimeter tumor. His surgeon was very clear. We appreciated and valued him, his apparent honesty, his friendly demeanor. His aura was trustworthy. Closer to midnight, he came out and said the surgery was very successful and he had taken out most of the tumor.

No pathology yet.

∾ SHEHER ∾

Rebecca and Andrew were friends since middle school. I introduced my best friend, Charles, to Andrew in 2009, and Rebecca joined the group in 2012. Andrew was spending a year abroad in Paris from 2014 through 2015. He lived in a dorm with a great view, had a private bathroom. He had made a set of wonderful friends. Rebecca and I visited him, and he took us to underground bars and the hippest restaurants and introduced us to his friends. We had the best time, going out dancing, clubbing, but some nights, we just stayed home, talking.

One incident is stuck in my head. It was our last night. We came back at 3:00 and had to leave for our flight at 5:00. Andrew asked Rebecca, "Can you do this one dish before going to bed?" She refused. He flared up, and he and Rebecca had a shouting match, calling each other entitled. But then it was over, and Andrew was the same loving self. He doted on Rebecca. He could be stubborn, obstinate, but fiercely protective of all his friends.

∾ KAT ∾

Two days after the surgery, they said it was a glioma, but they were not entirely sure yet. Then they said it was a grade 4 glioblastoma. My grandmother and I researched glioblastomas and found out how fatal they were. Mom and Dad did not even look. They could not. At New York General, he had some of the most painful experiences. He was paralyzed. He lost control of his bowels and bladder. He had to be disimpacted manually. He said it was the worst pain imaginable. They sent him to rehabilitation. He had to learn to walk again.

The doctors were very positive at this stage and said he was really doing well. Dr. C. wanted to do radiation and chemo separately, because simultaneously giving both could potentially cause too much inflammation, which would lead to other issues.

❧ SHEHER ❧

Six of us had a group chat. Andrew texted us. He started by saying, "Guys, I have a pinched nerve." Then, he texted, "Oh, it's some neuromuscular thing." And finally, "It's cancer." But he made it sound like everything was under control, even as he told us the diagnosis. He was very positive all along. I went to see him in the ICU before he had the surgery. He was already paralyzed, he could not move, but was very positive. He was more concerned about how Charles and I were doing. He was calm and matter-of-fact. "They have to do surgery and then radiation therapy, and chemo, but first I have to learn how to walk again after the surgery."

❧ KAT ❧

We sought a second opinion at another hospital. They said to give both chemo and radiation at the same time and deal with complications later. Andrew felt more comfortable at first. The doctors there were more hopeful and exhibited optimism. They started radiation. He did PT. Radiation was targeted to the regional spine, and the same area was repeatedly scanned to look for any recurrence. Afterward, my grandma felt that was negligent, that they took years away from him by not scanning his brain and spine routinely. Anyway, he was finally done with radiation.

He was so happy he was getting back on his feet. We were even able to go snowboarding that winter; after such an invasive spinal surgery, it wasn't clear if he could walk again. But when we tried to go a second time that winter, he couldn't. He started to get weak. He started getting really awful headaches. Doctors said maybe he had a sinus infection. It was the most ridiculous thing. They gave him antibiotics. He deteriorated very quickly, had to be rushed to the ER; he was throwing up nonstop. He looked totally green and was shaking. He spent another full day in the ER. They did a CT scan to see if there was bleeding. There was fluid built up that blocked off the ventricles. They did a full-body MRI and saw tumors all over the spine and all over his brain. Mom and I found out first in the ER. We were so terrified of sharing this news with him; thankfully, the doctors told him. Andrew was so stoic. All he said was, "That sucks," and then, "But what's your plan for fixing this?" They did another surgery and put in a shunt. They put him on high doses of steroids.

Dr. C. came to the ICU postsurgery. She was despondent and sorry and grim. She apologized a lot. I am not sure whether it was because she should have done a full-body scan or because she could not do anything to help now. She was very honest and told us that even though there were options, Andrew's chances of response were low and lower.

Andrew and my mom hated her being so honest. They decided to switch to the second hospital. He got assigned to the doctor who had done his second consultation. Dr. T. got along very well with Andrew and Mom. Dr. T. was very optimistic and said there were any number of experimental trials they could offer. Andrew would get sassy with Dr. T., and they would have a great time at every appointment, laughing and making jokes.

∞ SHEHER ∞

I first met Andrew in late winter 2009. Andrew had parties called the Slootsky Fest. His mom was very protective and insisted that instead of going out, he should invite all his friends over. She would be upstairs, and the kids partied in the basement. It was dark. Andrew was playing a band called Crystal Castles. I walked in, went straight to the iPod, and changed it to Mindless Self Indulgence. A voice in the dark yelled, "Why did you do that?" It was Andrew. The rest is history. The boldness of each struck the other, united and bonded us. I was a regular at the Slootsky Fest after that, and he was over at my place the rest of the time.

∞ KAT ∞

Andrew badly wanted to study abroad. Growing up in Brooklyn and staying in New York City for college, he longed to get out for a bit. Andrew almost always got what he wanted. He studied French all through school; Paris was the obvious choice for him. We traveled there as a family a couple of summers prior, and he thought it'd be a great place for a semester abroad. He left in late August of 2014. I wasn't really concerned about his experience there, since Andrew makes the most of everything instantly, easily making friends. My mom, of course, still needed to call as often as possible for her own peace of mind. She missed him. I did, too, but for me, it felt more natural. Sometimes when I get really sad now, I pretend that he's just living in Paris. It helps.

While in Paris, Andrew studied French and film. He was pretty much fluent after his time there. He always made fun of my pronunciations when I attempted to speak my very limited French. When he was admitted to the hospital for his cancer, a number of the patient care technicians were from French-speaking countries, and it was such a joy seeing him easily communicate with them in French. They had their own secret thing going on; it made anyone in the room smile. Mentally, Andrew was all there until the very end. One of the technicians, who was originally from Senegal, would always come find Andrew when he was admitted, even if Andrew was not assigned to his care—just to have a chat and see how he was doing. The technician stopped by on Andrew's last day and attempted to have a chat in French, but it proved to be difficult, not because of Andrew's loss for words but the morphine he was given made his tongue really heavy, and having a conversation was difficult. I remember the technician getting really emotional and leaving the room, which at the moment I couldn't understand and was angry about, but I can see more clearly why he did that now. Andrew's disease deeply affected him even though he dealt with terminal cancer patients every day. Andrew was different. They had a bond. He was one of the hospital staff members who came to the funeral. It meant a lot.

∞ SHEHER ∞

I remember a day in Berlin. We were trying to decide what to do. I wanted to go to the aquarium; Charles and Rebecca refused. They wanted to go shopping instead, but Andrew took me. We went into a room with insects, where ants were falling on our heads. We were screaming, running around. It was the best day I had on that trip. Andrew always paired up with me, and Rebecca with Charles, whenever there was a conflict in our plans. We would joke that people assumed he was my boyfriend. It had two advantages: boys didn't hit on me, and sweet Andrew carried my shopping bags. Besides, he was my designated fashion adviser. If he couldn't come, I sent him photos before buying anything.

∞ KAT ∞

Andrew mostly went to class, partied, and explored Paris with his newly formed group of friends. He interned at the Mary Katrantzou showroom during Paris Fashion Week. Since he was trilingual, he was able to communicate with their many Russian clients and translate Russian to French. He collaborated on a documentary film he directed with a friend from his program. The film documented Fashion Week through the eyes of their friend Yu attending some of the shows. Shopping was a favorite pastime. He was always on the hunt for something special. He got himself some classics thrifted in the Parisian boutiques.

∞ SHEHER ∞

When I first met him, Andrew wasn't into fashion. He dressed like a regular high school gay boy. In college, he developed a real sense of style. We were going to start a PR agency together. We used to throw big warehouse parties where kids could drink and dance. Both of us liked to dress well in college and executed the parties together. He was very artistic, always had a strong vision for things. Before I bought any bags, shoes, my statement pieces, I always got his approval first. He took great care to put together what he was going to wear. Kat is a photographer. He styled clothing for her. He loved

Prada, Dries Van Noten, Kenzo. Shoes and clothing both. He also looked for high-end obscure brands. He played with silhouettes, shadows. Even now when I dress to go out, I think of what Andrew would say. *Sheher, take that off right now.* Or would he approve? He was really into music. Just before the last time he went into the hospital, he demanded to live alone on Thirty-Ninth and Park in his grandma's apartment. He got this program called Ableton, which DJs use. He created a song. Rap, hip-hop, dance music, he loved it all. We argued a lot about who would play music at parties. Andrew would fight us but also protected all his friends with his life.

∾ KAT ∾

My mom and I went to visit him for his twenty-first birthday in December. We flew out to Paris and got an Airbnb near the history museum. Andrew abandoned his dorm to stay with us. We explored the city he now knew so well, guiding us around on bikes by memory. Then we rented a car and drove to the French Alps; we snowboarded, and our mom skied at Val d'Isère. It was such an amazing experience skiing in the Alps—vast open trails with endless peaks covered in snow every which way you looked. Andrew and I loved snowboarding, going as fast as we could, each trying to be the first one down, following closely on the other's tail. He would make playlists for us to sync up and listen to while flying down the mountain. Our mom always worried that we were going too fast, but we were having the most amazing time.

∾ SHEHER ∾

It was October of 2016. Andrew was much better. He was going out again, partying some. Mom, you asked me if one of my friends could video your keynote speech at the Development of Literacy gala where you were to be honored. Andrew jumped at the opportunity. He was so excited, went and rented the equipment, he rehearsed how to use the remote microphone. Sam, Andrew, Charles, and I arrived at Cipriani before the gala to scout the grand ballroom. Andrew set up his equipment and fitted you with the mic. It was a glamorous evening, and we had a blast, sharing drinks and jokes, dancing and living it up. He filmed you with great care and concentration. He never forgave himself for the sound. It was the one mistake he made; he forgot to turn the mic on when he fitted you.

∞ KAT ∞

Andrew was so much better. He was independent again. He went by himself to LA, then for three weeks to Berlin. He was on chemotherapy and then lots of clinical trials in sequence. In Berlin, he went to the hospital to get the blood work every week, which then had to be sent to Dr. T. Andrew was annoyed about spending a whole day at the hospital in Berlin. While in Berlin, he started getting weak again in the final days of his trip. He had an episode where he unexpectedly lost control of his bowels and was deeply embarrassed, but the people he was with were very nice about it. He was able to laugh it off. He had a way of making everyone feel better. In Berlin, while we were FaceTiming one day, I noticed that his sharp and chiseled face appeared bloated. We later realized it was due to the steroids he was on. He discovered the term for this condition was *moon face;* he was pretty upset about it but would always tell people that his face would go back to normal once he stopped taking the steroids. Later, his eyesight started to go, and in a way, it was a blessing, because he never really saw how drastically his appearance changed.

∾ SHEHER ∾

Andrew was very frustrated because his mom was very protective of him, very possessive, but he knew he could not be alone anymore. His close friends visited constantly, accompanied him to his appointments, sat with him in waiting rooms, tried to help as he threw up from chemo and developed the worst possible raw ulcers in his throat after the radiation. It was really awful to see him suffer so much. He could not eat much of anything; he could not swallow. Through the worst nightmarish times, Andrew never complained. He was the one asking all of us about our lives, always turning the conversation away from him, always cheerful, never complained. How is that possible, Mom? He was so sick. We could see it.

∾ KAT ∾

In late April or May, Mom and I were with him when he suddenly started talking gibberish. He had gone for a routine radiation treatment when this happened. They sent him for an emergency MRI, which showed a bleed in his head. Everyone thought he was going to die that night. They asked him to sign a proxy and to decide on a DNR. That was the night my parents finally realized he was not going to make it. He still woke up and lived another two months. When he woke up, he thought he was in Canada. Temporary lapse only. He rapidly returned to being himself.

This very young radiologist involved in Andrew's care was honest about how bad things were, but at least he was optimistic in his manner. He gave Andrew the choice to go ahead with the radiation or refuse it, calling himself the firefighter, putting out the immediate flame but not solving the overarching issue. He told Andrew frankly that it could help some of the symptoms but not do much for his survival. During that discussion, Andrew was very matter-of-fact: "Well, I don't want to die, so we've got to do the radiation." So they kept doing it until they couldn't. He was then sent to rehab because he had to try to get "stronger." At this point, within a month's time, he was quadriplegic. The insurance approved rehab because he had to learn how to exist in his current state, and my mom had to learn how to care for him. However, the rehab facility was nervous to have him because they were not equipped for handling him.

∾ Sheher ∾

I called you that night, Mom. Andrew started babbling in the radiation department. They did an emergency MRI and found a bleed in his head. Andrew's mother, Alena, asked me to call you and ask you to help. Everyone felt like this was it. He was dying. We were all with Andrew, taking turns going to the waiting room and crying, then we would panic and rush back to be with him. I called you at 1:00 a.m. and cried hysterically, begging you to do something to help him. It was so unbearable. I was really mad for once. I yelled at you, saying, "How is it possible that his mother survived breast cancer and Andrew is dying at twenty-three? How is this happening?"

I am sorry, Mom, but it was too much. The pain, his face, the fact that he was paralyzed. He could not do a single thing he liked doing. He could not even play video games. He was blind. I heard all my life that you and Dad helped cancer patients. You did not help Andrew.

∾ KAT ∾

The last week of August would be his last week of life, although we didn't know it yet. He could not see. He could not move at all, could not urinate or move his bowels. Next morning, he choked and stopped breathing. Mom responded quickly, a code was called, he was intubated and placed on a respirator. He was moved to the ICU. They weren't sure if his lungs were working on their own or not. They kept the tube down for twenty-four hours. My family was really nervous about them keeping the tube in for too long; they kept insisting on removing it. My grandmother, who is also a doctor, kept insisting they remove it. He was very frustrated, because mentally, he was all there. Then came a final blow. They told him he could not eat again, as his swallowing was gone. They offered a swallow test. Andrew took this test very seriously; he was very nervous and wanted to pass. Of course, he failed. He was so disappointed. He thought of it like a college exam: if he tried harder, he could do better the next time and possibly pass. He begged to be given a second chance. Knowing that the result would be the same, the hospital staff let him take the test again the following day. He failed again. That was when the doctors sat my parents and me down and suggested hospice care. This came as a total shock for my parents.

After the failed test, my grandmother and uncle insisted that if he could not swallow, we had to ask them to put in a feeding tube. One of the fellows who used to come on daily rounds was very honest and discouraged us from it, strongly.

He said he had another patient where they put in a feeding tube and it kept getting infected and was very painful. The medical team finally addressed the quality-of-life issue. Before that, it was all about "We will just keep fighting this disease." Then all of a sudden, they switched to "Let's do nothing."

The silver lining was that we could potentially do hospice at home. Even Andrew was happy at the prospect of being home. He always put up a brave front, especially for my mom's sake, and said to her, "Maybe they can't do anything for me now, but after a while, they are sure to have something." He never gave up. He could not.

My therapist recommended a really good book—Atul Gawande's *Being Mortal*—about modern medicine and how the medical field does not really know how to address the quality-of-life issues. Doctors don't know what to do when there is nothing more to do medically. The book helped me prepare for the hospice conversation. Hospice has a general negative association in our society; thanks to this book, I now understand how valuable hospice is. It helped me decide against the feeding tube. My uncle, the pediatrician, also insisted that we put in the feeding tube, and when I refused, he asked me pointedly, "Don't you want Andrew to live?" I said, "Of course I do, but not like this. The feeding tube will do nothing for him."

∞ SHEHER ∞

Some of our friends couldn't come to visit Andrew. For one thing, we didn't tell everyone just how bad things had become. But mainly it was because they couldn't face it. I talked to many of them, tried to tell them it would mean so much to Andrew. Andrew needed us all. He needed for us to be there with him. He always acted normal with us. On a few days, he was frustrated, upset; otherwise, we played music, played games, talked. His speech and hearing were fine until the end. Charles, Rebecca, and I were all working at the time, but we spent all the remaining hours we could being with him. The one time I saw him become extremely frustrated was with that stupid swallow test. Andrew became fixated on passing it, because he knew that literally his life depended on it. He looked so innocent, trying to succeed, but his mouth and tongue just refused to cooperate. His eyes, they reflected his torment briefly, and then he was fine again, even welcoming hospice care as a relief, to get out of the hospital and go home. He acted like it would be just for a few days.

∞ KAT ∞

In the final four months, Dr. T. did not come even once to visit Andrew. I was the one desperately researching possible trials. The hospital did not help us at all. They dropped the ball. It was a full-time job to do all that research. In the final month or two, I found out that they had never even done a genetic profile on his tumor.

People were not as compassionate as they should have been. I found one trial that required a blood test and a signed authorization from Andrew. He was in the rehab at his first hospital. Can you believe that it was impossible to get blood drawn there and get it to his second hospital? The bureaucracy of it all is so stupid when it has to do with human life. Most of the time, it was all about paperwork.

But then there were some amazing people we also met. The technician who would stop by and chat in French. John, Andrew's physical therapist, was so charming, sweet, and attentive to Andrew. When Andrew was sent back to the second hospital, John stopped by on his days off to hang out with Andrew and the posse of friends in the ICU during Andrew's last week. Another physical therapy assistant would come regularly to hang out with him. When I first met her, I assumed it was just one of his friends I hadn't previously met, when in fact they had just met a few days prior and were getting on as if they'd known each other for years.

The evening he died, we all met at a bar in Brooklyn to celebrate his life and remember him. A lot of the caregivers Andrew had met along the way showed up that evening and at the funeral a few days later. A therapist reached out wanting to do Cycle for Survival in Andrew's name. The little things people did were so touching.

∽ SHEHER ∽

In the hospital, I had a very upsetting evening with Andrew. He had relapsed, and there were metastases all over the brain and spinal cord. He had been in the hospital since May. Then he was sent to a second, pseudo–rehab center. He was getting physical therapy, people moved his arms and legs. He was mostly blind now and could only move one hand partially. He had several wisdom teeth taken out. He said it was the most painful thing, more than chemo. It was a week before he died. I was alone with him. I had just finished feeding him. He had to use a water pick to clean his mouth and get the food out of the gaping holes that were left in place of the wisdom teeth. Food would get stuck in those sockets. He was not allowed to use a toothbrush because his whole mouth was completely raw. He asked me to help. I filled the pick with water and handed it to him. He kept dropping it; he was too weak to hold it. I kept trying to grab it from him, saying,

"Andrew, let me do it." He got increasingly frustrated and finally yelled at me, "Please, Sheher! Can you just let me do this one thing for myself?" He tried so hard until that point to appear strong, as if he had no pain. In that moment, I could see the minute-by-minute agony he was going through more clearly than ever before. I waited until someone came to relieve me and left to bawl my eyes out. I sat outside and just cried and cried.

∽ KAT ∽

On the last day, there were forty or fifty people in and out of ICU. The hospital sent over a musical therapist who would stop by and have little jam sessions with us. Every person in the room got an instrument, and Andrew would be the conductor. That whole week, he had not eaten. There was the end-of-life team to manage the pain, giving morphine and making sure he had some relief. They let him break the rules: "You can eat whatever you want. But remember, you can choke." He needed to make a decision about whether he wanted to be intubated if he choked again. I was with him that evening, when the choice was presented to him, and I stayed the night. It was a quiet night; we fell asleep listening to Arcade Fire's new album. My dad stayed with him the next night, and it was horrible, and they were scared he wouldn't make it 'til morning. I remember my mom and me rushing to the ICU that morning, hoping to make it in time. That morning, before my mom and I got there, Andrew decided on DNR. I think it was easier for him to say it out loud without my mom and me present. He was alone with our dad. Andrew was always so stoic when my mom and I were there. It's my theory that he was protecting us, and by protecting us, he was also protecting himself from the truth.

∾ SHEHER ∾

He was so gaunt and so swollen at the same time. His body was wasted, but his face was puffy because he was pumped full of steroids. The shunt was draining fluid from his brain. His whole body was unrecognizable. He loved Brazilian jujitsu. He had lost his left arm soon after the diagnosis, but now his whole body was wasted. The fecal impaction was the worst; someone had to relieve him by hand. He did not want to ever go through that again. Or the spinal surgery. He said he would rather die.

∾ KAT ∾

They took him off all machines and put him on a morphine drip. I kept pressing the button for him even though he kept telling me he wasn't in pain. I later was told that the button was giving him a tiny amount more, and just the prescribed amount, and it was pretty insignificant, but by pressing the button, I felt like I was doing something in this excruciatingly helpless situation. He wanted to have Coca-Cola; Andrew loved a fresh, cold Mexican Coke in a glass bottle. On a little sponge, I gave him a tiny bit to taste. A few hours later, he developed strange, noisy, gargled breathing. I felt guilty that it was the Coke, and my boyfriend, Ed, kept reassuring me that it wasn't and that I didn't do anything wrong by giving Andrew a taste. As he got tired, he said to everyone in the room, "Please don't leave, just hang out. Don't mind me, I will sleep for a bit. Just don't watch me while I sleep." From ten to midnight, he got into a deep breathing and sleeping pattern. The whole hospice conversation had been for nothing. There was no way he was getting out of the hospital.

∾ SHEHER ∾

I had made a video in which he looks high because he was so sick. It was from the time when one of the tumors in his brain had hemorrhaged and he was making no sense. He looked so cute—innocent and bewildered. I have the video but cannot watch it. Andrew was very close to his mom; they yelled at each other a lot. He, his sister, and his mom, went on annual trips together. He adored Kat. That last night, we were all with him for almost fourteen hours. He did not want to close his eyes. He somehow knew that when he did, he would never open them again. He kept telling us to stay. Until the end, he was making total sense.

∾ KAT ∾

That night, after everyone left at midnight, I was sitting on the bed with him and holding his hand. Mom and her friend were sitting on the chair. I was talking about something silly, not even looking at Andrew. Mom's friend is a nurse, and she noticed that his breathing got slower and slower. We called the staff. They said Andrew was still with us; we could talk to him. We called my dad, who was in the waiting room. I felt like I had to tell Andrew it was okay for him to let go, even though I felt it was not okay. How could I tell him that? Suddenly, his hand went limp in my palm. I could not see him as I was sitting right next to him in bed, so I got up to look at him. It was the worst sight I've ever seen. Andrew's face had just fallen. His mouth open. I was devastated. I left the room instantly. He was gone.

∞ SHEHER ∞

We had just reached home after being with Andrew for fourteen hours when I got Kat's text. Andrew was no more. *Inna lillah e wa inna ilayhe rajeoun.* From him we came, and to him we shall return.

∞ KAT ∞

My dad and mom kept going back in to see him. I got frustrated, not understanding. "Why do you keep going in? There is only a dead body in there now. That's not Andrew anymore!" For some crazy reason, my dad became obsessed with Andrew's open mouth. What if it froze in that position as rigor mortis set in? He finally located some tape and managed to close Andrew's mouth and support his lifeless jaw.

◯◯

THERE WAS NOTHING else left to do for Andrew now. It was not even half an hour since he died, but his father's face had aged years. Your child's dead body can do strange things.

> *No, no, no life?*
> *Why should a dog, a horse, a rat have life,*
> *And thou no breath at all? Oh, thou'lt come no more,*
> *Never, never, never, never, never.*
> —SHAKESPEARE, *KING LEAR*, ACT 5, SCENE 3

A ghazal by Mirza Ghalib provides Urdu poetry with a new language for the elegiac; it articulates the anger of loss without in any way diminishing the intensity of passion. It addresses the dead son with the necessity of reproach. The poet declares that it was imperative that the absent should see his path again, and then asks a poignant question—why did you go alone?—and proceeds to state, "So stay alone, until some other day!" The couplet pierces because its sorrow is almost infantile in that it expresses the raw irritability of grief: there is no give-and-take in death; there is only a taking away.

> *Laazim tha kay dekho mera rasta koi din aur*
> *Tanha gayay kyoun, ab raho tanha koi din aur*
> —GHALIB: EPISTEMOLOGIES OF ELEGANCE

> Our paths had to cross again some other day
> Going alone, now stay alone, until some other day

THE FIRST THING Andrew said after his diagnosis, his mother, Alena, told me when I met her at the hospital, was, "Call Azra, Mom. She is on the cutting edge of cancer. I want her involved in my care. She'll make sure I'm okay." The words cut deeply and reminded me why I had quit my fellowship in pediatric oncology forty years before.

Two of my older siblings were already doing their residencies in Buffalo, New York, so I landed there on January 2, 1977. Three weeks later, Buffalo was hit by the Blizzard of '77. One hundred inches of snow fell within three days, and high winds blew the snow into drifts of thirty to forty feet. My brother and sister and their spouses got stranded in their respective hospitals. The two families lived in a duplex. Suddenly, I was the only adult, with five children between the two homes. We huddled in one living room, ate lots of bread and cheese, and watched *Roots* and *Welcome Back, Kotter,* which my thirteen-year-old brother, Abbas, was obsessed with.

When life returned to normal, I began making inquiries about finding work, as I had a six-month gap until the start of my internship in July. My sister Atiya, a third-year resident in pediatrics at The Children's Hospital of Buffalo, had done a rotation at Roswell Park Memorial Institute. When she told Arnie Freeman, the chief of pediatric oncology at the institute, that I wanted to be an oncologist, he offered me a fellowship for six months so long as I was at least half as good as my sister. So I began a pediatric oncology fellowship. Within a couple of weeks, it was obvious that I would not last, but not because I was incompetent. I could not handle dying children.

Judy Ochs, my attending physician and Atiya's close friend, had a serious talk with me one afternoon when she found me sobbing yet again in one of the back rooms. Frustrated, she marched me into the fourth-floor, windowless corner office of one Harvey David Preisler, chief of the adult leukemia program, and handed me over to him, saying, "Please give her a chance on your service. She might survive it. She has potential if she can face the pain." Harvey tried to conduct some kind of an interview, but I was too heartbroken over losing a four-year-old girl to leukemia that day. I did, however, report to work on his floor early the next morning, thus beginning my lifelong association with the man who would become my husband eight years later.

Shortly afterward, the famous Elisabeth Kübler-Ross, the author of the pioneering book *On Death and Dying,* came to give grand rounds at Roswell Park. She was the first to describe five distinct reactions to death, both in patients and their loved ones: denial, anger, bargaining, depression, and acceptance. The important point she made was that acceptance, though hard to achieve, brought a modicum of relief, a sense of tranquility, and may even lead to a sharper appreciation of the larger issues of life and death, a much-needed inner peace.

Kübler-Ross spoke thoughtfully and calmly and had such a compassionate manner that I mustered up enough courage to ask her a question at the end of her talk. "If you could give me one piece of advice about informing terminally ill patients how much time they have left, what would it be?" I asked. She thought for only a few seconds before replying, "Don't volunteer the information."

Throughout Andrew's sixteen months of illness, I agonized over the cruelty of the choices we oncologists offered. The issue became especially poignant when considering fundamental existential questions for Andrew. Is it less painful to let cancer kill him when experience and observation clearly indicate that the chance of recovery is practically nil, or should experimental drugs be offered with their attendant insufferable toxicities, prolonging survival by mere weeks at best? In the absence of experimental drugs, when the tumor began to invade organs, causing unbearable symptoms like the severe headaches and incessant, projectile vomiting, what was the right course of action? Palliation with pain medications and comfort care or aggressive attempts to produce remission with radiation and more chemotherapy, knowing that hope was nonexistent for any long-term remission?

Obviously, if there were even a remote possibility that a new experimental trial could help Andrew, the oncologists would have offered it themselves, but somehow, the patient and families have lost trust in their oncologists. His twenty-five-year-old sister searched desperately for any treatment strategy to help her brother, feeling, as many patients and their families do, that the burden of finding treatment rests with them. Why is this happening?

One reason relates to agency. On a daily basis, I have conversations with patients who are very, very sick. They want to have some control over what happens to them. Disease management, especially a chronic one, is truly a bilateral affair.

When treating low-risk MDS—a disease that requires complex long-term planning enacted on an evolving landscape of both illness and treatment—a patient's trust and confidence in a physician is directly proportional to the sense of ownership and agency the patient feels. The following patient is a perfect example of this empowerment when it works.

4-23-2018

> *My name is Donna Meyers and I am 80 years old. I was diagnosed with MDS almost twenty-five years ago when anemia was detected. I was told of its seriousness and that I had to find a hematologic oncologist. Of course I was scared and started interviewing doctors. I met Dr. Azra Raza at Rush University Hospital in Chicago and knew immediately that she was the one I could trust with my life. She, from the beginning, made me a part of the process and I knew this would be a partnership. For me feeling that I had some control over my illness gave me a feeling of hope and agency.*

My respect and admiration for Donna is directly proportional to the equanimity and poise with which she has handled, now for a quarter century, extremely challenging physical issues. A draining, sapping, wildly fluctuating profound anemia, weakness, uncertainty, the exhausting business of repeated recruitments into experimental trials with questionable benefits and unpredictable side effects. The burden of having to travel regularly to see me in Massachusetts and now in New York. Yet I have never heard her complain once about any of this. She quietly and calmly arranges everything in her life around the one thing she is certain of: the bimonthly blood transfusions. At the Northwestern University infusion center in Chicago, Donna has been a familiar face for decades; getting Procrit and Aranesp shots, receiving transfusions, undergoing added tests and treatments I prescribe long distance. Her wonderful local hematologist, Dr. Olga Frankfurt, and I remain connected via Donna's super-diligent mediation. She maintains records of her hemoglobin and iron levels, number of transfusions, and medications she is taking, all on her cell phone, which she whips out with equal ease in airless hospital rooms and fancy restaurants to update me on the latest numbers. You might be surprised to hear about the quality of her life in all these years.

Despite the constant intrusion of her disease's unpleasant reminders, Donna has been able to lead a very fulfilling life. She never stopped

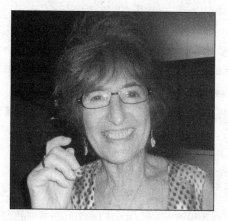

working in her profession and never stopped traveling. When in Chicago, she plays golf, has many hobbies, and has a ton of friends and family to socialize with. She enjoys her large family and travels extensively to see them. In short, she has more energy at eighty with her debilitating MDS than most healthy people have at forty. She refuses to let the disease dictate her daily activities, and she refuses to be pitied. Although her loving children and husband are always ready to accompany her, most of her trips to see me in New York are made by herself.

During all these years, every decision was jointly made by Azra and I; for 25 years we have managed my MDS together. There is a deep bond, a personal relationship, and love, we have developed over the years. I feel that this has been *our* journey. I am still alive at 80. I get up every day and say YES! I'm alive and I will do what I want and go where I want. Thank you to my family, my husband and to my wonderful friend, Azra, my doctor. I love you all.

Donna's story highlights the importance of agency in a chronic disease. One of my younger patients, Betty, suffering from a profound aplastic anemia, required multiple blood and platelet transfusions weekly. She looked exceptionally frustrated in clinic one day because of the long commute and inordinately protracted waiting times in the infusion center. She was exhausted to the point of crying. I asked her to inquire if we could arrange some of the transfusions in a facility five minutes away from where she lived. According to Tim, her doting husband, Betty was a different person within twenty-four hours. Because she had control of something finally—calling clinics, arranging appointments, making her wishes known, bargaining schedules—she was empowered. She was energized.

The concern with this bilateralism is the asymmetry between patient and physician. The patient's experience with cancer is singular. Their treatment from their own oncologist is supplemented by frantic literature searches, Dr. Google, and curbside consults with anyone and everyone remotely connected to the medical field. The problem is that even when patients are well informed, the one thing they lack is experience. Their knowledge is half-baked and creates false hope. When patients are not offered some therapy apparently successful in another type of cancer to treat their own, they feel cheated by their oncologists and start looking every which way on their own. Oncologists, on the other hand, have the benefit of having treated hundreds of similar cases in addition to years of rigorous training. This has earned them the right to make treatment suggestions. The responsibility of the oncologist when offering a choice between multiple courses of action to the patient is inversely proportional to the patient's experience and knowledge of the disease.

Another reason why patients and their families search frantically for treatments other than the ones offered by the primary treating oncologist is the way baby steps toward a new cancer treatment strategy are prematurely blown out of proportion by the media. Harvey and I experienced that firsthand in 1998 with an anti-angiogenic drug that showed efficacy against a variety of cancers in mice but zero response in human trials. More recently, this has happened for immune therapies. The success of one immune-based strategy called *CAR-T therapy*, in curing an extremely rare kind of childhood leukemia, is proclaimed from the rooftops as though it were the cure for all cancers. Bombarded with the massive coverage of these rare success stories in the media—contrasted with no mention of these therapies by the oncologist—patients begin to question the knowledge and intent of their doctors, start independent explorations of their own.

In addition to the sensationalized media reports of voguish therapies, there is yet another reason for this behavior. Cancer is a family affair, and not just for emotional reasons. Today, the traditional, paternalistic paradigm of medical treatment where doctors unilaterally made all treatment decisions is replaced with a more democratic system promoting autonomy and self-determination. Participation in treatment choice is a right of patients. This requires access to information, and online resources play a seminal role in this journey, especially for younger patients. Families are no longer the helpless bystanders, particularly as the end approaches. In their anxiety to assure that all is done for their loved ones, they question the expertise of oncologists, worry that they might not have received all the information to self-advocate. They search furiously, trying to find a reason to be hopeful in a desperate situation, knowing that nothing they choose is likely to work, yet unable to stop themselves from ceaselessly trolling the web.

⟋⟍

IS DYING A FAILURE?

In March 2004, I was in New Canaan, Connecticut, for a lecture. I happened to pick up a copy of the *Fairfield Weekly* and read a brilliant piece by Lorraine Gengo on the English artist Barbara Griffith, whose *New Canaan Observed: A Field Study* explored "how two individuals relate to the group and how we fit into society and what that takes out of us." In the article, Ms. Gengo discussed a painting by Ms. Griffith titled, *The Role of Synchronized Clothing and Movement in Evading Death.* This is how Ms. Gengo described it. The painting bears newspaper headlines:

TEA DANCE FIGHTS CANCER; TENNIS OUTING FIGHTS CANCER; POM-POM HATS FOR BATTERED WOMEN. The women in the painting appear as a "chain-gang of domesticity"; in their conformity, which Ms. Gengo describes as camouflage, she sees a "religious procession," the goal of which is the defiance of death. "As a marching body," she writes, the women "become a powerful organism which rejects any non-conforming cell to affirm its own health and virtue. The fallen woman (or non-conforming cell) is the statistical sacrifice, the one in five who must die that they may live. It is a poignant primitive rite to avert evil." It is a symbolic defiance of mortality through obsessive exercise by toned and tanned women jogging in groups.

Ultimately, the painting plays with themes that recur throughout our personal conversations and cultural discourse about cancer. Cancer is called a battle, a war, a fight; patients are the warriors, the foot soldiers, guided by the oncologists acting as their captains. The war is waged by groups comprising individuals, families, advocacy groups, industry, academia, and institutions, all joined in an effort to resist a malicious, evil adversary. The weapons used are surgery, chemotherapy, radiation therapy, and the occasional magic bullet. The individual patient is called upon to join the battle armed with a fighting spirit. This language is used by patients, doctors, families, the public, in formal meetings and informal discussions. It can serve as a positive reinforcement. Many patients take comfort in such militant metaphors; they put up a good fight, at least earlier on in the course of their illness. As the battle picks up and intensifies, however, the metaphor loses its power. The punishing, grueling, exhausting experience of dying is quite one-sided. No one feels heroic when they are throwing up or suffering from wearing, draining, unstoppable, persistent pain.

So it was for Harvey. In the second year of my husband's diagnosis, his condition worsened rather dramatically, and he required repeated admissions for unpredictable, unexpected complications. Within the space of some eighteen months, the man went through a series of bewildering neoplastic manifestations and paraneoplastic syndromes; a new onset of severe asthma; drenching night sweats; exceedingly painful migratory polyarthritis; disfiguring facial edema; DVT; shingles; facial paralysis; tuberculous meningitis; and multiple episodes of fevers of unknown origin.

Once, his three grown children, Sarah, Mark, and Vanessa, arrived during such an emergency admission. Harvey was extremely close to all three and spoke to each of them on a daily basis. When he would get really sick, they would come in from the East and West Coasts at short notice and do everything possible to help out, including taking charge of Sheherzad with utmost love, responsibility, and concern. One day, they cornered me. "Az, Dad never talks to us about his illness. The first we hear something is seriously wrong is when you call and tell us to come urgently. Can you please encourage him to talk to us so we have a better idea of what is going on?" That night, I broached the subject with Harvey.

He looked wistful. "What can I tell you? So much of talking to others is about asking for help. No one can help me. So why bother them?"

I persisted, arguing it would help them deal with the situation better. A scientist as he was, his response was quintessential Harvey. He rejected outright the added burden of trying to put others at ease. "Az, I cannot begin to describe to you the psychic energy I have to invest just to carry on with business as usual given the dizzying turn of events I am facing on a daily basis. I don't have energy left over to be concerned about how others are handling my illness. Even my own children. I want to, but cancer is draining in more ways than I imagined. You can talk to them if you want, but I honestly can't."

For a cancer patient, the only war is a war with one's own organs, where the self serves as a battleground. This battleground is unlike any other in that the body is both the theater of war and the combatant forces themselves. The fight begins as an inside job, a civil war. Cancer starts by attacking one organ and then expanding its reach. To fight this one enemy would be bad enough; unfortunately, the very weapons used to subdue the enemy and contain the civil war—chemo and radiation therapies—cause collateral damage, hurting the body indiscriminately, injuring organs, diseased or not. So how do we define this war when the body has to shield itself from internal and external aggressions simultaneously? It is a war for the body, on the body, by the body. The patient, held hostage by inside and outside forces, becomes aware of parts they never knew existed until unbearable pain and inflammation or a popping tumor or damage by chemotherapy unceremoniously bring them into the conscious realm. Caught in an incessant struggle between life and death, the body reluctantly yields a portion to cancer one day and to radiation and chemotherapy the next. Eventually, there is total confusion, and it becomes unclear whether organs need to be shielded from cancer or from the treatment. Total anarchy is the only endgame for such amorphous perversity. We say at this point that cancer is "winning" the war. But what is killing the body is as much the treatment as the cancer. So who is winning the war and who is losing? Cancer, chemo, oncologists, the cancer enterprise?

The very terms meant to empower end up detracting from the profound human experience of an individual facing mortality head-on in all its chaotic savagery, the physical suffering, anxiety, the grief. The patient, clinging obstinately to life, can only win this war by reconciling the body with death. They could achieve a more peaceful triumph if the mind were prepared to accept the need for such a reconciliation before the two sides—cancer and the insalubrious, noxious, vitriolic, awful treatments—locked horns in their violent, bloody struggle. Such thinking is entirely missing from the science of cancer, a tradition requiring urgent reexamination.

The terminology of positive thinking also stigmatizes by indirectly blaming the victim. When Miriam Hansen, one of my dearest, smartest, most brilliant friends, died, several friends and colleagues at her memorial service at the University of Chicago spoke about how she had fought the battle of cancer and survived, with a good quality of life for a number of years, because of her positive attitude, her willpower. Because of all the people praying for her. Her husband, Michael, rejected this. He categorically stated that his wife, Miriam, was able to live for twelve years with various cancers not because of willpower or positive thinking or prayers but because of her oncologists and the medical staff caring for her. To think otherwise is to say that those who died had no willpower, no positive thinking, and no one praying for them.

Harvey and Miriam, Omar and Andrew, and all patients facing terminal illnesses go through unspeakable suffering. They bear with unbearable grace whatever comes their way. There is no yardstick to measure their torment, no easier size to fit their grief, no scales to weigh their agony. No amount of analytic objectivity, no fancy subjective descriptions can contain their deep physical and psychological anguish. They may not have won the war on cancer, but dying was not a failure. In the end, there is no consolation, no answer. The science part can have an end in sight, but the human stories continue. Our patients need not be elevated in death, but remembered for what they endured. Lisa Bonchek Adams, who died of breast cancer in the prime of her life, rejected the stereotype, refused to be pitied, expressed the profundity of acceptance in these heartrending lines:

When I die
July 13th, 2012
When I die don't think you've "lost" me.
I'll be right there with you, living on in the memories we have made.
When I die don't say I "fought a battle." Or "lost a battle." Or
*   "succumbed."*
Don't make it sound like I didn't try hard enough, or have the right
attitude, or that I simply gave up.

When I die don't say I "passed."
That sounds like I walked by you in the corridor at school.

When I die tell the world what happened.
Plain and simple.
No euphemisms, no flowery language, no metaphors.

Instead, remember me and let my words live on.
Tell stories of something good I did.
Give my children a kind word. Let them know what they meant to me.
That I would have stayed forever if I could.
Don't try to comfort my children by telling them I'm an angel
   watching over them from heaven or that I'm in a better place:
There is no better place to me than being here with them.

They have learned about grief and they will learn more.
That is part of it all.

When I die someday just tell the truth:
I lived, I died.
The end.

⌒⌀⌒

THE STORY OF CAR-T therapy, its overblown reception notwithstanding, is remarkable. Scientific understanding rarely leads to successful, rationally designed treatments in oncology, a notable exception being chronic myeloid leukemia. More commonly, observations of a positive effect lead to a detailed examination of the molecular mechanism of response and not the other way around. The drug luspatercept is a recent example. This class of drugs was initially developed for a different purpose, but when healthy volunteers showed an unexpected improvement in hemoglobin, it was used to treat anemia in MDS patients. The precise mechanism of action is still being investigated but remains unclear. Immune therapies are an exception to this rule, representing an important revolution in medicine.

Manipulation of the body's own immune system to target the cancer is at least a century-old concept. A tremendous amount of knowledge generated regarding the intricate functioning of the immune system is only now starting to become translatable. Briefly, this is how it works. The job of T cells, key soldiers in the defensive army of the body, is to constantly inspect normal cells for expression of abnormal protein fragments or antigens on their surface. If detected, T cells latch on to the target antigen with talons and release toxic chemicals to destroy the offender. Cancer cells evolve strategies to deceive T cells by masquerading as normal cells, or expressing too many antigens, which confuse the attacking T cells. Another tactic cancer cells employ to evade the immune system is to turn off the "Eat me" signal on their surface so that cancer cells are perceived by the immune system as friend rather than foe.

Chimeric antigen receptor T cell, or CAR-T, therapy is a rationally designed, elaborate approach to overcome these cancer tricks. The question scientists asked was whether the body's own immune cells could be directed to attack the cancer. One way would be to find something unique on the surface of tumor cells, which T cells could latch on to and do their killing. The problem is that despite looking every which way for fifty years, no real unique cancer-associated antigen has been found. The same proteins that cancer cells express are also expressed on normal cells, just in different amounts. In the example of a B cell cancer, like acute lymphoblastic leukemia—ALL—the leukemia cells and normal B cells both express an antigen called *CD19*.

In a clever twist, the scientists who developed CAR-T decided to use the CD19 antigen as the target and send T cells armed with newly engineered claws to latch on to the CD19 antigen and kill all cells—normal and leukemic—carrying this marker in one fell swoop. It proved to be a smashing success for children with relapsed and refractory ALL and is now an FDA-approved treatment for this indication. The problem was that the treatment killed all normal B cells along with the leukemia cells. The function of normal B cells is to produce antibodies to fight infection—immunoglobulins. Ordinarily, one cannot live without B cells, but B cell function can be replicated by infusing immunoglobulins. Possibly, replacement therapy might be necessary for the rest of their lives, because CAR-T cells live for a long time and would keep destroying any emerging normal B cells. What this type of replacement therapy will mean in the long run for the patients is, at present, completely unknown.

CAR-T therapy has not become a universal treatment for all cancers for a host of reasons, the most important being that not all cellular functions are replaceable like the immunoglobulins for B cells. Furthermore, CAR-T therapy comes with its own set of serious and life-threatening toxicities. To start with, before engineered CAR-T cells can be infused into patients, marrow must be emptied to some extent to make room for them. This calls for treatment with very high doses of chemotherapy similar in intensity to the preparative regimen for a stem cell transplant. This step immediately precludes older patients with comorbid conditions from being considered for CAR-T therapy.

The second problem relates to the antigens expressed by cancer cells coming from different organs. The cancer-specific mutations affect proteins working inside the cell, while CAR-T recognizes only proteins expressed on the outside of the cell surface. Cancer cells express normal antigens on the outside, and these antigens are unique to cells belonging to different tissues or lineages within the same organ. For example, while all B cells express CD19, all myeloid cells (precursors of red blood cells, white blood cells, and platelets) express CD33. If we wanted to treat acute myeloid leukemia (AML) with CAR-T therapy targeting the antigen CD33, then all myeloid cells would be sought and killed by the superefficient engineered T cells. Unfortunately, there is no rescue of myeloid cells possible like there is for the B cells (with immunoglobulin infusions). A novel approach using CD33 CAR-T cells is being developed where all myeloid cells in an AML patient would be destroyed along with the leukemia cells, and then the patient could be transplanted with donor stem cells from which the CD33 antigen has been removed through genetic engineering. This may work; CD33 is not known to have any vital function as of yet. It is possible that donor myeloid cells lacking this antigen can repopulate the recipient marrow and lead to production of normal myeloid cells sans CD33 while AML cells that expressed CD33 will not be able to survive. If successful, a similar approach could be extended to other cancers as well. But once again, this therapy would only be an option for patients who are candidates for a bone marrow transplant, automatically excluding older individuals over seventy years of age.

Then there is the issue of off-target killing. Researchers describe how CAR-T therapy can backfire in a review article in the *Journal of Immunology Research:*

> The first fatal adverse event due to off-tumor recognition by a CAR occurred in a patient with colorectal cancer treated with high numbers of T cells expressing a third generation CAR targeting ERBB2/HER2. The patient developed respiratory distress and cardiac arrests shortly after the T cell transfer and died of multisystem organ failure 5 days later. It was postulated that the CAR T cells recognized ERBB2 expressed at low levels in the lung epithelium, leading to pulmonary toxicity and a cascading cytokine storm with a fatal outcome. Predicted on-target off-tumor toxicity with depletion of normal B-cells has been reported in nearly all patients treated with CD19 CAR T cells, and depending on the CAR configuration, B-cell aplasia lasts from months to years.

Perhaps the most dreaded complications of CAR-T therapy are the tumor lysis and cytokine release syndromes. Because of the extreme competence of CAR-T cell therapy, billions and billions of leukemia cells are destroyed in one swift blow. Tumor lysis syndrome arises when such massive cell death produces an immense amount of debris— choking up the kidneys—along with release of toxic material from the dying cells as they undergo lysis—that is, as they break apart. This constitutes a true medical emergency, as patients can die of multiple organ failure within hours if the syndrome is not recognized and treated early. Cytokine release syndrome is essentially an overstimulation of the immune system, and it can also be fatal. Financial toxicity is also enormous, costing anywhere from half a million dollars to much more, depending upon the level of complications encountered. The company Novartis has a deal where payment is due only upon proof of success a month after therapy.

CAR-T therapy in a very small subset of cancer patients with lymphoid disease is fantastically successful, albeit causing severe short-term toxicities and many known and unknown lifelong side effects. It is clear that much work lies ahead before this strategy can be scaled up for general use. Yet the hype surrounding CAR-T is such that practically every patient questions me about why they are being deprived of the magic cure. The results are not always magical:

Despite high-target, cell-specific killing in vitro and encouraging preclinical efficacies in murine tumor models, clinical responses of adoptively transferred T cells expressing α-folate receptor (FR) specific CAR in ovarian cancer were disappointing. No reduction of tumor burden was seen in the 14 patients studied. The absence of efficacy was ascribed to lack of specific trafficking of the T cells to tumor and short persistence of the transferred T cells.

The CAR-T hype is similar to the attention CRISPR (clustered regularly interspaced short palindromic repeats) is receiving. This laboratory tool, known popularly as *molecular scissors,* was described in detail just a few short years ago but has already led to the creation of commercial entities trading in hundreds of millions of dollars, institutions fighting nasty patent wars for its use in custom-designing babies to curing every genetic disease and, of course, cancer. Numerous panels debating the ethics of using this technology to alter human embryos have been conducted before any proof-of-principle studies. Several publications finally emerged. First, the news arrived that CRISPR is efficient in cells lacking a functional copy of the protein p53, that famous "guardian of the genome" and a favorite target of cancer research.

Then came another bit of bad news: when CRISPR was used to cut specific areas of DNA in human cells, it resulted in large segments of DNA being lost—thousands of base pairs away from the cutting site—strongly suggesting that CRISPR can cause mutagenesis and cancer. Why had it taken several years to show something so essential and basic before all the publicity? Why all the mad rush to commercialize before undertaking even the most fundamental science? If it were a matter of technology, then why so much advance promotion? Such are the vagaries of our field. Beautiful science. Not so, the scientists.

෨෨෨

WE FAILED ANDREW. In countless ways. As oncologists, first and foremost, we failed to provide a cure for his extremely malignant, exceedingly painful cancer. We added insult to injury by offering confusing choices—you can take this therapy or not; either way, it makes no difference. He died a tormented death, and his family had to stand by and watch it happen minute by minute. His sister frantically searched for treatment options. From a distance, I did what I could to connect her to whomever she asked to be in touch with. I knew how futile it was, but when she asked me about CAR-T options, I called Jasmine Zain and Steve Rosen because City of Hope had a CAR-T trial for glioblastoma. Steve put me in touch immediately with the principal investigator of the trial and offered his personal help in every way possible. Jasmine was exceptionally kind and considerate toward Kat, answering every e-mail with not just detailed medical answers but doing so with deep empathy and compassion. How fortunate we are to have such amazing colleagues. Andrew was not a candidate for the CAR-T trial because of the shunt. Kat continued e-mailing protocol sponsors, trying on her own to get his blood tested for genetic mutations, maneuvering the absurd legalities of institutional red tape to get a tube of blood sent from one hospital to another, following up on every lead to secure new treatments for her baby brother.

For most patients with advanced cancers, the end is extremely painful whether the disease is the killer or the treatment. The experimental trials we offer prolong survival by a few months at best, at the cost of incalculable physical and financial toxicities.

Did Andrew ever ask to be told his chances of survival? Did he and his family even want to know?

Was honesty a choice?

Let us, with deep humility, admit that, alas, we failed Andrew Slootsky.

ⓢ

❧ KAT ❧

Andrusha. You were the most incredible baby brother I could have ever wished for—I only would have wished for so many more years. But I'm truly lucky to have been your big sister for twenty-three years.

I can't possibly have a favorite memory—they will all be my favorite.

Your laugh will be one of the hardest things to live without. Its evolution over the years. As a baby, you had this old-man laugh, like Santa: "Ho ho ho." It would keep reinventing itself throughout the years; it always got younger and younger. I would love your laugh so much that I'd tickle you to tears. And you'd warn me that people could die from laughter, and I wouldn't believe you. But I guess in the most beautiful way, you were right. On your last day in the hospital, the room was full of laughter—mostly you making all of us laugh. That's why I'm trying my hardest to just keep laughing and smiling these past few days—I keep telling everyone who starts crying that we should laugh instead. It's what you'd have wanted us to do.

You were so good at living. You really had it down without any second thoughts. So now everything I do, I'm going to try to do it better, the way you would have. You always believed in what you put your mind to, and that's why everything you did was so beautiful and effortless. It just came to you so easily because you cared about it so deeply. You wanted to learn to play something from *Amélie* or Grizzly Bear or Metric on the piano, and you'd do it. You'd make incredible mixtapes. You made hilarious movies with friends just for fun as a kid, then you'd end up making thought-provoking beautiful films for school. You wanted to live in Paris and learn French—you made it all happen. And we were all so proud of you. In your final days, you'd speak French with some of the hospital staff who found out that you were trilingual, and it was so beautiful to hear you speak and connect with everyone so effortlessly.

I want to share with everyone what outfits you have with you in whatever Berghain heaven you are partying in at the moment: Andrew is wearing his black Dries blazer with the flower patch at the label, Marni white button-down, black jeans, and his new Pradas he got in LA a few months ago. He has his Saint Laurent sunnies, a blue hat that Carol gave him just a few days ago that says DOING THINGS. He wanted to point to it when people asked what he was up to. It was hard to pick a single outfit for Andrew, so I decided he needed to have a spare. So he also has his moss-green wool suit babushka got him a few months ago, with a Junya Watanabe–print button-down tee we got together at Tokio 7.

Andrush, I hope you are happy with these two outfits. All your clothing is amazing, but I got to pick this time, and these were my favorites.

I'll love you forever.

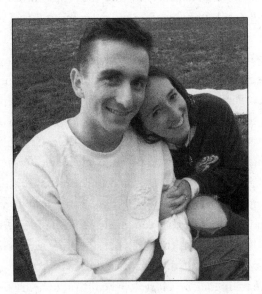

| # HARVEY

Death Stared Him in the Face, and He Stared Right Back

The Moving Finger writes; and, having writ,
Moves on: nor all your Piety nor Wit
Shall lure it back to cancel half a line,
Nor all your Tears wash out a Word of it.

—OMAR KHAYYAM

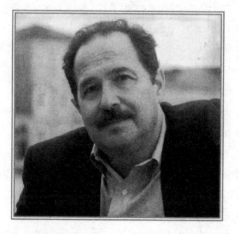

HARVEY DIED ON MAY 19, 2002, AT 3:20 P.M. THE CAUSE OF death was follicular lymphoma / chronic lymphocytic leukemia. Death had already approached him once: at the age of thirty-four, he was diagnosed with his first cancer. After years of living under the shadow of a relapse, when he was over the fear, death loomed again. Harvey faced both his cancers with courage, remaining astonishingly calm and at peace even as he lay dying.

Harvey became impatient with "holy men" when they appeared to counsel him during his frequent hospitalizations, especially in the last eighteen months, because he drew no consolation from visions of an afterlife. I saw him waver only once.

In 1996, our daughter, Sheherzad, developed a high fever and a severe asthmatic attack at the age of two and a half. Harvey's anxiety was palpable. After hours of our taking turns in the emergency room, rocking and carrying her while her little body was connected to the nebulizer, she finally dozed off. Harvey asked me to step outside. In the silence of a hot, still Chicago night, he said in a tormented voice, "If something happens to her, I am going to kill myself. If there is even a remote chance that those fundamentalists are right and there is a life after death, I don't want the little one to be alone."

For himself, Harvey faced and accepted the truth. When I would become upset by the intensely painful nature of his illness, he was always calm and matter-of-fact. "It's the luck of the draw, Az. Don't distress yourself over it for a second." It was an acceptance of the human condition with almost inhuman composure. "We are all tested. But it is never in the way we prefer, nor at the time we expect."

W. B. Yeats was puzzled by the question: "The intellect of man is forced to choose / Perfection of the life, or of work." Fortunately for Harvey, it was never a question of either-or. For him, work was life and life was work. The two were inseparable. Once, toward the end, when I asked him to work less and maybe do other things that he did not have the time for before, his response was that such an act would make a mockery of everything he had stood for and had done until that point in his life. Work was his deepest passion outside of the family. Three days before he died, Harvey had a lab meeting at home with more than twenty people in attendance, and he went over each individual's scientific project with his signature boyish enthusiasm. Even as he clearly saw his own end approach, Harvey was hopeful that a better future awaits other unfortunate cancer victims through rigorous research.

It all started on a gorgeous Chicago morning in February 1998. We had just returned from Hawaii. With his newly acquired tan after a week of reading and relaxing on the beach, playing with four-year-old Sheherzad in the water, Harvey looked the best I had seen him in a long time. Several months prior, he had suddenly become conscious of a few extra pounds he had put on, and he had placed himself on a strict diet. His running partner, Henry Black, a fellow New Yorker and one of Harvey's best friends, was forced into longer and more frequent jogs by the water on Lakeshore Drive. Harvey was lifting weights in the gym in our building on Fullerton Avenue, and so pleased was he with the results that he asked me to go shopping with him for new, better-fitting clothes. I was pleasantly surprised. Normally, I would have to nag him for weeks before he agreed to go within a mile's radius of a mall. That morning, however, Harvey did not come out of his study for a long time. Sheherzad was getting late for her kindergarten class, just down the road from us. Harvey loved to walk in the mornings with her and often left work in the afternoon for a couple of hours to bring her home and play with her. Finally, I went searching for him. He was sitting at his desk, his feet propped up, looking out the glass windows that lined two walls in his study.

Words are not necessary when you have been with someone for almost twenty years; his body spoke volumes. My heart missed a beat.

"Are your children okay?" I asked. Harvey was extremely close to Sarah, Mark, and Vanessa, his three grown children from a previous marriage.

"Yes, and so are my parents," he said, anticipating my next concern.

"Then what's wrong?"

In a hundred years, I would not have suspected what he said next: "I have an enlarged lymph node in my neck."

After confirming that there was indeed a small, hard presence in the left anterior cervical area, I said, more to reassure myself than him, "It's probably an infection you picked up in Hawaii."

"No," he said. "It has grown slowly over the past couple of months. I can't ignore it anymore."

Ever since he had survived one cancer, Harvey had developed a fatalistic streak, convinced he would die young. He detected a tiny growth on his arm a few years before, a self-diagnosed malignant sarcoma, and immediately began putting his business in order, preparing for a swift end. When I took him to the dermatologist, who essentially told him what I had been saying—that it was a sebaceous cyst—Harvey wanted to know how long it had been since the dermatologist had finished his training. I regularly made fun of Mr. Hypochondriac. But this node, it was a different story. It didn't feel right to me, even to touch.

I called our internist at Rush University and made an appointment to see him later that afternoon. All of us agreed that in the absence of any infection, instead of a course of antibiotics and another few weeks of anxious watching and waiting, we should just take the lymph node out and be done with it. For the first time, I saw Harvey demur. It was as if he did not want to know. Convinced he was fretting over nothing, I insisted on urgent action. He finally agreed when I said he was going to make my life miserable until we knew. Still, he went into the OR reluctantly. I scrubbed and went in with him on March 4, 1998. As soon as the neck was sliced open, I knew for certain that it was not an infection. Behind the superficial growth was a chain of pea-sized lymph nodes dotting the lymphatics with irregular regularity, up and down the neck, creeping their way behind the supraclavicular area and disappearing into the chest. The surgeon, Dr. William Panje, looked concerned but maintained a stoic silence. He carefully dissected out the largest node and closed the wound with aseptic efficiency.

I sat with Harvey in the recovery room. As I called the babysitter to make sure Sheherzad was picked up from school, a nurse came over and whispered that I was wanted on the phone. It was Jerry Loew, the best hematopathologist at Rush, and by now a dear friend. "Azra, I think you should come look at this."

A while later, he ushered me into the frozen-section lab. One look at the slide in Jerry's double-headed microscope evaporated any hopeful delusions that it was an infection. There were sheets of monotonous, small, round lymphocytes, looking deceptively innocent but announcing their malignant nature by their sheer number, constricting sinuses, distorting the nodal architecture, effacing crowded follicles. Jerry looked over the microscope. "I'm sorry. Not sure yet about the exact type, but it does not look good. Lymphoma. Let us wait for the permanent sections."

Standing alone in the sanitized hallway of the pathology lab, unconsciously registering the sharp, pungent smell of formalin, I made two calls. First, to Steve Rosen, the best oncologist I knew in Chicago, and one of our closest friends. He was the director of the Northwestern University Cancer Center. The second call was to my sister Atiya in Columbia, Maryland. She is a superbly trained pediatric oncologist with the reputation of being the best general clinician in the Raza family. "I think Harvey has c—" I could not pronounce the *c*-word. That choked-up feeling I experienced in the first few lonely minutes of Harvey's initial diagnosis would stay with me, off and on, for the next four and a half years. Both wanted to come over immediately. I stopped Atiya. Steve dropped everything he was doing and was by my side within half an hour. I did not want to tell Harvey what we suspected just yet on the off chance that the permanent biopsy sections, due out in a week, would show that this was reactive hyperplasia after all. Harvey did not ask. Steve agreed with me, but he came in to say hello to Harvey anyway. "I'm not here for you. Azra was nervous, so I came over to hold her hand," he said, putting his arm around me.

Harvey relaxed over the next few days. Removal of the physical lump brought a measure of psychic relief. A cloud lifted. No more obsessive fingering of the neck, gauging the size of the node, its shape, level of tenderness. I was anxious, but Harvey looked so good that I allowed myself to slip into a hopeful fog. Anyway, there was not much else to do but wait.

A week passed by, and it was time for the appointment with the internist, who would give us the final pathology report. If Harvey was anxious, he did not show it. Instead, he did his best to make me relax.

Of course, the one thing we are trained as doctors to avoid at all costs had to happen to a doctor who is suddenly a patient. Harvey found out his diagnosis of cancer in the worst possible manner. In the corridor. On our way to the internist's office, we exited the elevator, coming face-to-face with the chief of pathology, who, assuming that of course we already knew, blurted out, "Harvey, I am so sorry about your lymphoma. Please know we are here to help you in any way possible." He refused to see the internist after that. We returned to Harvey's office and called Jerry Loew. Jerry confirmed the diagnosis. It was a chronic lymphocytic leukemia, follicular lymphoma. After I hung up, Harvey said, "Let's go for a drive." We sat in the car by Lake Michigan for a long time, silently holding hands. We were both oncologists. We knew pretty much what was coming. He finally spoke. "This I can take. I'm glad it's me and not you or Sheherzad. That I could not handle."

∽

Even in our sleep, pain which cannot forget
falls drop by drop upon the heart
until, in our own despair, against our will,
comes wisdom through the awful grace of God.

—AESCHYLUS

After Harvey was diagnosed with cancer, we prepared ourselves for all sorts of eventualities, but even we were taken aback by the unexpected intensity and recurrent nature of the pain, appearing in wholly unpredictable places and forms. Masquerading as arthritis one day and a neuralgia the next, it showed up as venous thrombosis, assaulted nerves, skin and bones, digits and muscles, mucous membranes, glands, organs, and limbs in a series of reckless tsunamis. No tissue was spared. These were all manifestations of the collateral damage resulting from a twisted, misguided tug-of-war between the body's confused immune system and the lymphoma, and all were accompanied by intense pain.

After several months of scorching and blistering its way through practically a quarter of Harvey's visible joints in a sequential, syncretic, episodic wrecking storm, the lymphoma finally seemed to reach a pact of coexistence with the immune system in his ravaged body. Harvey started thalidomide, and four weeks later, the symptoms had vanished as suddenly as they had appeared. The agonizing combat seemed spent. By that time, Harvey had lost more than twenty pounds in the short space of three months. The skin on his arms, gorgeously toned just months earlier, sagged. He looked gaunt, emaciated. An unhealthy pallor covered his entire body. Cancer became visible, announcing its residence through the unmistakable wasting, a sudden and dramatic loss of fat and muscles. His exterior began to reflect the deadly mayhem of the unstable interior. He felt drained as never before.

> *After great pain, a formal feeling comes—*
> *The Nerves sit ceremonious, like Tombs—*
> *The stiff Heart questions was it He, that bore,*
> *And Yesterday, or Centuries before?*

> —Emily Dickinson

It took him months to regain a fraction of his old vigor and humor, but we both knew the calm was temporary. He was sitting on a time bomb. We said little about the subject, but both of us were helplessly suspended in a state of harrowing apprehension, not knowing when and how the lymphoma would rear its ugly head, what organ was the next target of its indiscriminating malice.

In June 2000, I went to Atlanta for a four-day medical conference. On the third morning, I made my presentation. Shortly thereafter, I received a call from our program's administrative executive and beloved friend, Lakshmi. She sounded grim.

"Dr. Raza, no need to worry, but now that your talk is done, perhaps you can return earlier? No, no, Sheherzad is fine, and it is nothing serious with Dr. Preisler, but he is developing a rash and not feeling great."

I flew back the same afternoon, landing in Chicago around 6:30 p.m. Heading home from O'Hare, I stopped to order takeout from Maggiano's, Harvey's favorite Italian restaurant in the city. Armed with breaded veal cutlet and his favorite pasta, I walked in to find Harvey lying in the family room watching *The Sopranos*. Breathing a sigh of relief, I walked over and was horrified to see that half of his face was covered with red, papular lesions, some of which were already evolving into vesicles and bullae.

"Where else do you have the rash?" I asked.

He stuck his tongue out. This is one time when I almost fainted. Half the tongue was studded with the angriest-looking raised pustular rash; some lesions weeping and oozing pale, thick secretions, others bleeding. The distribution of the rash—its restriction to one side of the face and tongue—left no doubt that this was herpes zoster or shingles, one of the most painful conditions imaginable. Even I had never seen shingles of the tongue before. Harvey's equanimity in the face of such punishing displays of cancer's malevolence was decidedly saintly. He looked at the Maggiano's carryout bag and managed a smile. "Thanks, Az. Guess I will be giving this a miss tonight. I know you will want Pakistani food after being away for three days. Better send this down to the doorman. Tony loves Maggiano's."

Harvey had started antiviral therapy two days prior, but at that point, things seemed to be worsening instead of improving. The pain and discomfort was frightful. The next morning brought another terrifying development. It was Sunday. I had barely slept and finally, giving up at 4:00 a.m., had come out to do some work on my laptop in the family room. Around 6:30 a.m., Harvey emerged from the bedroom. He did not look like Harvey. He had developed facial paralysis. The asymmetry in those early hours of onset was dramatic. One half of his face drooped, sagging helplessly. He could not completely close his mouth, and saliva dripped from the side. The paralyzed cheek flapped, out of sync, as he tried to speak. The facial lesions were coalescing, the tongue simply unbearable to look at. This man, who was strikingly handsome, slumped into the chair, unable to blink, smarting from itching in the dried-up, perpetually open paralyzed eye, slurring his speech, drooling, twitching, wincing as the lacerating pain sliced and throbbed its way through his palate and tongue, singed his ears, scorched his breath. Master of supreme meiosis that he was, Harvey managed a single sentence. "I guess I'm a mess."

> *They say, the tongues of dying men*
> *Enforce attention, like deep harmony;*
> *Where words are scarce, they're seldom spent in vain;*
> *For they breathe truth, that breathe their words in pain.*
>
> —SHAKESPEARE, *RICHARD II*, ACT 2, SCENE 1

As the day wore on, I obsessively inspected Harvey's torso and limbs, and by evening, I had located a few new lesions on his back. He now had disseminated shingles, something seen in individuals with a compromised, suppressed, weakened, malfunctioning immune system. It can be deadly. I panicked and called up Harvey's oncologist, our good friend Steve Rosen. We agreed that Harvey should be admitted. Harvey refused. Steve came over to the house, reviewed the long list of medications, added some, subtracted a few, and held my hand. By the time he left, I felt reassured, thanks to his calm and confident bedside manner. The next morning brought a fresh crop of lesions to various areas of Harvey's body, but as I decompensated, Harvey maintained his calm. Days progressed at an agonizingly slow pace into weeks. Round-the-clock pain medications helped, and eventually, he was able to tolerate a semiliquid diet. He could not shave from that point on. The facial lesions continued to seep, which made him very uncomfortable. Over the ensuing weeks, he gradually improved, but until he died almost two years later, the facial asymmetry remained a particularly disagreeable, disfiguring, visible reminder of cancer's vengeful ferocity.

If one is to get cancer, a diagnosis of lymphoma usually brings a modicum of relief since it is treatable with a decent chance of cure. In fact, Harvey did quite well for a while. In June 1998, after treatment with Rituxan, we harvested stem cells from his blood to save, in case we decided on an autologous transplant at some point. I think it was more for our psychological benefit than of any practical value, but the transplant team went along with our request. By 1999, things started going downhill quite rapidly. He developed deep-vein thrombosis, asthma, the migratory polyarthritis, night sweats, infiltration of subcutaneous tissues with the lymphoma cells. I was particularly shocked by the en masse migration of lymphoma cells from one compartment to another, waking up one morning to find his spleen had enlarged and another to discover lumps in the neck and armpits.

He started thalidomide and responded, but after a few months, he developed extremely uncomfortable and painful symptoms of peripheral neuropathy. He was switched to Revlimid, and he experienced much relief for a while, but then that drug proved quite toxic for the marrow. When his platelet count dipped into the teens, we had to abandon this approach. He was eventually started on chemotherapy. I don't know how much effect all these treatments had on the lymphoma, but they essentially destroyed Harvey's immune system. He became exceedingly prone to repeated infections, landing him in the hospital frequently. Were he alive today, Harvey could have benefited from the drug ibrutinib, which is proving to be fantastically successful in several types of lymphoid cancers.

It is still uncertain whether the lymphoma came first and affected the immune system or a defect in the immune system enabled the lymphoma to appear. Harvey suspected the latter because he had already suffered from testicular cancer before and the lymphoma was a second primary cancer, rather than a recurrence or derivative of the first. And then, of course, there is always the question of the endless treatments he received, which played havoc with the immune system in unknown, destructive, suppressive ways. Whatever the case, the failure of his immune system caused sepsis after sepsis until the treating physicians sat me and his adult children down and advised hospice care, gently suggesting that I not rush him to the ER when his next infection appeared. We were to let nature take its course now. Harvey had been suffering from a tuberculous meningitis at that point and unable to make an informed decision by himself.

It was a relief to bring him home, both for him and for all of us. He recovered from the meningitis eventually, regained his full intellectual vigor, and, while on hospice care at home, conducted regular lab meetings with his scientific colleagues. I sent Mark, Harvey's son, to fetch Harvey's parents from Florida. Lenny and Estelle, both in their nineties, stayed by Harvey's side the entire time he was on hospice care at home, providing their love and care until the last moments of his life. One of the hardest things for me in those days was to face his mother. I always took a few moments to compose myself before I emerged from our room, because I knew how anxiously Estelle would scrutinize my face, scan my body language. Harvey was their pride and joy.

∽∾

HOW MANY OMARS AND ANDREWS WILL IT TAKE?

Why did we only diagnose Harvey when his lymphoma was widespread throughout the body? Or Omar when his sarcoma was already spilling cells into blood vessels, invading surrounding muscles, settling in lungs and limbs, or Andrew's tumor only when it had grown to a nine-centimeter mass, threatening to choke the spinal cord, making him quadriplegic within days of the initial symptoms? Why are we not doing more to detect the earliest sign of cancer instead of chasing after the last cell with draconian treatment options? This leads to the question of why would anyone be looking for cancer in a twenty-two- or a thirty-eight-year-old man? Of course, no one is immune to cancer at any age. Every individual has to be monitored for it on a regular basis. The science and technology must be developed to make this happen. Cancer must be prevented at a precancer level. I am not the only one saying this.

It is universally acknowledged that early detection is the key to the cancer problem. This is why screening procedures were set into motion decades ago and early detection has reduced mortality by at least 25 percent. Now we need to trace our way to even an earlier detection of cancer cells, prior to their appearance on scans. So why is it that only 5.7 percent of the total budget of the National Cancer Institute is allocated toward this critical area of research? Why is 70 percent of the budget funding research that concentrates on advanced malignancies conducted on animals and tissue culture cells that will lead to clinical trials with a failure rate of practically 90 percent? Why isn't it just the opposite, with the majority of support going to detect cancer at its inception?

How many Omars, how many Andrews, will it take?

What would it have taken to cure Harvey? There are many cancers curable by surgery, chemotherapy, radiation therapy, and stem cell transplants. Which cancers are curable hasn't changed much in recent years. Most advances in cancer treatment have been incremental and have focused largely on better identification of the patients who are likely to benefit from each. Of the cancers resistant to these approaches, little progress has occurred in the past five decades. Targeted therapies and individualized precision medicine approaches benefit a small percentage of patients by adding a few months to their survival while costing enormous physical and financial burdens. Immune therapies have been in trials since 1910 in various forms and sporadically help subsets of patients.

I have already argued that a major part of the problem is the reliance on unreliable preclinical testing platforms and animals for preclinical research. I am not against the use of animal models across the board. In biologic research using these same models, great progress has occurred in understanding cancer at the molecular level. Most of these advances have occurred through careful study of tissue culture cell lines and animal models, be they the fruit fly, zebra fish, worms, rodents, or apes. But they have been useless as preclinical drug-development platforms.

If we continue in the same direction, spending precious resources to improve the same models, it will take us another few hundred years to arrive at a meaningful solution for cancer.

Contrast the putative scientific gold standard of a reproducible animal model with the known fact that every patient's cancer is a unique disease, and within each patient, cancer cells that settle in different sites are unique. When a malignant cell divides into two, it can produce daughter cells with the same or radically different characteristics because during the process of DNA replication, fresh copying errors constantly occur. Even if two cancer cells have identical genetics, much like identical twins, their behavior can differ depending on genes expressed or silenced according to the demands of a thousand variables, such as the microenvironment where they land, the blood supply available to them, and the local reaction of immune cells. The resulting expansive variety of tumor cells that exist within tumors are unique within unique sites of the body. Multiply this complexity further by adding the host's immune response to each new clone and you get a confounding, perplexing, impenetrable situation in perpetual flux.

Disease complexity is not restricted to cancer. Jon Cohen reported in *Science* on the failure of an anti-inflammatory antibody in having any benefit for human HIV after a study demonstrated cures in monkeys intentionally infected with the simian form of the AIDS virus. Attempts by an independent team to replicate the results in a second set of diseased primates also failed. The conclusion by the head of the National Institute of Allergy and Infectious Diseases, and a coauthor on the study, was that the original monkey results "might be a fluke." While such an unusually candid admission is laudable, the question I have relates to the path forward. What steps has the agency taken to shut down animal studies of this nature susceptible to unpredictable happenchance? Despite these findings, why are we continuing to invest hundreds of millions of dollars into animal studies with the delusion that the next one will provide clinical guidance for humans? Why are we, the public, not demanding more accountability about the way our resources are being allocated? Who are the beneficiaries of these resources, and why? The patients certainly are not.

The ultimate aim of all cancer research is to find better therapies, yet the means we have employed for the study of human tumors are grossly inadequate, especially the drug-testing platforms. We remove a few cancer cells extracted from a minute sliver of the tumor, plate them in dishes or inject them in mice, and expect them to recapitulate the vast heterogeneity of the evolving, expanding, transforming, invading, regressing, recovering, transmuting population of malignant cells in vivo. Whatever grows out cannot be representative of even that small sliver because upon removal from their normal habitat, cells change characteristics as they adapt to new environments. There is more than ample evidence to show that cell lines growing in vitro resemble each other more than the tissue of origin (liver, lung, pancreas) from which they were derived. They manifest a uniform "transcriptomic drift" in that the majority of genes expressed by all cell lines are ones needed for survival ex vivo. How can scientists, who demand great precision in everything they do, simply turn their eyes away from such fundamental fallacies?

So what is the solution? The first step is to descend from our high horses and humbly admit that cancer is far too complex a problem to be solved with the simplistic preclinical testing platforms we have devised to develop therapies. Little has happened in the past fifty years, and little will happen in another fifty if we insist on the same old same old. The only way to deal with the cancer problem in the fastest, cheapest, and, above all, most universally applicable and compassionate way is to shift our focus away from exclusively developing treatments for end-stage disease and concentrate on diagnosing cancer at its inception and developing the science to prevent its further expansion. From chasing after the last cell to identifying the footprints of the first.

⚭

BY THE TIME of diagnosis, one centimeter of the tumor contains roughly three billion cells. This is far too many cells needing elimination. A millimeter of tumor carries three million cells, and a 0.1 millimeter tumor approximately three hundred thousand malignant cells. The future lies in developing technologies to detect the presence of very few cancer cells through telltale footprints. What are these footprints?

The science of surrogate marker detection is in its infancy. Cancer cells die at a rapid rate, jettisoning revelatory biologic markers. Pieces of DNA, RNA, and proteins shed in a drop of blood, traces of cancer, can be detected as molecules exhaled in the breath. Or through recording changes in magnetic fields caused by the presence of very few cancer cells, or using antibodies that bind and reveal femtomoles of proteins (a billionth of a millionth mole, or very minute fractions of a gram).

As seen repeatedly so far, a major problem with cancer is its silent, surreptitious nature. Tumors can replace a large portion of the organ in which they are growing without causing any symptoms. It is exactly what happened in the case of Suketu Mehta, Omar, and Andrew. Suketu lucked out by being diagnosed with lung cancer serendipitously, but by the time cancer in the other two was detected, the game was already over. I had been working with deadly cases of AML for many years until I realized the hopelessness of chasing after so devious an enemy and turned my focus to early detection. I have been studying preleukemia for this purpose for thirty years, but since MDS can also kill with the vengeance of AML without ever becoming AML, I have also been committed to screening normal, seemingly healthy individuals for the earliest sign of MDS, AML, or cancer in general.

Efforts to diagnose cancer early are as old as the declaration of war on cancer. Unfortunately, population-based, conventional screening programs costing astronomical sums of money have not yielded the dramatic success that was expected. Moreover, the assumption that early detection and therapeutic intervention would lead to cures has also been challenged through cautionary tales associated with these attempts.

For one thing, screening can result in overdiagnosis and overtreatment, and this could harm patients and be an added financial burden on the health care system. Cancer begins in a single cell, but given the variability in growth rates, it can take decades to become clinically apparent, one study suggesting that the journey for breast cancer could be starting in utero. With the time line spreading over decades for some common tumors, the contention that finding a tumor and eliminating it urgently at some point in its natural history is the only way to cure it is clearly misplaced. It is therefore no surprise that many cancers detected early—say, through imaging or tumor-specific antigen tests— have proved to be of nonlethal varieties that would have responded to treatment even if detected at a later stage once they became clinically apparent.

Of the aggressive cancers detected early, the news was also less than encouraging: the majority had already disseminated anyway, offering no advantage for early diagnosis. In breast cancer, for example, early detection of tumors with favorable molecular signatures was not helpful because the tumors would have grown so slowly as to be inconsequential within the life span of the patient, and even if they progressed to a clinically detectable state, they would be amenable to standard available treatments. Early detection of more aggressive breast cancer was not helpful because by the time the tumor appeared on a mammogram, it had already spread and was incurable. A review of multiple large population-based studies from several European countries examining the role of mammography as a screening tool led to a depressing conclusion by P. Autier and M. Boniol: "The epidemiological data point to a marginal contribution of mammography screening in the decline in breast cancer mortality. Moreover, the more effective the treatments, the less favourable are the harm-benefit balance of screening mammography. New, effective methods for breast screening are needed, as well as research on risk-based screening strategies." The US Preventive Services Task Force recommends biennial screening mammography for women aged fifty through seventy-four, the current evidence being insufficient to assess the benefits and harms of screening mammography in the other age groups.

As far as affecting mortality of prostate cancer, a meta-analysis of multiple studies also failed to show substantial improvement through PSA screening, D. Ilic and colleagues concluding that "at best, screening for prostate cancer leads to a small reduction in disease-specific mortality over 10 years but does not affect overall mortality. Clinicians and patients considering PSA based screening need to weigh these benefits against the potential short and long term harms of screening, including complications from biopsies and subsequent treatment, as well as the risk of over-diagnosis and overtreatment."

If there is one situation where early detection markers are urgently needed, it is ovarian cancer; notorious for being a killer of fourteen thousand women annually in the United States, the disease is generally diagnosed when it is already beyond the grasp of curative therapies. Cancer antigen 125 (CA-125) produced by as many as 80 percent of epithelial ovarian cancers, detectable in the blood with a simple test, was hailed as a welcome advance. Screening studies, however, revealed fundamental problems with the test, calling its use as a screening tool into question. First, the amount produced by early, small tumors is undetectable in the blood, and by the time blood levels increase, the tumor is already far advanced. Its levels seem related more to the tumor burden since 90 percent of women with stage II ovarian cancer tested positive as opposed to only one-third to one-half with stage I disease. Second, CA-125 is not always a harbinger of malignancy, present in rare cases of benign, inflammatory situations. This may be why a Swedish study found only 6 cases of ovarian cancer (with 2 out of the 6 at the targeted early treatable stage) from 175 exploratory surgeries following random screening of 5,500 women. CA-125 measurement is more suited to monitoring the efficacy of a given treatment in established cases of cancer since diminishing levels relate to regressing tumor burden. Clifton Leaf, in his excellent book *The Truth in Small Doses,* concludes about CA-125: "The point of diagnostic screening is to alter the outlook for many individuals while keeping the cost of unnecessary intervention low. This biomarker, as with hundreds of other well-touted candidates, managed neither."

Based on minor successes compared to the enormous investment of resources since 1980 in population-based, conventional screening measures, Hans-Olov Adami and colleagues have called for an end to such studies altogether since "population-based early detection screening for cancer has not fulfilled our expectations, and indeed induced considerable harm to a large population of healthy individuals." They propose saving early detection screening measures for populations at high risk of developing cancer, either because of genetic susceptibility or through lifestyle risks and exposures.

On the other hand, screening has helped save lives of colorectal cancer patients. These cancers start out as benign adenomas and progress in a stepwise manner from stage I through IV so that early detection is helpful. Similarly, screening for cervical cancer, which also progresses through distinct stages from dysplasia to stages I through IV, worked dramatically, as deaths from cervical cancer declined substantially when the Pap test became common practice. Despite the many pitfalls in screening measures, the 25 percent decrease in overall cancer mortality between 1990 and 2015 is largely due to high-quality screening for breast (down by 39 percent) and colorectal cancers (down by 47 percent in men and 44 percent in women). Of note, most of this screening is preventive screening and not early detection of an established, bona fide cancer.

To summarize, early detection screening tools available thus far are helpful in preventing cancers that evolve in well-defined stages but fail to benefit cancers of unpredictable potency. The latter would include thyroid, prostate, and some breast cancers, where size may not correspond directly to metastatic potential—a small tumor potentially capable of shedding cells early in its development, while larger ones may follow a less aggressive natural course. The challenge is how to improve detection of precancers through minimally invasive tests before they become cancer.

Improved cancer treatments have helped only a fraction of the 1.7 million patients diagnosed annually, resulting in 600,000 deaths in the United States. Through early detection and preventive measures, we can save the lives of 120 million, one-third of the population slated to get cancer in their lifetime.

⟨∞⟩

IMAGINE A MACHINE that automatically images your entire body while you are in your morning shower. Or a smart bra that has two hundred tiny biosensors built in to monitor micro-alterations in temperature and texture; worn for an hour a week, it generates sufficient data on an accompanying app to show distortions created by the presence of very few cancer cells. Or taking a pill whose contents are absorbed preferentially by cancer cells, excreted in the urine, and detected by a Fit Loo. Or receiving a cocktail of reporter genes whose protein products can be imaged with handheld devices to pinpoint cancer cells anywhere in the body. How about yelling at a cancer using ultrasound, compelling it to reveal its presence and its lethal potential as the tumor is forced to shed more markers into the blood when hit by waves at the right frequency? Or exhale deeply into a device that accurately recognizes the earliest footprints of cancer. Or simply prick your finger periodically to provide a drop of blood to a magneto-nano-sensor that identifies surrogate markers of malignancy instantly.

The above are not scenes from *Fantastic Voyage*. These are real-life technologies in various stages of development today, heralding the dawn of a new era in cancer research. Sanjiv Sam Gambhir at the Canary Center at Stanford University is at the forefront of this revolution in early detection of cancer from blood, urine, stool, saliva, breath, and tears, using a host of genetic, sonic, and imaging methods. The emergence of these groundbreaking technologies is a direct result of collaboration between experts coming from many disciplines— geneticists, biomedical engineers, radiologists, oncologists, molecular biologists, nanotechnologists, AI experts, computer scientists, and bio-informatics wizards. Even in sports, teamwork and cooperation win the day, so why not in cancer?

Here is one scenario for the future. Everyone from birth to death is regularly screened for the first appearance of cancer cells in the body. Once detected, protein markers would be identified, providing a zip code for the cancer cells. A tube of blood from the individual would be obtained, and T cells would be isolated, activated, and armed with the address for the cancer based upon the unique protein bar code and the RNA signature it expressed. These CAR-Ts can be injected back into the individual to seek out and kill every cell with that address. None of the toxic effects seen with the present CAR-T therapies would be an issue because the tumor mass would be minuscule compared to what we target now. Eventually, we should not even have to draw blood for screening. Rather, every infant would be fitted with an implantable tiny device at birth that would constantly monitor for such a mishap, send signals in a timely manner so that confirmation, validation, and treatment could swiftly follow. The ideal is to find every cancer at the precancerous stage through perturbations in disease-prone networks detected via dynamic monitoring by implanted devices. Of course, this is the dream scenario and far from current practices. There are a thousand slips betwixt this cup and lip, but we will never get there if we don't start. Besides, I have great faith in the ability of humans to step up and innovate rapidly as long as they have a goal and are financially incentivized to do so. The goal now should be spelled out in no uncertain terms. We are to stop developing minimally effective therapies and go for nothing less than a humane cure that will be applicable globally. The best cure will be prevention.

To detect the first cancer cell's footprints, a map of early biologic markers of cancer has to be constructed. This is what our resources should be targeting. Thankfully, the race has already begun. We will all benefit from cooperation at the deepest level. Heed the advice of an anonymous sage who said, "If you want to be incrementally better: be competitive. If you want to be exponentially better: be cooperative."

ᘐᘗᘖ

For the life of a creature is in the blood.

—LEVITICUS 17:11

It began at the junction of the mother and child: the placenta. The question was whether congenital diseases in a growing fetus were detectable by seeking their footprints in the mother's blood instead of the amniotic fluid. The embryo is known to exfoliate cells that cross the placenta and enter the mother's bloodstream, but capturing and examining these fetal cells for detailed molecular analysis proved to be a challenge because they were so few. The quantity issue was resolved when fetal DNA, known as cell-free fetal, or cff-DNA, was found circulating in the maternal blood during pregnancy. Shed by the placenta in large enough quantities, cff-DNA was promptly utilized for noninvasive prenatal screening (NIPS) of congenital diseases in the developing fetus. NIPS, using a few cubic centimeters of blood drawn from the mother, has proved to be the most sensitive method for prenatal diagnosis of Down syndrome.

Analysis of cff-DNA has displaced amniocentesis. Can similar techniques be developed whereby surrogate markers released into the blood by a growing tumor are detected? This would provide not just early cancer diagnosis but also save the patient from undergoing an invasive biopsy procedure. In healthy individuals, cell-free DNA, or cf-DNA, is found in the blood but in very tiny amounts. In cancer patients, however, circulating tumor DNA, or ct-DNA, derived from dying cancer cells, is detectable in higher quantities even in early stages of tumor formation because immune cells fail to clear it efficiently from the blood. This ct-DNA can be subjected to molecular profiling and serve as the noninvasive "liquid biopsy" comparable to NIPS. Much effort has been devoted to developing liquid biopsies that can noninvasively identify the presence of genetic material from cancer cells in the blood or molecular markers in urine or saliva to diagnose cancer at its inception or even precancerous lesions. What are these surreptitious, clandestine, cloaked, surrogate markers?

One is the mutated DNA discarded by dying malignant cells. The second is transcripts of messenger RNA transmitting instructions for abnormal protein synthesis or the proteins themselves. All three can serve as biomarkers for malignancy, all three can be detected in the blood. While germ line DNA is exactly the same in all cells of an organism, the transcriptome and proteome differ depending upon cell lineage. The transcriptome and proteome of a white blood cell would be different from that of a brain cell, whereas DNA in both would be the same. Early signs of a cancerous growth could be traced through mutations in the DNA or abnormal expression of sets of RNA and proteins. Ideally, a measure of all three will be combined in the future for a truly comprehensive picture using no more than a single drop of blood, urine, or saliva. The population-based screening trials to establish the clinical relevance of these approaches would require massive cooperation between academia, institutions, industry, and oncologists.

There is much exciting work going on in the area of detecting the first rather than the last cancer cell. Large-scale, population-based studies are being conducted by several commercial entities to test the accuracy and clinical utility of their methods of screening, and the results are regularly posted in the public domain. It is the responsibility of government institutions to provide a coordinated, collaborative approach designed to systematically study the common deadly human tumors and provide a road map for progress in a timely fashion. In the following sections, we will briefly look at some of the ongoing attempts in this area.

MicroRNAs are small regulatory RNAs that don't code for proteins. They are frequently dysregulated in cancer, and because they are present in human plasma in a remarkably stable form, they can provide robust information on otherwise unrecognized malignancies. A comprehensive database showing unique profiles important for different types of cancers remains to be assembled, but serious research is already under way at multiple levels in this area. Using digital microfluidics—a decentralized, automated, and affordable platform called a *lab on a chip* that requires only one drop of blood to do its work—microRNA diagnostic signatures of various common cancers, such as lung, ovarian, and gastric tumors, are being generated. At present, only 1 percent of endoscopies yield a diagnosis of cancer. A full 99 percent are performed in vain. With this blood test, only a selected few would need to undergo the invasive procedure, resulting in tremendous cost savings also. A panel of eight microRNAs demonstrated robust diagnostic accuracy in not only tissue specimens but also in the plasma specimens from stage I ovarian cancer patients. Similarly, microRNA signatures serving as diagnostic, prognostic, and predictive biomarkers for early breast cancer are being formalized. MicroRNA signatures for lung cancers exist. Preoperative plasma levels of four microRNAs (specifically, miR-29a, 200b, 203, and 31) can serve as potential prognostic biomarkers in colorectal cancers, and detection of miR-31, 141, and 16 levels in the plasma herald recurrence during colorectal cancer surveillance. The microRNA field is practically in its infancy but will receive the attention of researchers if the funding agencies make it their priority.

Detection of circulating tumor-derived DNA (ct-DNA) from the blood could provide a safe and reliable platform for early detection of cancer. Former vice president Biden's Cancer Moonshot initiative is undertaking the Blood Profiling Atlas in Cancer project, which will collect data on cancer signals in the blood. Because ct-DNA carries the somatic alterations of the tumor, it is a more reliable test but presents challenges related to the number of genes that would have to be sequenced to cover the most frequent mutations seen in common cancers. The depth of sequencing would have to be dense also to distinguish small amounts of ct-DNA from much higher levels of cf-DNA shed by normal cells. A reference library of cancer mutations versus those found in matched healthy donors is under creation now. This ten-thousand-plus-subject study, called the Circulating Cell-Free Genome Atlas (CCGA), will be the largest database of mutations found in the blood of cancer patients.

Once ct-DNA is detected, the next challenge is to identify the organ source from which it is derived. The specific mutations would be helpful in tracing the tissue of origin since the patterns of somatic alterations for specific tumor types have been well described. To prevent overtreatment, it would be critical to separate the aggressive tumor types from less invasive ones. Recognition of unique associations of lethality with ct-DNA profiles on serial sampling would help refine these distinctions. Even if the tissue of origin is traced and the tumor removed in a timely fashion, there is no guarantee that occult metastases are not already operating elsewhere. In patients at risk of developing certain cancers like those with mutations in BRCA1 or BRCA2 genes (at risk of breast and ovarian cancers), or smokers at risk of lung cancer, the ct-DNA results can be supplemented with organ-specific tests and imaging. Finally, if detectable after tumor resection, presence of ct-DNA is associated with a high risk of recurrence in patients with breast and colon cancers, as well as with non-small-cell lung cancer. In these cases, ct-DNA can be used to monitor the success of therapy.

The ability to distinguish a cancer patient from a healthy individual is not enough; some tumors grow so slowly that detecting them early and treating them aggressively could be more of a health hazard for the patient than simply letting the cancer grow. Ideally, a biomarker for early detection of cancer should be able to provide clues to the source organ and the potential aggressiveness of the disease. In other words, the information has to be actionable. Detection of proteins unique to a tumor cell would be the ideal biomarker, as they would provide both diagnostic information and serve as a therapeutic target. Tests to measure blood-borne proteins, such as PSA, CEA, and CA-125, have been available for decades. They are helpful in early detection, but for even earlier detection, a collection of antigens—or what might be called a *protein signature* of an occult tumor, as opposed to a single protein—is likely to provide a more comprehensive view. Proteomics is not as well developed so far as the study of genomes or transcriptomes. There are many reasons for this related to sampling errors, lack of technology, and bioinformatics support. To detect large numbers of proteins, well-characterized antibodies have to be available. A new method using antibody microarrays is now available for this purpose. Large-scale studies for protein signatures have not been conducted yet. The Cancer Moonshot initiative could help in this area.

Another interesting biomarker is the exosome. These are small vesicles pinched off from cells and shed into body fluids like blood, saliva, and urine, and they carry signals for intercellular communication. Their role in cancer, in coagulation, and in waste management is well recognized; exosomes can serve as biomarkers of many diseases. They are collected from blood and analyzed for their cargo. Those derived from cancer cells can provide clues to their cells of origin. They serve as the advance party, deployed to scout fresh target organs for the metastatic spread of cancer. They carry oncoproteins, RNA, DNA fragments, and lipids from malignant donor cancer cells to recipient host organ cells in local and distant sites, preparing the microenvironment, making it suitable to receive and house the arriving cancer. Exosomes help create the premetastatic niche in new areas and promote disease progression. Proteomic, transcriptomic, and genomic analysis of exosomes has led to the identification of markers that can serve as liquid biopsies for a variety of solid tumors like colorectal cancers, brain tumors, and breast and prostate malignancies. High-throughput platforms for clinical utilization of exosome-based diagnostics have been developed. One microfluidic device can profile exosomal microRNAs. Exosome-based diagnostics provide more specific information in comparison to other liquid biopsy biomarkers because they are more stable. Finally, exosomes can serve as vehicles to deliver cancer drugs and vaccines.

Following the exosomes preparing new sites for metastasis are the cells that tumors release in the bloodstream. Like exosomes, these circulating tumor cells (CTCs) can be captured through liquid biopsies to help in early cancer detection. They can also serve as prognostic markers and to monitor response to treatment and early relapse. As few as one abnormal cell can be detected from a cubic centimeter of blood using technologies such as the isolation-by-size-of-epithelial-tumors (ISET) methodology. Captured on filters, these rare circulating cells can be studied using immune markers and histochemical stains for further characterization. In one study, no CTCs were detected in the blood of six hundred healthy volunteers, while all patients with diagnosed cancer showed the presence of CTC detected with the ISET technology, CTC counts being higher in more advanced cases. With further technologic refinement in accuracy and specificity, CTC monitoring can become a part of routine periodic checkups in healthy individuals.

The heyday of reductionism, looking for one culprit gene at a time and searching for the one magic bullet, is over. The era of big data, cloud computing, artificial intelligence, and wearable sensors has arrived. The study of cancer is evolving into a data-driven, quantitative science. Merging information obtained from liquid biopsies (RNA, DNA, proteomics, exosome studies, CTC) with histopathology, radiologic, and scanning techniques, aided by rapid machine learning, image reconstruction, intelligent software, and microfluidics can—and will—revolutionize the way we diagnose and prevent rather than treat cancer in the future. The ideal strategy will emerge from harnessing cutting-edge technology for a multidisciplinary systems biology approach through a consilience of scientists with expertise in molecular genetics, imaging, chemistry, physics, engineering, mathematics, and computer science.

Leroy Hood has done precisely this with his Institute for Systems Biology in Seattle. He has initiated a novel concept designed to detect disease in its earliest stage through health care that is predictive, preventive, personalized, and participatory (P4). By using detection of disease-perturbed networks in otherwise healthy individuals and finding solutions early, Hood is pioneering a new health care discipline termed *scientific wellness.* Through application of systems biology and P4 strategies, cancer care can finally be personalized in its truest sense.

The challenges after an abnormal cell is detected early are to determine the organ it is coming from, its malignant potential, and finding the means to eliminate it immediately. At least for MDS and AML, we are well equipped to begin the exploration using the tissue repository. Selected samples studied by panomics to understand the natural history of the preleukemia and its transition to acute leukemia would lead to an understanding of changes at the RNA, DNA, and protein level involved in the transformation. Studies of microRNA, cell-free DNA, and exosomes from the serum as well as the clonal response of immune cells as the disease progresses are of critical value in defining stage-specific markers of disease perturbations. Once we have the early markers of disease transition from preleukemia to acute leukemia, these markers can provide the missing "address" of cancer cells to the body's immune cells. As already noted, when cancer cells are detected at such an early stage, the first issue is to determine whether the tumor is aggressive or not because nonaggressive ones may as well be left alone. This research is ideally conducted on banked samples where the outcome for the patients over a period of a decade or more is known. For example, MDS patients whose serial bone marrows are stored in the repository can be studied for markers that identify patients likely to progress to leukemia and die early versus those who lived with MDS for more than ten years.

Once we have the biomarkers to identify its potential lethality, attacking the cancer early will be lifesaving. The strategy to eliminate early cancer has to be a better one than the traditional slash-poison-burn approach. The presently evolving cellular therapeutics would be ideal for targeting those few abnormal cells with laser-like precision.

Advances in our understanding of the immune system have led to therapies based on using the body's own soldiers, such as T cells and natural killer cells, to target cancer from the inside. The supreme efficiency of CAR-T cells becomes a problem in treating advanced cancers because of their overefficiency—they kill off any cell expressing the marker they are seeking, including normal cells. With more discriminating addresses being developed to target cancers, this supreme competence can be turned to our advantage by directing the CAR-Ts to cancer cells when their number is low. This would avoid all the life-threatening cytokine storms and tumor lysis syndromes associated with destruction of large hunks of tumor tissue. In the case of MDS, as soon as an early marker is detected—waving a red flag that the first acute leukemia cells have arisen—the markers can be used to arm and activate immune cells to home in on their target. The same strategy of identifying markers on the earliest cancer cells of all types—breast, lung, prostate, GI—is now being developed. Elegant studies, especially those coming from Bert Vogelstein's group at Johns Hopkins University, have already elaborated various aspects of this proposal.

Research is also ongoing in all these areas funded by the National Institutes of Health, but the investment remains paltry compared to funding provided for studies conducted on cell lines and animal models. Through redirection of intellectual and financial resources from the same old grant proposals to grant incentives for early detection using actual human samples, and by posing exciting challenges to competitive scientists, progress will be accelerated dramatically. The piece that is missing from the equation is an admission of failure of current strategies and a willingness to take a 180-degree turn to start all over again. We already invest a lot of effort to find minimal residual disease. Why not apply the same rigor and focus to minimal initial disease?

From the perspective of my lab, with the tissue repository at its disposal, this new approach to investigating cancer would start with a focused, systems biology approach to interrogate the first thousand samples of serum and bone marrow from patients who either died early (within two years) or late (after five years). So far, we have compared small numbers of patients in these types of sets using one or at most two of the omics technologies—for example, quantifying the messenger

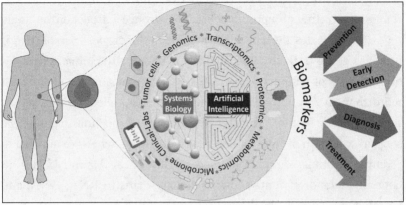

Courtesy of Dr. Abdullah Ali

RNA for gene expression profiling and/or sequencing the DNA to look for mutations in targeted genes. Studying large numbers of patients simultaneously using every technology available to examine RNA, DNA, and protein expression in multiple compartments (blood, bone marrow, buccal smears, circulating T cells) is more likely to yield complex signatures with strong clinical associations than have been discovered with limited samples. This discovery-set data, examined exhaustively by the latest technology, would then be used to characterize the next group, a test set of another few thousand samples from the tissue repository, for confirmation of the biomarkers. The refined signatures would then be used in a prospective validation set of samples for final and ultimate application to the clinical setting of living, dynamic patient populations. Such a thorough, retrospective analysis of the tissue repository studied through a systems biology approach has the best chance of yielding clues to perfect our diagnostic, prognostic, and therapeutic capabilities. Novel targets will emerge when important proteins or gene mutational profiles together suggest activations of heretofore unsuspected signaling pathways.

This pluralistic approach using actual human tissue is far more likely to be high yield compared to the reductionist approach prevalent for the past fifty years comprised of tweaking one or two genes at a time in the setting of mouse models. The strongest aspect of the tissue repository, besides the physical samples, is the clinical perspective it provides going back to 1984, making it possible to compare samples of thousands of patients who died early with thousands who survived more than five or ten years or longer. Sample collections started in the last decade cannot provide this unique retrospection. Imagine the staggering wealth of information that will emerge when we are able to examine multiple samples obtained serially at regular intervals from large numbers of patients showing biologic drifts in RNA, DNA, and protein expression as the disease evolves through its natural history. In addition, we can have a detailed understanding of how the patient's immune system responded to these tectonic shifts since T cells from the peripheral blood of patients are simultaneously obtained and preserved in the tissue repository, cells viably frozen, which can be thawed out, regrown, and studied. The biomarker signatures thus developed can then be applied for early detection of MDS and AML in our aging population, the prime target of these diseases. But where is the support?

❧

AND HOW MANY ZAINEBS?

I landed at the Qaid-e-Azam International Airport early one crisp December morning in 1992. I grew up in Karachi and moved to the United States immediately after graduating from medical school. As long as my parents were alive, I returned home frequently to see them. Each time I arrived back home at Gulistan-e-Raza, my mother would hand me a list of patients she had lined up for me to see. On the ride home during this particular visit, Ali Asghar, our driver, warned me that the list this time contained an emergency. "Begum Sahib is very anxious about a young woman dying of blood cancer, and she wants me to drive you there as soon as this afternoon." Sure enough, my mother broached the subject within hours of my arrival. "Zaineb is only thirty-five-years old," she said. "Her husband died in an accident last year. She has been doing cleaning jobs to support herself and her children. Suddenly, she got very weak and sick, and the government-run dispensary has been of no help to her. Poor thing cannot even get out of bed anymore. I heard of her through Bazm-e-Amna"—a charitable organization my mother was active in—"and offered your help. Please go see her today."

As I arrived in the slum area and made my way to her little shanty, I was greeted by the sight of three skeletal little girls ranging from five to nine years outside the hut. The eldest looked particularly pale and listless. I asked her if she was okay, and she shook her head. I was scared to ask the obvious: if she had eaten. My older sister Atiya is not only a first-rate pediatrician and pediatric oncologist, she is also the president of the Human Development Foundation. She is on a mission to improve health care and primary education in deeply poverty-stricken areas of Pakistan and had asked one of the little girls in the school the same question: "Have you eaten today?" The six-year-old replied, "No. It was not my turn to have breakfast today." That answer rang in my ears as I faced the three little ones outside Zaineb's hut. Probably none of them had had a "turn" for any meals. For days, even.

How does one go in and talk to a thirty-five-year-old woman for whom dying from leukemia is only her second-biggest problem?

Cancer treatments such as CAR-T and other targeted therapies, stem cell transplants, and immune manipulations cost hundreds of thousands of dollars. They are bankrupting affluent, developed nations of the world. They are absolutely beyond the reach of someone like Zaineb. We cannot neglect our responsibility as a global society to develop an affordable answer that is universally applicable for the nearly eighteen million people diagnosed with cancer around the world each year.

Samuel K. Sia, professor of biomedical engineering at Columbia University, wants to do just that: develop an affordable diagnostic platform. Sam created a microfluidic chip that tests for multiple diseases, including sexually transmitted ones, and is eminently affordable, costing pennies. Referred to as the mChip and no larger than a credit card, it is a handheld device that takes a drop of blood and analyzes it for quick diagnosis of a variety of diseases. It has already received approval for diagnosis of prostate cancer in Europe. Our two labs at Columbia University are collaborating in an effort to develop an implantable chip that can be inserted under the skin for constant surveillance, detection, capture, and destruction of the first cancer cells. Early detection is the most compassionate and humane solution for the cancer problem.

∽

LAURA AND THE IMPORTANCE OF ETIQUETTE

Between May and October of 2002, both Harvey Preisler and Per Bak were dead. The aftermath of Harvey's death included a painful awakening about how inappropriate most people are when offering their condolences. One friend, while crying her eyes out, began by offering to take me out to a singles' bar. A surprising and recurring comment, also supposedly well meaning, but one that left me baffled about how to respond, was, "Sorry to hear Harvey died. But you are looking well." Perhaps the most patently absurd was a message left on my answering machine by a colleague saying how sorry she was that my husband was dead, but "don't worry, you will join him soon, and then the two of you can live happily ever after in heaven."

I wish they had read Laura Claridge's insightful and engaging biography, *Emily Post: Daughter of the Gilded Age, Mistress of Manners.* Laura, introduced to us by my brother Abbas as a brilliant professor of English, rapidly became a beloved family friend. She makes two points very clear in this book: first, from birth to death, we humans need constant guidance about how to behave; and second, minding our manners can overcome even some of our most glaring deficien-

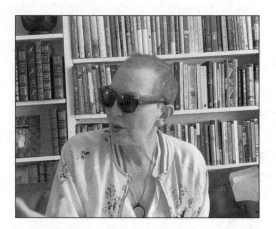

cies. One early review of Post's *Etiquette* captured her spirit perfectly with the quotation from Mathew Arnold: "Conduct is three-fourths of life." As Laura put it succinctly, "The subject hardly mattered: funerals or flower arrangements, broken hearts or broken glasses, Emily held her audience in esteem, and she meant to teach her readers, would-be 'Best People,' whatever their background, race or creed, to do likewise." Deep down, the real meaning of manners, according to Ms. Post, is a demonstration of sensitivity to the feelings of others. "Best Society is not a fellowship, nor does it seek to exclude those who are not of exalted birth, but it is an association of gentle-folk [in which] charm of manner . . . and instinctive consideration for the feelings of others, are the credentials by which society the world over recognizes its chosen members."

A few months after Harvey's death, I received a brief but deeply sympathetic note from Harvey's ex-wife, Angela. Beginning in 1977 when I first met Harvey, all the way up to 2002 when he died, I had met Angela only a handful of times and not seen her since 1982. I only have positive memories of her. The letter was remarkable because of its profound kindness and also because it contained a check for rather a large amount of money. Apparently, Harvey had not changed the name of the beneficiary in his retirement plan at Roswell Park Memorial Institute so that once his death was registered, the check was automatically sent to Angela. "This rightfully belongs to you and Sheherzad," she simply said. Such are the acts of extraordinary decency, civility, and etiquette that Ms. Post is talking about.

I remember distinctly the evening when I was getting ready for Harvey's memorial service, just a little over twenty-four hours after his death. The opaque, intricate mundanities of living were already starting to emerge in unexpected places. I picked up my wedding band and looked to my sisters for guidance.

"Should I still wear this?" I asked.

Sughra, my younger sister, who had been silently crying as she watched me getting ready, snatched up the ring and slipped it firmly on my finger.

"Yes, you will wear it tonight and for as long as you wish!"

As Laura writes, "Only Emily Post understood the power of routine to hold one's raw emotions at bay." No wonder *Etiquette* was "second only to the Bible as the book most often stolen from public libraries." Post counseled the bereaved wisely with these words: "At no time does solemnity so possess our souls as when we stand deserted at the brink of darkness into which our loved one has gone. And the last place in the world where we would look for comfort at such a time is in the seeming artificiality of etiquette; yet it is in the moment of deepest sorrow that etiquette performs its most vital and real service."

While Laura was working on the Post biography, she was diagnosed with a particularly lethal form of brain tumor with little chance of survival beyond a few months. Despite the bleakest of outlooks (at one point, her ICU physician called me to request that I counsel the family to "let nature take its course with Laura now"), Laura not only defied all odds by surviving, she restarted her work on the book in a miraculously short period of time after her surgery. Even as her brain was being regularly assaulted by the insults of radiation and chemotherapy, Laura found her own grounding in meticulously researching and recounting another great woman's life story. The book *Emily Post,* supported early for its merit by Harvard's Nieman Foundation, is not only a fantastic personal achievement for Laura, it also stands as the finest testament to the indomitable sublimity of the human spirit. Both Post and Claridge transmuted tragedy into constructive pursuits, representing the best behavior in good times and bad.

Laura did not have a primary brain tumor. She had a lymphoma with multiple lesions in the brain. She underwent several surgical resections, repeated rounds of chemotherapy, radiation therapy, targeted therapy, and an autologous bone marrow transplant. Throughout these difficult times, Laura has continued writing; indeed, she writes now with greater clarity and verve than ever. Her latest book, *The Lady with the Borzoi: Blanche Knopf,* was published to great acclaim in 2017. She is now working on her first book of fiction.

Harvey died of the lymphoma. RIP, Harvey.

Per died from the complications of a stem cell transplant. RIP, Per.

Laura is alive with a lymphoma sixteen years after the diagnosis. She survived the stem cell transplant.

Laura is the reason oncologists don't give up. We can't give up.

Long live Laura.

◈

MARK AT HARVEY'S MEMORIAL SERVICE:

Our dad was not a sentimental man. He was ever the scientist. Emotions clouded reason . . . and if you cannot see reason, you may as well be blind. But Dad did have a side few were lucky enough to see. While he was always practical, he truly was an emotional man. He stood up for his beliefs, and he never backed down. One of those beliefs was that it was important to die with dignity. No complaints, despite all the pain. He didn't want to be a burden to his children or his wife. He never was. Azra said it best: taking care of him was an honor, never a burden. There's a quote he often spoke of: "Death stared me in the face and I stared right back." Dad, you certainly did.

More than anything, our father was a family man. He cherished us, and we cherished him. He often thanked us for all the days and nights spent by his side, but I told him there was no need for thanks. None of us could have been anywhere else. He and I often discussed his illness. He once asked me why he should keep fighting . . . what good was there in it? I told him his illness had brought our family much closer together. He smiled and said he was glad something good came of it.

Azra, he adored you. He often told me it was love at first sight. You two shared a love that only exists in fairy tales. Dad could be unconscious but still manage a smile when you walked into the room. I have never seen anything like it, and I feel privileged to have witnessed your devotion to each other. The way you took care of him is inspiring. You never left his side, and you refused to let him give up. No one could have done anything more for him, and he knew it. He was very lucky to find you.

While going through his wallet, I was shocked to find a piece of paper folded up in the back. On it were two quotes written in his own pen. I'd like to share one with you. "There isn't much more to say. I have had no joy, but a little satisfaction from this long ordeal. I have often wondered why I kept going. That, at least I have learned and I know it now at the end. There could be no hope, no reward. I always recognized that bitter truth. But I am a man and a man is responsible for himself." (The words of George Gaylord Simpson.) Our father died Sunday, May 19, at 3:20 in the afternoon. His family lives on with a love and closeness that will make him proud. Pop, we love you. You were our best friend. We will miss you every day.

IN HONOR OF Harvey's lifelong dedication to science and to finding a solution for his cancer patients, an annual lecture was started in his name. Below are remarks from Sheherzad at the Tenth Harvey Preisler Memorial Symposium in 2012:

> I recall that last morning on May 19, 2002, as he lay dying. At 7:00 a.m., my mom came into my room where I was sleeping with my sister Sarah and told us that Dad wanted to see us. I ran into his room with the sinking instinctive certainty of an eight-year-old that all was not well, only to find him sitting up in bed, smiling and stretching his wasted arms out to hug me. We spent the next several hours with me alternately reading to him from my various favorite books, jumping on his bed, running away with his walker, having a serious discussion with him about Madagascar frogs, and taking his "tenchapur" with the thermometer I loved to play with. And each time, he would oblige me by smiling sweetly. Finally, Vania, a family friend came and took me out to the park with his daughter and my best friend, Salpi. This was the last time I saw my father.
>
> It was only several years later that Mom told me how Dad had woken up at 5:00 a.m. that morning, saw that he was bleeding from multiple sites, recognized that he had DIC (disseminated intravascular coagulation), and announced calmly that he was going to die that day. After Mom cleaned him up and changed his dressings around the port, all he wanted to do in the last hours was to spend time with the family, even as he got more and more short of breath and his lungs filled up with blood. Dad calmed himself in those last hours by watching me play, listening to me chatter on endlessly, reading, and discussing biological facts about my pet frogs.
>
> *Amor Fati* at its best.

◌

AND THUS HARVEY lived, and thus he died. Proud to the end. He took his last labored, agonal breaths in my arms on a clear, sunny May afternoon in Chicago. His composure and his comportment until the final conscious moments was nothing short of heroic.

Stop all the clocks, cut off the telephone,
Prevent the dog from barking with a juicy bone,
Silence the pianos and with muffled drum
Bring out the coffin, let the mourners come.

Let aeroplanes circle moaning overhead
Scribbling on the sky the message "He is Dead."

— W. H. AUDEN, "FUNERAL BLUES."

GIVE SORROW WORDS

NAHEED. ALENA.

Some sorrows are unfathomable, language incapable of expressing them. What combination of letters could possibly speak the unspoken thoughts of the mothers Naheed and Alena as they bid unhurried farewells to the serially dying parts of the creatures they birthed and nurtured for decades? The anguish has no beginning and no end, no relief, no ascent or descent, no respite, collapsing past, present, and future into one bottomless pit.

A new language needs invention to encompass the defenselessness, the vulnerability of these two mothers who, with utmost delicacy, eased their boys into the grave, one piece at a time, each over a period of sixteen months, tormented until their child's last breaths about how to make the bewildering segmented departure less painful. Omar had seven surgeries to remove slices of arms and lungs, a cancer-filled shoulder. In Andrew's case, first the limbs went, followed by the bowel and bladder, then his eyesight, and in a final insult, he could swallow no more. To dare to mourn with Naheed and Alena, one must own the sorrows of the universe. No linguistic hyperbole can do justice. Language itself becomes speechless, vocabulary held hostage by the raw agony of such incalculable scales. The infinite care with which Alena washed, scrubbed, and dressed the wasted, limp body of her twenty-three-year old, or the relentless, whacking, blistering, piercing, frightful terrors haunting Naheed in every waking hour, and in sleep, deplete the hubris of death, elevate the status of motherhood to where the stars lower their gaze. One spark of pain in the heart of these mothers eclipses the glory of the sun. Dust raised by their agitation conceals deserts, their tears forcing a river to recede, dragging its forehead obsessively in front of their grief.

> *Hota hay nehaan gard mein sehra meray peechay*
> *Ghista hay jabeen khaak pe darya meray aagay*
> —GHALIB: EPISTEMOLOGIES OF ELEGANCE

Next to me, the wilderness is shamed into hiding in dust
The servile river grovels in the dust before me

ꙮ

OMAR AND ANDREW:
WHAT WERE THEIR CHOICES?

Classic Greek canon places great emphasis on choice. In the *Oresteia* by Aeschylus, every character had a personal choice to make. Agamemnon did not have to kill his daughter Iphigenia. Clytemnestra did not have to kill Agamemnon in revenge for her daughter's murder. Orestes did not have to kill his mother Clytemnestra to avenge his father Agamemnon. Everyone had a choice.

The Greek term *pharmakon* combines three meanings—remedy, poison, and scapegoat. Aeschylus uses the term in the *Oresteia* to refer to a drug that can either be remedy or poison; it gets rid of illness either by killing the disease or killing the diseased. When Agamemnon sacrifices Iphigenia, his act epitomizes the dual-edged *pharmakon* since it cured the problem of winds needed to drive his ships but ended up causing death of the whole family.

The *pharmakon* we offered both Omar and Andrew encompassed all three meanings. Prescribed to fight the tumor, chemotherapy and radiation therapy would serve as both remedies and poisons simultaneously. Basically, the treatment would destroy the tumor in one area as new ones erupted in a hundred others in brutal acts of ruthless, diabolical, vicious reciprocity. Of course, there was no hope of any improvement in survival. The poisonous side effects would land them in the hospital for weeks and months, with their mouth and esophagus one big, raw, open wound. The third meaning of *pharmakon* refers to the ritual of human sacrifice. By testing experimental drugs in humans, knowing little about the risks and benefits involved, yet, hoping to learn from observations made on the current subjects, were we not turning the societal demands, inner desires, conscious concerns, and capricious, arbitrary violence on Omar and Andrew in order to secure a better outcome for others in the future?

We gave those awful treatments anyway, because the alternative would be no less agonizing. Allowed to run amok, cancer is one of the most painful, horrifying diseases. The fundamental question for both Omar and Andrew related to making this impossible choice—succumb to the ferocity of cancer, or seek refuge in palliative treatments that temporarily control a growing tumor but come with their own set of excruciating side effects? Die from the disease or die from the treatment?

Which would you choose?

Why are these two the only choices?

⟡

WHAT IS PAST IS PROLOGUE

In 2005, Elisabeth Kübler-Ross published her final book, *On Grief and Grieving,* in which she suggested that families go through the same five stages of denial, anger, bargaining, depression, and acceptance, not necessarily in that order, as do patients given the diagnosis of a terminal illness. The problem turned out to be more complicated, however, as the bereaved suffer emotional bedlam in unpredictable installments rather than an orderly, stage-defined, specific progression, at all times attempting to readjust their place in a new world devoid of the loved one. Being part of the disquieting, vexing, confounding action as the disease flamed and burned its way with primeval savagery, all the characters seem larger than life, observations seem disproportionately significant, every question—no matter how inconsequential—worthy of an answer. The necessary issue ultimately relates to choice. And when the choice involves life-and-death situations, both the potential risk and individual responsibility demand intense emotional, psychological, rational, spiritual input. Was some choice—made under such intense pressure, caught in the whirling vortex of a rapidly progressive, unmistakably fatal disease—the right one? Would clarity come from looking back years later?

But then hindsight can also pose a problem, as retrospection tends to interpret events in rosier terms, to bring intellectual order to the impossible practical disorder of life. Consider the famous Robert Frost poem "The Road Not Taken," which addresses this question of choice examined in hindsight. The last, most famous lines of this poem, "Two roads diverged in a wood, and I—I took the one less traveled by, and that has made all the difference," appear to define the essential characteristic of the intrepid, bold, self-reliant, daredevil, quintessential New Englander. The ideal American, who goes against the grain, exerts individuality by choosing an unusual, risky, unknown, seemingly untrodden path. The key to the poem lies in the middle, where Frost describes the two roads. Being entirely covered with fallen leaves, they were basically indistinguishable. It is only when the poet looks back years later and reflects on the events of his life "ages and ages hence" does he decide that he made the best choice since "that has made all the difference." Of course, it made no difference at all, but hindsight allows the poet to bring order to randomness, as if the decision that made the difference were rational, logical, evidence-based.

Although it posed the risk of rationalizing irrational events, I asked a few of the family members of the patients we have met in this book to cast a backward glance on the events. I had them read what I have written about their loved ones, about the gaping holes in our scientific understanding of cancer, about the draconian measures offered as palliation or treatments, about our failure as a society. Knowing all of that, I asked them how they might have reinterpreted or come to view the choices that were made differently. My hope is that given the benefit of reappraisal, reexamination, the information can be methodically re-reviewed, decisions made under intense pressure can be calmly and systematically sifted, reconsidered, questioned, alternate possibilities imagined. From this perspective, the what-if questions might finally be addressed, especially as related to what pain and suffering could and should have been avoided, what can be prevented in the future should such situations arise again and affect the living, understanding what choices would be altered, how to balance external contingencies with inner compulsions. The hope in reliving tragic situations is that it brings a modicum of relief to acknowledge the randomness of life—to concede that no matter how hard one tries, it is impossible to make any sense of the profound anguish their loved ones went through, to allow one to face the unintelligibility of disease, to face death. To accept that the only answer is that there is no answer.

⚬∾⚬

OMAR

May 9, 2018
Naheed (Omar's mother)

> *What I say with complete truth is that at no time . . . not for*
> *a second did I allow myself to believe or think that Omar would*
> *actually die . . . go away from me forever. He takes me to a sofa, sits*
> *down and in a casual tone announces that the doctor he consulted*
> *suspects something . . . some "grunge . . . or maybe a tumor."*

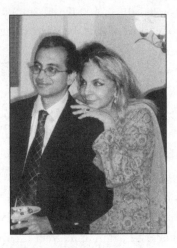

What happened to me from that moment to the very second that I realized the labored breathing sound was no longer coming from him and, in my hope-filled heart, assumed it could only mean that he had beaten whatever had been bothering him. That he was now better . . . he had been cured . . . he was alive . . . I cannot explain any of this rationally.

The truth of the matter is that "hope" as much as the cancer is an affliction . . . of the heart and head in the first case, of the body in the second. Hope latches on to you, crawls in and burrows deep inside your heart and your head. Once it goes, it leaves a cavity behind, a hole that can never ever be filled . . . and it is this hole, this nothingness, one needs to live with for one's entire life . . . and it is this emptiness within this hole that we cover with the proverbial "patthar" [stone].

Omar would never have accepted any option that required him to accept his fate without fighting it every inch of the way. If it meant chemotherapy, radiation, experimental trials . . . he would go for it.

Do you remember how a few hours before he died he discussed a new therapy . . . stem cell or some other drug that you had discussed with him earlier?

And as for being told cold mathematical percentages of possible survival for treatments and experimental drugs . . . there was never

*a moment of doubt that he would be, must be, had to be counted
among the survivors. And why not? Miracles happen, don't they?*

*He might have had his own thoughts that were less happy, but
he never conveyed them to me. Except for the single time when he
asked me to learn to take care of my own finances . . . that was it . . .
never after I told him that I would do no such thing and that he
would be there to do it for me.*

*Should the doctors have held out hope to Omar? . . . Yes. After
all, it took nothing away from him. Yes . . . it meant painful treatments but it did not mean that there was no possibility of survival.*

*I feel that a patient must decide . . . with or without the family.
Unless a patient is suffering beyond the limits of the human body
he should be allowed to live in his own universe.*

*What researchers must do is what researchers should. They must
work and work and think and feel like a patient or the family . . .
they have to create new medications. New tools for isolating these
cells and new concoctions to kill them. If the present laboratory is
not equal to the challenge more research is needed . . . I was struck by
how cells from one dish can jump into another in spite of stringent
controls . . . how and why. Cancer is not infectious, is it?*

*In the end I think everything that happened to Omar had to
happen but for the weak chemotherapy he was given by that first
doctor. If any single mistake was made in Omar's treatment,
that was it.*

ଔ

June 15, 2018

Farid (Omar's younger brother)

Dear Azra Apa,

*Thanks for your message. Each of these questions is harder than
the next, but I will try my best to answer them.*

*Was my brother ever told that his chances were zero? The an-
swer to this one is a resolute "no." We definitely weren't told that
his chances were zero. Not only that, the question of chances was*

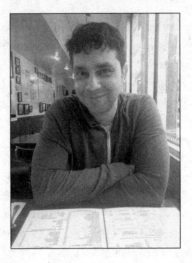

studiously avoided by the vast majority of my brother's doctors,
down to the very end of the process. To be fair to them, this was a
question I avoided myself in all my heated inner dialogues. It is not
that I didn't know that his chances were, in fact, exceedingly low.
In fact, I was extremely surprised when he was given, at the very
first meeting, a prognosis of 85 percent. Perhaps the doctor wanted
to make him feel better? Unless her confidence was a matter of
honor—the honor of medicine in the face of disease. In either case,
it had the effect of momentarily boosting his confidence and casting
doubt on what I had gathered.

We went on a walk, he told me not to worry: he was going to
fight this thing, he said. Did he really believe this in his heart, or
was this an act of fraternal compassion? Or is it that these two
possibilities really cannot be separated? In either case, two months
later, he was completely shaken upon being told (by his oncologist
at NY Hospital) that the actual figure was 75 percent. In many
ways, this figure was even more inaccurate than the 85 percent that
was given to him at NY General Hospital since, in the in-between
period, it had become quite clearly apparent that the methotrexate
wasn't working. Why, then, did the doctor give him that figure?
Was this blatant lie an act of kindness? And why did it not achieve
its effect? I remember Mursi asking him what the difference was

between 85 and 75 percent. But in his mind, that 10 percent plunge in life chances required a categorical adjustment.

It is strange the effect that numbers can have. Numerically, at least, I knew more about his chances than did others, but still I was enraged beyond words when friends or family would say he was "dying." I was enraged on his behalf and enraged because it was emotionally unrealistic even though it was manifest that the cancer was invading his body—cell by cell, organ by organ—to suggest that my brother was "dying." Here was a man who produced a list of "100 Books to Read Before You Live"—because (as he said) "'before you die' is just too depressing." This was also a man who insisted on going to see The Cherry Orchard—not a cheerful play exactly—knowing that his days were numbered. "No point in not living while I'm still alive," he said when this choice was briefly questioned. Which is to say that this was a man whose idea of living wasn't to be cheered up but to face life in all its intensity. Another reason why the bucket list wouldn't have worked. My point is that he was in his prime—married to the love of his life, surrounded by loved ones in the place that he loved more than any other place in the world. He refused to be pitied or mourned pre-emptively by those who loved him. And yet, of course, he was very much dying, if that word has any meaning at all.

All this is to say that had his doctors refused him treatment, he would have fought back and refused their refusal. The thing is: at least for him, he—his life—wasn't the only thing at stake. Also at stake was science and medicine, scientific progress, and the scientific method. To give up on himself was to give up on science—and that wasn't really possible in his case. He wouldn't have enjoyed his bucket-list world tour knowing not only that the end was coming, but also knowing that science had failed. Sometimes I wonder if one of the reasons that he didn't follow the advice for a far more radical approach was because that advice was, in a way, an admittance of that failure.

I do think it would have been the ethical choice to tell him that his chances were nil. Perhaps the emotional pain of hopelessness would have been even more excruciating than that long succession of horrific surgeries? Still, I have to wonder why his doctors were quite so ready to operate if they knew that his chances were actually nil. I have to wonder even more why they couldn't have told him clearly that a radical surgery or amputation was the only real chance for survival. Even if that chance was a fraction of a fraction, it would have helped to hear it from them. Did his surgeons really not know this? If not, why not? If yes, then why did they stick to their protocol? And why did they become so condescending—even aggressively mocking at times—at any point this decision was questioned?

I am sorry to answer your questions with questions. As for all the other Omars, it seems to me that the ethical choice would be to inform the patient of their certain death. But if that death is all but certain, it behooves the institution to let them know that the course they're following has no chance of succeeding. But more than anything, the ethical choice is to accept, at the deepest level, the fallibility of institutions and the imperfection of epistemologies that are cherished and defended aggressively. After all, it is this fallibility which explains why these protocols are even needed.

Love,
Farid

∽

October 29, 2018
Sara (Omar's sister)

One of my last conversations with Bhaya [brother] was in Brooklyn. We were standing at a vantage point, the vista of Prospect Park before us—he turned to me and said, "Do you think Heaven looks like this? I can't imagine anything better."

As his "Little Sis," I probably read him differently from others; it is of course the prerogative of all younger siblings to be able to read through their older ones. I believe that Bhaya knew his

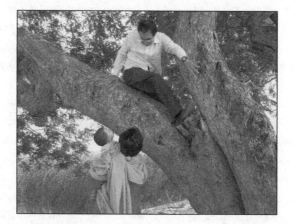

prognosis, he knew the chances of survival were very small, and he knew the chances of imminent death were high. He knew that radical surgery was his best chance of survival. The complexity of human relations does not of course translate this knowing on his part in any linear way to the decisions that he made for himself.

This is partly because there is one quality of Bhaya that defined how he dealt with his illness and his loved ones through this time in his life—it is a very rare quality but one which defined who he was in a very profound way—the ephemeral lightness with which he could be selfless, loving, protective, generous. Please don't think my brother was a saint; he was as exasperating a sibling as can be, but he was an exceptional human being in so many ways, and this was one of the ways. If we had acknowledged this quality vocally, if it had been part of our narrative about him and how he was coping, perhaps we would have given him a chance to have an honest conversation with us.

I wonder sometimes, what would he have chosen to do if we were the kind of family that spoke collectively and openly—imagine us sitting around a dining table, his family and friends there, and his family saying to him: "Beloved, think of yourself and not of us. Here are your options. Option 1: radical surgery. Option 2: palliative care. Option 3: multiple surgeries and chemo and radiation. This is what all three mean for you. We are here to support you in *whichever one you want to do. We are here to support you if you change your mind. We love you enough to not only help you fight this, but to also support you if you choose not to fight this. You tell us what you want to do. We are here for you. Talk to us, please. Share your fears and thoughts."*

I would like to say to families, friends, doctors, nurses, and social workers out there—have that conversation. Nobody dies because of a conversation. Nobody chooses physical pain over death because of a conversation. No one will give up on life, because you have put choices before them. Please don't be a coward.

Don't do what I did, waiting for someone to bring up palliative care and even assisted suicide, for me to share the research and options I had explored for him, to give me a crutch, an opening to have that conversation.

For me, we all failed Bhaya. Collectively, we forgot the most important quality of love—selflessness and compassion.

൚

July 10, 2018

Mursi (Omar's wife)

It never occurred to us that Omar would die. We did not talk about him dying ever. If we knew how hopeless his prognosis was, we would have decided to have children. I did not want kids. He did. One month before his diagnosis, we discussed the topic and decided to have kids. But then he was diagnosed even before we got married, and then of course too much was happening to talk about it. If we knew he had no chance of survival, we would have thought about kids.

A second thing we would have done differently, had we known, is travel more. In 2008, after multiple lung surgeries, we decided to go to Greece for our honeymoon. Omar didn't even want to tell the doctors because he did not want to be told not to go. They would have said his immune system was suppressed and it was too *dangerous for him to travel. We had a wonderful time! He never complained throughout the trip even though of course there were days when he had pain, but the joy we had was unparalleled. We should have taken more trips like that.*

Another thing is related to all the surgeries he had. After the very first one, we were told the cancer cells were already in the veins. That means it had already spread. Yet the doctors did not tell us what that spelled as far as his prognosis went. We were always talking about chances; one day it was 85 percent, and next time it had slipped to 75 percent. Even if they did, it did not regis-ter. Omar definitely, and all of us also, had all this hope. This one more treatment might do the trick. This is why we kept going. The later surgeries and pneumonia were terrible for him. At some point after the seventh or ninth surgery, we questioned why he needed so many operations. Thinking back, I can say for sure that if I was in his shoes, I would not have gone through so many surgeries. They were too painful.

⚭

KITTY C.

June 18, 2018
Conor (Kitty's son)

As far as my experience, I can't quibble with the medical ele-ment. My mom always had glowing reviews of you and the other doctors who treated her—or to be more accurate, who she worked with. My mom was an incredibly giving person and, as a friend of hers told me casually but poignantly, "She really gave you a good life." This is absolutely true, and I realize it more and more every day—she gave everything she could possibly give to me. Indeed, she even didn't want to burden me with the knowledge of her disease for the first several months she was sick, until my aunt Helen persuaded her to tell me. Even then, somehow she shielded

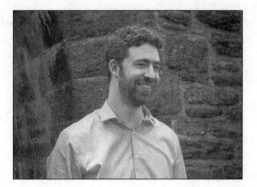

me from the worst elements. Helen and I became sleuths who tried to put together the bits and pieces of the progression of her disease and her treatments, to try to form a complete picture of what was happening in her life. In the weeks after she died, Helen and I wondered, had she held out for me? Was she looking at all the chaos in my life saying to herself, "I can't die just yet because he needs my support"? We still tease her to this day for the copious notes she left on funeral parlors and cremation services, as if, even in death, she had to carry her weight in the family. We always tried to take that weight from her, but to no avail.

Well, I believe our last days with her may have eased my mom's passing into the unknown. No matter how much you try to give back to someone like this, it never feels like enough. My last moment with her was two nights before she died. She was lying in her favorite spot on the couch in our living room, thin and frail, curled up like a child. I sat with her and ate a late dinner as Eulalee, her aide, took care of the intangibles. This may sound dark, but I think of Eulalee almost as a midwife of death, a kind of shaman who steps in at the end and guides people through the fear and sadness of dying, helps them remain present and accept it, and even guides their loved ones through it all. Like my mom, Eulalee was incredibly giving. She knew exactly what was needed to ease the transition. After engaging with my mom in what limited chat she was capable of, I was getting ready to leave for my apartment and Eulalee told me to give her a hug. My mom was a fiercely independent person, and she often shied away from overt affection, so it was difficult for her to signal when she needed it. But I obliged. Since my mom was not able to even sit up at this point, I sat down next to her and reached my arms under her, feeling her boney back and weak limbs. I saw an elated smile on her face, a feeling of satisfaction as she exclaimed, "You're so great! You're so great!"

Was that enough for a lifetime of self-sacrifice and kindness to a son who was sometimes clueless of his mother's own struggles? No, it's never enough. But by showing this gratitude, I sent my mom the message that her struggles were not in vain. She was proud and happy that she had raised a partner who could be there in the moment when she needed someone most.

The next day, Helen visited her as she drifted in and out of consciousness. She was traveling, as Eulalee said. Helen, her sister and best friend, gave her the strength to embark on this mysterious voyage. She reassured her, "I've got the pearls"—some storied family jewelry—which gave them both a nice laugh in the waning hours. I called from work in the afternoon and spoke to my mom. She was so happy to hear from me. She had no idea where I was or what day it was, but she conjured up a setting where she imagined me in my element. She said, "You're at the protest? Are there a lot of people there?" I was confused, but I went along with the fantasy and was happy of how proud she was.

The next morning, I got the call from Eulalee that my mom was in the throes of death. When I arrived, she was breathing heavily but not conscious in any apparent way. Helen and Eugene, my half brother (who has the same father), came up to the apartment, and we waited it out. Eulalee knew to the minute when it was coming and told me to lie in bed with my mom and hold her hand. Again, I obliged. I gave her some parting words as she drifted away.

To my surprise, I went into a rage that she had abandoned me. But as I write this, the loving kindness that she gave me is all that I feel. And I take solace in the freedom she must have felt in those last moments to travel by herself, like the bird she always wanted to be.

❧

ANDREW

Alena (Andrew's mother)

How do I even think about what happened, and did we do the right things? Do we know even now what would have been better? What eats me is his last radiation therapy. The radiation therapist came in and said, "It's your choice. You can do it or not do it." I was so confused. I asked him, "What would you do?"

Did he stop swallowing because of tumor or the radiation? I spoke to someone whose nephew was dying of cancer at twenty-nine. They told him, "You will have a month to live." Right before the doctors told him, he was full of life. After that, he broke and died in twenty days. Andrew had no chance of surviving. Would he have died before sixteen months if he was told that? As a mother, I would take every day. Every extra minute he could live and I could see him. An older man I know in Israel also has glioblastoma, and he is alive, though in a wheelchair, six years later. I would accept a wheelchair for Andrew as long as he could live.

I wish I knew what gave him a better quality of life—to treat or not to treat him? When given a choice, until the last day, Andrew said, "I want to live and will do everything to beat this cancer."

Azra, I have to tell you, no one was honest with me. No one told me. But even if they had, what would I do?

Even my friend who stayed with me the last night said, "It is time to let him go." I couldn't. I always had hope. When he asked me, "Ma, is this it?" what did I say? He was still walking, getting radiation treatment, but walking with a cane. We were coming out of the apartment. He just turned to me and said, "Looks like I just got the bad lottery ticket. I'm not gonna make it." I said, "No one knows. Perfectly healthy person could get hit by car and die."

His father was more accepting.

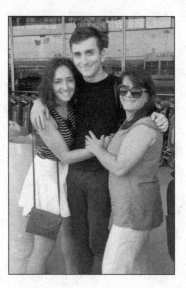

Andrew did not lose hope. Even when he failed the swallowing test, he wanted to take it again.

I keep thinking about this: If he had no chance to live and telling him would take away his hope and kill him faster, could we give him placebo instead of that terrible treatment with chemo and radiation therapy? At least he would have kept thinking he was getting treatment, not lose hope, and it would not kill him faster. Why make his life more miserable with those poisons?

When he started with the terrible headaches after the first round of surgery and chemoradiation therapy, we called NY General Hospital and were not getting any satisfactory answers. They told us it is probably a sinus infection, he should take antibiotics. He had no relief and the headaches were killing him. We called a few times, and they made us feel like they didn't want to be bothered. When I called a few more times in a row that he was having terrible headaches, they seemed annoyed. Finally, they told us to go to the ER. By then, he was throwing up and almost losing it. In the ER, scans showed tumors all over. When Dr. C. found out Andrew had metastases all over, she was very upset. Then we went to NY Hospital, and she never called once to follow up to ask about what happened to

Andrew, was he even alive. We just never heard from them again. It still bothers me to think of how they treated Andrew. Sure, we need hope, but we also need more compassion. It's great they follow the books to do things, but compassion is not in their books.

And what of NY Hospital? His oncologist just disappeared after he came once, joked a little, and left. That was it. After that, he just never bothered. For more than three months, Andrew was admitted, going through hell, but the oncologist, he never came.

∾

Kat (Andrew's sister)

Because Andrew never accepted he would die, I cannot. Looking back, his condition was so brutal. He was receiving special pills from California with THC. He was taking a very strong dosage. He did not like taking it because he would wake up high and drowsy, and anyway, we couldn't tell if it was helpful at all. Only twice I saw him scared. Once after the first surgery when he was in rehab. One morning when I arrived, he started sobbing, "Why is this happening to me? Am I going to die?" I did not know what to say. Should I say, "Yes, you are dying"? Instead, I said, "We are all dying." At the end of Andrew's life, Charles and Rebecca wanted him to acknowledge that he was dying. Sheher did not. Andrew liked attention but not pity. He did not want to admit dying because then people would pity him. That was Andrew.

The second time, he was depressed for a month or so when things started going downhill. Mom moved in with him and wanted to be there all the time. He was trying to negotiate his personal space. He felt she was taking away his privacy and independence. Once when he felt better and they were having lunch, I talked about something in the future, and Andrew said, "You know I am always going to have to deal with this."

He showed sadness and disappointment every time doctors told him bad news. He would always respond by saying tomorrow would be different. He understood how much it would hurt me and Mom so he made it seem like it was not as bad as it really was. The thing that hurt us the most was how he was abandoned by his oncologists both at NY General and Special Hospitals.

☙

Sheher (our daughter)

(Opening remarks at the Fifteenth Harvey Preisler Memorial Symposium, November 14, 2017)

On my mother's side of the family, we have the sweet custom of being welcomed into the world at birth with an adult whispering the Azaan, or the Islamic call to prayer, into the newborn's ears. When I was born and being handed over to my mother's older sister for this ritual, my father intercepted. He snatched me from the nurse and repeatedly whispered into my ears, "Quantum gravity, quantum gravity!" Believe it or not, the first letter of the alphabet my dad taught me was G, for "glavity," as I pronounced it. This was my dad: a scientist to the core, one who harbored an unmatched respect and appreciation for seeking answers to the wonders and mysteries of the universe through a serious commitment to the pursuit of knowledge.

The truth mattered to my father more than anything else. This is what has motivated me at a deeply personal level to devote myself to multimedia journalism as a venue to uncover the secrets of science, technology, and medicine. My childhood is filled with memories of evening excursions to the Lincoln Park Zoo, the Shedd Aquarium, and the countless at-home experiments and science fairs my father and I participated in together. And after studying premed and working in Dr. Siddhartha Mukherjee's lab for the last few years, I've found my calling in science journalism.

Following my father's footsteps, my biggest hope is to improve the lives of others. That is what my dad devoted his own life to. He grew up in Brooklyn, the child of parents who had migrated from Eastern Europe, escaping the Holocaust. He took an IQ test in high school: it was off the charts. He didn't have to take any science courses during his last two years of high school because he knew the syllabi better than his teachers did. And at fifteen, he made the decision to dedicate his life to cancer research. He never looked back.

What a cruel twist of irony it was that as he was directing the Rush University Cancer Center in Chicago, he was cut down in the prime of his life by the very disease he had dedicated his life to curing. I was only four when he was diagnosed and eight when he died. My parents took great pains to never mention the c-word in my earshot and yet most of my memories of Dad are related, at least in part, to the presence of this nameless "other" in our lives.

Even though I was too young to know what was going on at any tangible level, I had some sort of instinctual knowledge that something was terribly wrong. I could sense my mother's struggle as she was navigating through stages of optimism, pain, dread, despondency, and eventually hopelessness as my dad underwent a seemingly endless stream of experimental treatments. These stages are what most cancer patients and their caregivers experience.

Another example is Andrew, one of my best friends. In the spring of 2016, he developed numbness and tingling in his arm, which made him exercise more vigorously. One afternoon, while visiting family upstate, he felt weakness in his right arm. He was driven to the NY General Hospital emergency room. Within days, Andrew was quadriplegic: a nine-centimeter tumor was found in his neck. During the emergency operation, neurosurgeons couldn't completely remove the glioblastoma multiforme that had already enveloped several upper vertebrae.

The year that followed was characterized by a mixture of hope, fear, anxiety, panic, pain, more pain. Too much pain. Andrew received round after round of chemotherapy, radiation therapy, immune therapy, more surgery, placement of a shunt, and then more chemotherapy and more radiation and more immune therapy. Throughout all these treatments, Andrew experienced indescribable agony and discomfort from the side effects, yet the tumors continued to multiply. He lost his battle on August 25, 2017. Andrew

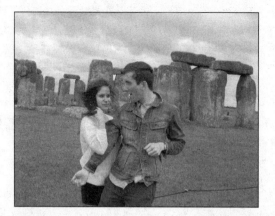

was twenty-three years old. What struck me the most throughout his ordeal, during which our friends and family never left his side, was his positivity and selflessness. He never lost hope that he'd get better, and spending time with him—even in the ICU—felt like we were just hanging out. He rarely—if ever—complained and always went out of his way to ask everyone else about themselves and shifted the focus away from himself.

Some of the best times of my life involve traveling through Europe with Andrew and our other two best friends, Rebecca and Charles. We had a great time clubbing in Berlin, visiting Versailles and the Louvre in Paris, fighting over bunk beds in London. Throughout his illness, we sat with his mother and sister, his grandmother and father, at NY General Hospital and at NY Hospital, laughing with Andrew, crying among ourselves in the waiting room, choking over food at night thinking how Andrew could not even swallow his own saliva, and staying up night after night in a cold sweat, dreading the worst.

Andrew and I shared December birthdays. Alas, neither Andrew nor my dad will be with me to celebrate my twenty-fourth this year. Picking up a yellow rose petal from Andrew's grave and handing it to my mother for safekeeping forever, I realized that both my childhood and entry into adult life have been marked by the intrusion of this "other": cancer. I have been forced to look at life itself through a prism of psychological and physical suffering *caused by this deadly disease, for which there seems to be no solution. For me, life can never be business as usual.*

I stand here today and entreat you not to forget what Harvey Preisler and Andrew Slootsky went through and what thousands of cancer patients are going through every day. I am deeply humbled by the courage and nobility of endurance I witnessed firsthand in my father and in Andrew. Let us pledge to work together at all costs to help all cancer patients.

〰

I HAVE TOLD the stories of men and women facing death. These remarkable souls continued to inspire and humble their caregivers by their poise, their dignity, their grit, right to the very end. Death is not a failure, pervasive societal denial is. Greek gods could not accept mortality. Humans do.

Immortals are mortal, mortals immortal,
one living the others' death, and one dying the others' life.

—HERACLITUS

THE DAWN
HAS ALREADY
ARRIVED

MY OLDER SISTER AMERA, MY BROTHER TASNIM, AND I TOOK OUR mother shopping in Buffalo one sunny summer afternoon in 1988 when she was visiting from Karachi. Tasnim, a cardiac surgeon at Buffalo General Hospital, had already performed hundreds of coronary bypass surgeries, and his group was leading the charge in heart transplants in western New York. It was impossible to walk fifty feet in the mall without being stopped by one of his cured patients, pumping his hand enthusiastically, beaming at our mother, awash in gratitude because her son had heroically saved their lives. Of course, at home, Tasnim was less eulogized, we siblings refusing to let him develop the God-complex of surgeons. We teased him mercilessly at family gatherings. My sister Sughra would innocently ask, "Aps, what do you call two cardiac surgeons looking at an EKG?" I would reply, deadpan, "A double-blind study!" Thankfully, no one likes a joke better than Tasnim, who would gleefully address the pediatrician (my sister Atiya), radiologist (my sister Sughra), and oncologist (me), "Statistically speaking, nine out of ten injections you ladies give are in vein." He loved calling us by an acronym that we reserved for some of our ex-boyfriends—"Hello, sisters, what is the NATO group up to this evening?" (*NATO* being our code word for No Action Talk Only)—or he would ask us sweetly if we had heard of the mechanic, working on the heart surgeon's motorbike, who said, "So, Doc, look at this engine. I open its heart, take the valves out, repair any damage, and then put them back in, and when I finish, it works just like new. So how come I make $40,000 a year and you get $40,000 a month?" The surgeon replied smugly, "Try doing it with the engine running."

As we were returning home, my mother asked the question I had been dreading.

"You have been in Buffalo for almost ten years. I have never met any of your patients. Why are heart patients doing so much better than cancer patients?"

She had put her finger on the heart of the matter. Tasnim and I often had the same conversation. Our conclusion—heart doctors recognized that the only effective treatment was prevention and early intervention. The equivalent of cancer in heart disease would be a heart so severely damaged that the only possible treatment would be a transplant. Advanced cancer is like this end-stage heart disease, where only extreme, heroic measures have the potential for saving lives.

"So why don't you find ways to diagnose cancer early also?" my mother asked. She was pleased to hear that devoting my life to understanding and treating MDS was my attempt to do precisely that—catch the leukemia early. "I am glad you are living in America, then. You will have an easier time convincing your colleagues to alter their attitudes. In Pakistan, the systems would be impossible to change in one lifetime."

She regularly inquired about my progress in MDS, and when she died less than three months before Harvey in 2002, I sat by her coffin-draped body in the Defense Housing Society Imambarda in Karachi, feeling strangely orphaned in an intellectual sense. I discovered at a deeply experiential level how much strength I had derived from her super-confidence in me, how much I looked forward to our weekly long-distance conversations over the phone, talking about everything under the sun, but especially about my work, which she found fascinating. There was a good reason why we called her the rocket scientist of the family.

> *Kis ko ab hoga watan mein aah! mera intezar?*
> *Kaun mera khat na aanay se rahay ga beqarar?*
> —ALLAMA IQBAL

> Now who will wait for me, alas! In my homeland?
> Who will agonize when my letter does not arrive?

∽

SO WHY DON'T WE FIND WAYS TO DIAGNOSE CANCER EARLY?

Arrogance. Overconfidence. Contempt.

These are the words of Robert Weinberg. He is a founding member of the Whitehead Institute for Biomedical Research at MIT, the recipient of the National Medal of Science and the Keio Medical Science Prize. He used these words to describe the attitude of molecular biologists who arrived like knights on white horses to solve the cancer problem through their reductionist approach back in the mid-1970s.

> We were, after all, reductionists, who would parse *cancer cells* down to their smallest molecular details and develop useful, universally applicable lessons about the mechanisms of cancer development. We would somehow develop logical order out of the phenomenological chaos that the traditional cancer researchers had been accumulating for more than half a century.
>
> Arrogance like this is never appreciated, and so we tried to keep it under wraps. We were aware of the sensitivities of the ruling barons of cancer research and tried to be non-confrontational. We couched our work in molecular biological terms that were unthreatening for

those who had toiled for generations without making much headway into the simple questions of what cancer was and how it began. We knew, all along, that simple answers to complex questions would be greeted with mixed feelings by the large community of more traditional cancer researchers. After all, if we succeeded, we might put many of them out of business.

I suppose our self-confidence was necessary to make our way through the endless complexity represented by neoplastic disease: We needed to ignore the objections that the old-line cancer researchers repeatedly tossed into our path; they said that cancer was really much too complicated to be understood through simple molecular mechanisms. Indeed, they portrayed our reductionism as simplistic if not simple-minded.

We have seen that the current cancer landscape is worse than it was in the 1970s. Even today, 95 percent of experimental trials continue to fail. The 5 percent that do succeed extend life of patients by a few months at the cost of millions of dollars. These are roundly touted as paradigm-shifting treatments, game changers. The situation is, both morally and fiscally, profoundly irresponsible. By law, the FDA can only take safety and efficacy data into account when reviewing a drug for approval, not its price tag. On the other hand, Medicare has to cover the cost of a more expensive drug with the same efficacy as a cheaper one if both are FDA approved. My colleague Antonio Fojo, a researcher and oncologist who worked at the National Cancer Institute for three decades, provides a sobering calculation of the cost of health care while reviewing several trials for new cancer treatments:

In the lung cancer trial, overall survival improved by just 1.2 months on average. The cost for an extra 1.2 months of survival? About $80,000. If we allow a survival advantage of 1.2 months to be worth $80,000, and by extrapolation survival of one year to be valued at $800,000, we would need $440 billion annually—an amount nearly 100 times the budget of the National Cancer Institute—to extend by one year the life of the 550,000 Americans who die of cancer annually. And no one would be cured.

I had a recent experience underscoring the truth of Robert Weinberg's criticisms of oncology researchers. I got a call from a young PhD scientist who was preparing to submit an application for an NIH grant. Apparently, he had been studying a gene in animal models, and now it looked like the gene could have a role in abnormal signaling seen in MDS cells. He was preparing a request for a three-year grant. In the first two years, he proposed to examine the role of this gene in a mouse model of MDS. If this showed any relevance, he would like to test human samples. Would I be willing to provide him those samples?

Of course, I want to help MDS patients in every way I can, which means that I will support any and every researcher interested in studying their disease. I pointed out that I would like to work with him as an equal intellectual partner and collaborator, not as a source who blindly hands over the extremely precious samples. Obviously, I am concerned that the samples I have collected at great financial cost to me and great physical pain to the patient may be squandered on thoughtless experiments by an inexperienced researcher. Further, I would like to decide with him what and how to study the samples. There are absolutely *no* mouse models or tissue culture cell lines that even remotely recapitulate the human disease. Why spend an enormous amount of resources for two years trying to determine if this gene was important in human MDS by studying absurdly artificial systems? It would make more sense to examine the human tissue first and see whether any follow-up studies were worth pursuing.

Sadly, several things became clear. The young man had no idea about the human disease MDS, nor did he care to know more about it unless his mouse model showed it could be relevant for his research. I offered to meet so we could discuss what is important for MDS patients and determine how his research interests could align with those patient needs. He again politely refused. All he wanted was an official letter of support from me that could be clipped to his grant application attesting to the fact that he would have access to human samples in year three of his grant. Most grant applications follow the same trajectory, leading to an enormous waste of resources.

After a few decades of accumulating strangeness in the field, we have come to a point when there is little connection between where we started and where we have arrived. To change a situation, one has to first lift the blinders and dare to see the situation for what it is. By trying to fit an impossibly complex problem into a straightforward, simplistic, linear narrative, cancer research has reached a new reductio ad absurdum milestone. There is a crisis in the field. The bizarreness of things we are doing both in clinical and basic science research is effectively cloaked under important-sounding terms, conveying a reassuring sense of objectivity—best practices, evidence-based medicine, precision oncology, genetically engineered mice. Mostly we have euphemisms to sweeten the bitter truth that we don't really have better treatments than what we were offering fifty years ago.

In 1980, I was briefly at George Washington University and frequently had lunch with Dr. Ayub Ommaya, the great Pakistani neurosurgeon who invented the Ommaya reservoir for delivering drugs into the brain. He was obsessed with everything to do with the brain. I once asked him what he thought would be the final level of reductionism needed to sight the root of consciousness. "Azra, taking apart the Taj Mahal brick by brick to discover the source of its beauty will yield only rubble. It is the same with the brain. The emergent complexity from simple individual parts accounts for its essential mystery." It is also the reason why cancer will not yield its secrets through a reductionist approach.

Cancer, when it appears, is sudden. And yet it is also the result of a gradual accumulation of small changes, intricately tied to aging. Each perhaps is inconsequential by itself, but each contributes toward the eventual instability of the system. I talked about a growing pile of sand and how the concept of critical states explains the way a single grain can set off an avalanche. In a similar manner, the biologic disturbances bubbling under the surface in an aging body tip the system toward entropy in a slow, unrelenting manner, such that cancer can arise suddenly from what, in other circumstances, would be an inconsequential event. Self-organized criticality develops both inside the cell and in its microenvironment with age. Reductionism calls for finding the "cancer gene." But what tips a system into cancer isn't necessarily a particular mutation but the last mutation that causes the avalanche, a catastrophic phase-transition into cancer. That mutation may be no different in lethality from thousands of others, which the cell's DNA sustained over the years. Similarly, the one senescent cell whose appearance tips the garbage-collecting system, causing the soil to become pro-inflammatory, too toxic for healthier cells, is no different from the million others before it. With age, the entire system, the seed and the soil, like a growing pile of sand, becomes more and more prone to unpredictable, abrupt collapses. The question should really be why cancer does not occur in *every* old person. The answer is because juxtaposition of the immortalized mutated seed with the appropriately poisoned soil, the perfect "fitness landscape," happens rarely.

Cancer and aging are two sides of the same coin. Understanding one, in all its granularity, can automatically reveal the secrets of the other. This is how complex cancer is. It is pure arrogance to think the problem can be solved by a few molecular biologists if they put their minds to it. Cancer is a perfidious, treacherous, evolving, shifting, moving target, far too impenetrable to be deconstructed systematically, far too dense to lend itself in all its plurality to recapitulation in lab dishes or animals.

⚭

MDS CAN BE a deadly disease by itself without necessarily transforming to leukemia. I became interested in identifying individuals at risk of developing this preleukemic condition, a pre-MDS state. In fact, we do know of at least one such high-risk group—patients previously treated with chemoradiation therapy for other cancers have a very small (1–2 percent) chance of developing MDS, sometimes many years after having received the toxic agents. My idea was to identify MDS-susceptible individuals by monitoring cancer survivors through twice-yearly "liquid biopsies" and look for the appearance of markers associated with MDS. In 1998, I began to obtain blood samples from patients treated previously for breast, prostate, lung, and GI cancers and lymphomas. We collected and stored hundreds of samples along with accompanying clinical information on these patients in the tissue repository. I applied for a grant, formally starting the TIME Center (Therapy Induced Malignancy Evaluation), and received incredibly generous support from the Women's Board of Rush University.

After Harvey died and I moved out of Chicago, I was able to transfer the entire tissue repository with me. However, as the accompanying research charts of patients were being loaded on the moving truck, despite having all the requisite permissions of the institutional review board, hospital lawyers, and a hundred administrators, an uninvolved nurse supervisor arrived on the scene and decided to take matters into her own hands. She informed my program directors, Dr. Naomi Galili and Laurie Lisak, PA, supervising the move that some of the research charts looked thicker than actual patient charts from which they were copied so she could not let them leave the university premises until she made sure that every chart was an exact duplicate. The majority of them were the charts of the TIME Center patients. Of course, there was an obvious reason for this discrepancy. Because of the chaos following Harvey's prolonged illness and death, we had not yet computerized the research charts, and all the research data were also present in those actual physical hard copies along with the duplicated clinical records. She was not willing to listen to any explanation and directed the movers to unload hundreds of research files, promising prompt release once she had cleared her confusion. Needless to say, despite trying for years, I have been unable to overcome the institutional red tape. It was always about the two institutions involved in legal issues of intellectual property rights and data ownership. Long letters of appeal not just to the chair of the IRB and chair of medicine at the university but even to the FDA to intervene have been in vain. As a result of the university's recalcitrance, the TIME Center charts are rotting in a warehouse in Chicago and the samples in my freezers at Columbia. We can do nothing with the samples without the accompanying clinical information.

While I have been unable to make use of these precious TIME Center samples, I was delighted to see a study led by Pinkal Desai, who found somatic mutations in blood samples obtained as part of the Women's Health Initiative, sometimes years before the appearance of acute myeloid leukemia in some of these individuals. This study validates my concept of the TIME Center inaugurated two decades ago. It is critical to study our TIME Center samples today because many of those individuals must have developed MDS by now, and we are missing a golden opportunity to understand what is unique about them. It is also the type of biomarker information needed to design strategies for detecting the first cell. But once more, bureaucracy became, as James Boran pointed out, the glue that greased the wheels of progress. A system has evolved geared more toward protecting institutions and less toward protecting patients. Another example of this is the "Informed Consent Form" for experimental trials. Nowadays, these can run up to dozens of pages and contain paragraph after paragraph of confusing, cut-and-paste language, demanded by the NIH, FDA, IRB, and trial sponsors, which has little relevance for the patient. Most patients look baffled when presented with these forms. By law, we also have to insist that they read every word of the document before signing. One of my patients threw up his arms in utter desperation. "Dr. Raza, first I need to hire a lawyer to explain this to me!"

❦

BECAUSE I HAVE been speaking and writing about cancer and its discontents for years, I am familiar with the common misunderstandings that arise in the minds of my audience. I am *not* saying that all scientific research on animal models should be abandoned. What I am saying is that animal models are misleading and harmful for *cancer drug development,* because the disease cannot be reproduced in such simplistic, artificial systems. I am *not* saying that all cancer research should stop except that related to early detection. What I am saying is that more resources have to be dedicated to this area. I am *not* saying that technologies like CRISPR are all hype. What I am saying is that the discovery of CRISPR as a tool in molecular biology is truly revolutionary, but its application in fixing human cancer cells by cutting and pasting DNA needs years of careful study before commercializing it into billion-dollar companies. I am *not* saying that advances in cancer treatment are entirely absent. What I am saying is that they are too few, occurring in an incremental manner, not curative, extend survival by months at best, and at this rate will take too long to make a substantial difference in decades to come. I am *not* saying that immune therapies, especially CAR-T cell therapies, are universally overrated, empty promises. What I am saying is that so far, they have only benefited a subset of highly select patients. They are a long way from becoming the routine in clinic because of their dreadful physical, psychological, emotional, and financial toxicities, as well as the lack of suitable, specific target identification. I am *not* saying that cancer researchers are insincere and driven only by personal greed. Of course mostly everyone is sincere and has good intentions. What I am saying is that the cancer paradigm has reached a grotesque, unrecognizable, destabilized end point. The entire society needs to pause, think deeply about the overall complexity of our challenge, and admit that presently, we lack even the conceptual archetypes for solving so dense a problem. The public needs to demand that more of their tax dollars support researchers developing strategies for early detection of cancer that don't require detailed, intricate understanding of every molecular signaling pathway in a cancer cell.

I COULD NOT have written this book when I was thirty years old. After being in this field for all of my adult life, I am even more invested in demanding a complete overhaul of the current cancer culture that has evolved. I know that mine is a small, relatively lonely voice in the field, but I refuse to be silenced. I received a lesson in the power of individual engagement quite early on in my career. An international conference was organized in the United States, to which, despite strong opposition and threats of a boycott, researchers and oncologists from an apartheid-ridden South Africa were invited. The protesters were warned not to make a brouhaha, because there is no politics in medicine, cancer is a universal issue, and the platform being provided to the presenters was critical for precisely this reason—racially diverse cancer patients could be compared in an international setting. Tensions were high in the cavernous hall where the white South African team presented their data showing that the incidence of esophageal cancer in the Bantu natives was higher than that in the white population. At the end of the presentation, there was total silence until one young African American oncologist raised his hand, stood up, and calmly asked in a loud, controlled, powerful voice, "Dr. Johnson, do you think that the incidence of esophageal cancer in the Bantu natives is high because of swallowed pride?"

There is no activism without despair, no despair without hope. Despair can be as powerful an engine for change as hope. In the cases of Omar and Andrew, there was no best decision. The question for them was not what to choose but how to achieve a balance between hope and despair. Once it became known that the primary tumors were not removed in their entirety, their choices were to die of the cancer or of the treatment. Which was less painful? False hope and positive narratives are not the answer. Barbara Ehrenreich in a telling passage writes about her diagnosis of breast cancer: "The trick, as my teen hero Camus wrote, is to draw strength from the 'refusal to hope, and the unyielding evidence of a life without consolation.' To be hope-free is to acknowledge the lion in the tall grass, the tumor in the CAT scan, and to plan one's moves accordingly."

If hope can help individuals survive seemingly impossible odds, despair can galvanize efforts to seek solutions. The practice of Sufism consists entirely in welcoming and enduring affliction precisely for this reason. Negative emotions can be useful if they influence the future by serving as a motivation for transformation. In an ontological leap, affliction and despair lead to agency, seeking explicit solutions, exploring possibilities for a radically different future. An accounting of cancer's unresolved scientific complexities alongside the toll of human suffering should serve as a tool with which to pry open new ways of critical thinking, a grander global vision, a positive outlook toward our world. A hope that of all possible outcomes in the future, alleviation of pain and distress from cancer can and will happen, positive change, both individual and societal, will occur.

The burden of this book, from its opening paragraphs, has been to chronicle the intimacies of cancer kept confident by those who experience its anguish. The conceit is my absolute conviction that the engine driving social and scientific progress in quantum leaps, rather than in unbearably slow increments, is one fueled by empathy. Only the profound suffering of cancer patients has the power to ignite a brand of compassion necessary for demanding urgent and dramatic change. Only empathy can break the foolish consistency that is the hobgoblin of oncology and little minds. The future is in preventing cancer by identifying the earliest markers of the first cancer cell rather than chasing after the last. I have been saying this since 1984, and I will continue to say it until someone listens.

For the individual with eyes, the dawn has already arrived.

—ALI IBN ABI TALIB

KHATAM SHUD

Acknowledgments

I WROTE THE INITIAL DRAFT OF *THE FIRST CELL* IN THREE MONTHS. My nephew Asad Raza pointed out, "Achi, you have been writing this book for thirty years. You just downloaded it in three months." True. I owe *TFC* entirely to the profound impact that patients have had on my life for the past three decades. Sadly, for all the commitment and dedication, I have very little to show for it in terms of improvement in their treatment outcomes. So I begin this section by acknowledging my failures and apologizing to all the patients for not having done more to help.

But tried I have. Every chance I got, I have spoken up about these issues, written extensively on various problematic aspects of the current cancer paradigm, appeared on radio and television, delivered a TEDx talk, given interviews and podcasts. To what end? I have not managed to change many minds. Everyone listens to me sympathetically, and then they go back to doing whatever they were doing before. I finally had a little break when I answered the 2014 annual Edge Foundation question, "What scientific idea is ready for retirement?" My answer—"Mouse models are the real elephants in the room"—was noticed by the media. It grabbed attention because of the controversial nature of my claims. Even a negative reaction is better than no reaction. Oscar Wilde said, "There is only one thing worse than being talked about, and that is not being talked about." I was invited on NPR. I was interviewed on *Freakonomics Radio*. Sporadically, I started to receive notes of support. Alan Schechter from NIH and Robert Perlman from the University of Chicago applauded my efforts to unmask the problems with the reductionist approach and use of mouse models in cancer drug development.

John Brockman, founder of the Edge Foundation, who "runs the world's smartest website," brought his wife, Katinka Matson, for dinner to my apartment one evening. "You want better answers for your cancer patients. You want researchers to stop fooling around with mouse models. You want oncologists to treat patients differently. You want nothing less than a paradigm shift in cancer studies and treatment. Write a book. Only someone like you, an insider in the field, can raise these issues. The public will take note if your message is compelling enough. A conversation could begin," said sweet Katinka, gently encouraging me. John, on the other hand, known for his brutal bluntness, and not one to mince words, patted my back affectionately. "Put up or shut up, kid. Send us a proposal. By next week."

My first instinct, given the hectic work schedule I keep between seeing patients and supervising a very busy cancer research lab, as well as teaching and administrative duties, was to tell my story to a professional writer. I called Zara Houshmand, a dear friend, who has ghost-written several hugely successful books, and she talked me right out of it. Thanks, Zara!

I wrote to my younger brother Abbas in Italy for advice. Abbas is the founder of the website 3 Quarks Daily. More importantly, he is my most trusted editor in chief. I have published original pieces at 3 Quarks Daily over the years, parts of several of which are included in this book (including Omar, Per, War on Cancer, Harvey, and Laura; a small portion of Lady N. appeared in the *MDS Beacon*). Abbas is extraordinarily well read and has an unparalleled instinct in matters related to both science and literature. He said, "Aps, I had to think really, really hard about your question of whether to listen to John and

Katinka or not. For exactly three seconds. Yes. Of course they are right. Get on with it immediately." Asad, the author of several amazing books on art and artists, said, "Achi, it is a badly needed book. From my experience, I can tell you it will take approximately eighteen months. Please start right now. Just write what you have been telling us over the years. That's all. Do it." I did. Here we are. Thanks, John, Katinka, and Max Brockman. Thanks, Abbas and Asad.

When I was considering thalidomide for Harvey, I called Owen O'Connor, the chief of lymphoma service at Memorial Sloan Kettering Cancer Center in New York, to seek his advice. I had never met or spoken to Owen before, but after I told him the reason for my call, he gave me his home and cell numbers, urging me to call any time of day or night if I needed help. This was the reaction of practically every colleague around the country I contacted for advice throughout Harvey's illness. Extraordinary compassion, incredible willingness to help, unconditional offers of their time and expertise. We traveled to Boston to see John Gribben at Dana-Farber and Bruce Chabner at Mass General; we consulted Ron Levy in California and called Harvey's beloved, longtime best friend, Kanti Rai, in New York. Kanti found reasons to come to Chicago many times in the ensuing years, providing not just expert medical advice but much-needed and much-appreciated comfort at a personal level.

Despite our habit of sorrow in those days, moments of such radical kindness and consideration from oncologists around the country and, more locally, from the nurses and medical staff, secretaries and lab assistants, scientific colleagues and administrative officers at Rush University lit up our lives with the comforting radiance of their acts. My deepest gratitude is owed to Lakshmi Venugopal, Sairah Alvi, Vila Ravanam, Suneel Mundle, Laurie Lisak, Minnie King, Beverly Burge, Chris Kasper, and Naomi and Uri Galili, who were ever present to help Harvey and to hold my hand and take care of business when Harvey and I were indisposed because of his illness. I cannot recall one single instance in almost five years of Harvey's illness—innumerable tests, hundreds of clinic visits, and dozens of hospitalizations later—when we registered a complaint of even the slightest significance against the medical establishment, either privately or publicly. Everyone stepped up to do more than we'd expected. Drs. Steve Rosen, Hans Klingemann, Parameswaran Venugopal, Jamile Shammo, Seema Singhal, Jayesh Mehta, Stephanie Gregory, Sefer Gezer, Raphael Borok, and Phil Bonomi took care of Harvey as if he were a family member. Leo Henikoff, the president of Rush University, and his brilliant wife, Carole Travis Henikoff, were sources of extraordinary friendship and support at every level. Most loving and helpful was our dear friend, colleague, and an all-around wise person, the chairman of medicine at Rush, Stuart Levin. The manner in which Stu calmly and quietly provided strength and solace to both Harvey and me during five years of Harvey's illness can never be repaid in words. As Harvey was taking his last breaths, the person I called was Stu. He was by my side in minutes. He stayed until the death certificate was signed and all the formalities were taken care of.

Sol Barer, the founder of Celgene, and Jerry Zeldis, the chief medical officer, two visionary leaders who would transform the little, unknown company worth a few million dollars into a global biopharmaceutical behemoth worth tens of billions, stepped up to help when I most needed them by providing thalidomide and Revlimid on a compassionate basis for Harvey. They have remained dear friends these twenty years later, as has their successor, the talented and deeply empathetic Mark Alles. Mohamad Hussein at Celgene has been a rock-solid friend for decades.

Seema and Vania's presence was a godsend. They shared the happiest of times with us in Chicago and saw us through the heartbreak right to the end. Harvey gave instructions for his cremation to Vania. On the home front, I could not have survived in America without the unconditional love, nurturing, and benevolence of my beloved brother-in-law Tariq Khan, a superbly trained surgical oncologist with a second career as the best ER physician. In addition to Sarah, Mark, Vanessa, and my siblings, all of whom kept in touch constantly and made frequent visits to Chicago to see Harvey, it is to Irshad and Muhammad

Mumtaz that I owe a profound debt of gratitude. The concept of daily existence without them in my life does not exist anymore. No one did more to help with Harvey when he became incapacitated than these two devoted souls.

Early readers of the book to whom I am greatly indebted for invaluable feedback include my siblings Amera, Atiya, Tasnim, Javed, Sughra, and Abbas Raza and my sister-in-law Nazli Raza. Other early readers in the family and beloved friends include Zaineb Beams, Jaffer Kolb, Musa Raza, Zehra Raza, Carol Westbrook, Kanti Rai, Bob Gallo, Mary Jane Gallo, Naomi Galili, Seema Khan, Siddhartha Mukherjee, Darryl Pitt, Connie Young, Nermeen Shaikh, Stavroula Kousteni, Ellen Cole, David Steensma, Steve Rosen, Candi Rosen, Rafia Zakaria, Shan Rizvi, Nancy Bachrach, Susan Bates, Tito Fojo, and Anisa Hasan. Laura Claridge read the first chapter, gave me the green light, and has since supported me throughout. Ivana Cruz and Darryl Pitt helped clarify my thinking about the jacket design by producing some gorgeous alternate versions.

Abdullah Ali is the son I did not have and, fortunately, the director of the MDS translational research program at Columbia University. He read the earliest version of *TFC* and gave brilliant suggestions, as did Naomi Galili, my most trusted, beloved friend and scientific colleague and the previous director of the MDS research program. Abdullah provides me with the strength to continue in my single-minded quest for the first cell and is equally motivated by the philosophy of only pursuing what is best for the patients. He is my right hand and my go-to scientific compass on a daily basis. I can never thank Abdullah enough, so I thank my lucky stars that brought him into my life when I was heartbroken over Naomi's retirement. Naomi is supremely talented in the sciences and possesses a profoundly sensitive soul. She was a joy to have as a colleague in the lab, someone who got the centrality of the patient in even our most basic research endeavors.

At Columbia University, I am grateful for the strong support I have received for a decade from the chairman of medicine, Don Landry; the dean, Lee Goldman; and, since he arrived, the chief of the division, Gary Schwartz. They have protected me from unnecessary bureaucratic entanglements and have wholeheartedly cheered my efforts on behalf of the patients. I am also deeply grateful for the collegiality and excellence of my medical and scientific colleagues. Over the years, some have become close personal friends: Greg Mears, Stavroula Kousteni, Connie Young, Emmanuelle Passegue, Joe Jurcic, Mark Heaney, Nicole Lamanna, Craig Blinderman, Hamza Habib, Riccardo Dalla-Favera, Emerson Lim, Chuck Drake, Susan Bates, Tito Fojo, Abbas Manji, and David Diuguid. A big thanks to the incredible staff of our offices and clinics, the nurses and administrative assistants, whose devotion and compassion for the patients strike awe in hearts. After the cancer patients themselves, it is to these selfless, dedicated medical staff that I owe the inspiration to write this book.

Siddhartha Mukherjee and Sarah Sze are like family, or as Sid says, "Azra, you are a cross between my mother and my editor." Writing a book about cancer after *The Emperor of All Maladies* is almost heretical, especially because I am Sid's biggest admirer. It is one of the greatest joys in my life to spend time with Sid, whether we are batting scientific ideas back and forth, arguing in lab meetings, laughing at Bollywood jokes, or transported into ecstasy by Sid's divine renditions of Indian classical vocals, accompanied by my adopted son, the great Ustad Ikhlaq Hussain, on sitar, lasting into the early morning hours.

My dearest friend and coauthor of *Ghalib: Epistemologies of Elegance*, Sara Suleri Goodyear, read the earliest drafts, talked me through many difficult decisions, gave thoughtful, incredibly helpful suggestions, and gave me moral support when I was overcome with grief periodically while writing some parts of the book.

I want to acknowledge the women who have influenced my way of thinking greatly over the course of a lifetime; my mother, Begum Zaheer Fatima; my younger sister Sughra Raza; my friends Seema Khan, Maliha Hussein, Sara Suleri Goodyear, and the great Urdu writer Qurratulain Hyder (Aini Apa), whose friendship meant the world to me. The four teachers with the biggest impact on my early thinking include Qamar Jehan, Farhat Aziz Muazzam, Nikhat Afroz, and Afroze Begum.

Karachi life is unthinkable without my cousin Qasim Raza; my sister-in-law Arfa Raza; my friends Seema Khan, Anisa Asim Haider, Mansoora Ahmed Sheikh, Meher Fatima, Nigar Khan, Anisa Hussain Hasan, Shakeela Khan, Farrukh Seir, Tahir Alvi, Mehro Hamid, Tariq Shakoor, Rashid Jooma, and Sheena and Jamil (Jimmy) Malik.

New York felt like home from the moment Sheherzad and I moved here in 2007 because of the friendship, warmth, and protection provided by Anees and Rafat Mahdi and Marina and Shaukat Fareed.

At Basic Books, Liz Stein edited the first draft of the book, and I thank her for her incredible effort and sympathetic reading. Liz Wetzel, Kelsey Odorczyk, Rachel Field, Melissa Veronesi, and my copy editors Sara and Chris Ensey have been unbelievably thorough and supportive.

TJ Kelleher, my editor, recognized that the patient stories were worth telling, the message compelling and timely, from the moment he read my book proposal, all the way up to this final version, overseeing every aspect of editing. While I was regularly astounded by the depth of TJ's scientific understanding, it is his exquisite sensitivity that helped me polish some of the rust off dense sentences upon many rounds of rereading and editing. Lara Heimert, our publisher, is sui generis; incredibly brilliant, she is quick to spot the good and the bad. Lara stepped in at crucial moments to weigh in with suggestions, commands, and appropriate hand-holding as required.

Thanks to all the present and future patients who continue to humble us every day with unparalleled grace. Know that there are thousands of devoted oncologists ready to listen to you, advocate for you, and thousands of scientists moving heaven and earth to find solutions to your problems. Thanks to all the clinical and basic cancer researchers and the incredibly hardworking, dedicated oncologists spread throughout the country, working night and day to help cancer patients. I have had the great good fortune to interact with many extraordinary colleagues in these last three decades. So much of what this book says is owed to what they have taught me.

My best teacher, one who shaped my personality and my thinking in profound ways, is of course Harvey. I was fortunate to find so unique a mentor when I was barely twenty-four, one who insisted that the only things that matter are excellence and a serious pursuit of truth, and that after all is said and done, the most beautiful thing in life is still an adult intimate relationship.

Lastly, I thank my daughter, Sheherzad, whose unconditional love for and confidence in me and whose intellect and courage are so totally Harvey that it is frightening. She has sustained me through some rough patches in the last two decades. Above all, Sheher has witnessed the ravages of cancer at a deeply personal level, as she watched her father and her best friend succumb in excruciating and painful installments to its exacting malevolence. Here's to hoping she will continue to promote the mission of her parents by serving cancer patients in every capacity possible and always with sensitivity and humility.

Bibliography

NOTE: Sources in the bibliography coincide with the order in which they appear in the text.

INTRODUCTION: FROM LAST TO FIRST

DeVita, Vincent T., Jr., Alexander M. M. Eggermont, Samuel Hellman, and David J. Kerr. "Clinical Cancer Research: The Past, Present and the Future." *Nature Reviews Clinical Oncology.* 11, no. 11 (2014): 663–669.

Horgan, John. "Sorry, but So Far War on Cancer Has Been a Bust." *Scientific American,* May 21, 2014.

El-Deiry, Wafik S. "Are We Losing the War on Cancer?" *Cancer Biology & Therapy* 14, no. 12 (2013): 1189–1190.

Davis, Devra. *The Secret History of the War on Cancer.* New York: Basic Books, 2007.

Scannell, J. W., et al. "Diagnosing the Decline in Pharmaceutical R&D Efficiency." *Nature Reviews Drug Discovery* 11 (2012): 191–200.

Chandrasekar, Thenappan. "Why Are We Losing the War on Cancer?" 2018 European Society for Medical Oncology Congress (#ESMO18), October 19–23, 2018, Munich, Germany. www.urotoday.com/conference-highlights/esmo-2018/esmo-2018-prostate-cancer/107789-esmo-2018-why-we-are-losing-the-war-on-cancer.html.

Ehrenreich, Barbara. *Bright-Sided: How the Relentless Promotion of Positive Thinking Has Undermined America.* New York: Metropolitan Books, 2009.

Baldwin, James. "Letter from a Region in My Mind." *New Yorker,* November 9, 1962.

Döhne, Hartmut, et al. "Diagnosis and Management of AML in Adults: 2017 ELN Recommendations from an International Expert Panel." *Blood* 129 (2017): 424–447.

LeBlanc, Thomas W., and Harry P. Erba. "Shifting Paradigms in the Treatment of Older Adults with AML." *Seminars in Hematology* 56, no. 2 (2019): 110–117.

Goldman, J. M. "Chronic Myeloid Leukemia: A Historical Perspective." *Seminars in Hematology* 47, no. 4 (2010): 302–311.

Lo-Coco, Francesco, and Laura Cicconi. "History of Acute Promyelocytic Leukemia: A Tale of Endless Revolution." *Mediterranean Journal of Hematology and Infectious Diseases* 3, no. 1 (2011): e2011067. doi:10.4084/MJHID.2011.067.

Mak, I. W., N. Evaniew, and M. Ghert. "Lost in Translation: Animal Models and Clinical Trials in Cancer Treatment." *American Journal of Translational Research* 6, no. 2 (2014): 114–118.

Wong, Chi Heem, Kien Wei Siah, and Andrew W. Lo. "Estimation of Clinical Trial Success Rates and Related Parameters." *Biostatistics* 20, no. 2 (2019): 273–286. https://doi.org/10.1093/biostatistics/kxx069.

Lowe, Derek. "A New Look at Clinical Success Rates." *Science Translational Medicine,* February 2, 2018. https://blogs.sciencemag.org/pipeline/archives/2018/02/02/a-new-look-at-clinical-success-rates.

Nixon, N. A. "Drug Development for Breast, Colorectal, and Non–Small Cell Lung Cancers from 1979 to 2014." *Cancer* 123, no. 23 (2017): 4672. www.nature.com/articles/nrd1470.

Hay, M., D. W. Thomas, J. L. Craighead, C. Economides, and J. Rosenthal. "Clinical Development Success Rates for Investigational Drugs." *Nature Biotechnology* 32 (2014): 40–51.

"95% of Promising Cancer Research Fails." Dying for a Cure, July 10, 2016. http://dyingforacure.org/blogs/95-promising-cancer-research-fails/.

Davis, C., et al. "Availability of Evidence of Benefits on Overall Survival and Quality of Life of Cancer Drugs Approved by European Medicines Agency: Retrospective Cohort Study of Drug Approvals 2009–13." *BMJ* (2017): 359. https://doi.org/10.1136/bmj.j4530.

Kola, I., and J. Landis. "Can the Pharmaceutical Industry Reduce Attrition Rates?" *Nature Reviews Drug Discovery* 3 (2004): 711–716. www.bmj.com/content/359/bmj.j4530?_ga = 2.220433373.434514445.1555067451-1576958994.1555067451; https://www.nature.com/articles/nrd1470.

Hay, M., et al. "Clinical Development Success Rates for Investigational Drugs." *Nature Biotechnology* 32, no. 1 (2014): 40–51.

Thomas, D. W., et al. *Clinical Development Success Rates, 2006–2015.* www.bio .org/sites/default/files/Clinical % 20Development % 20Success % 20Rates % 202006-2015 % 20- % 20BIO, % 20Biomedtracker, % 20Amplion % 20 2016.pdf.

Siegel, R. L., et al. "Cancer Statistics 2018." *CA* 68, no. 1 (2018): 7–30.

Siegel, R. L., et al. "Cancer Statistics 2019." *CA* 69, no. 1 (2019): 7–34.

"Cancer Death Rates Vary Greatly Among US Counties." American Cancer Society. www.cancer.org/latest-news/cancer-death-rates-vary-greatly-among -us-counties.html.

Mokdad, A. H., et al. "Trends and Patterns of Disparities in Cancer Mortality Among US Counties, 1980–2014." *JAMA* 317, no. 4 (2017): 388–406. doi:10.1001/jama.2016.20324.

Maeda, Hiroshi, and Mahin Khatami. "Analyses of Repeated Failures in Cancer Therapy for Solid Tumors: Poor Tumor-Selective Drug Delivery, Low Therapeutic Efficacy and Unsustainable Costs." *Clinical and Translational Medicine* 7, no. 1 (2018): 11.

Fojo, T., and C. Grady. "How Much Is Life Worth: Cetuximab, Non–Small Cell Lung Cancer, and the $440 Billion Question." *Journal of the National Cancer Institute* 101, no. 15 (2009): 1044–1049.

Kantarjian, Hagop M., et al. "Cancer Research in the United States: A Critical Review of Current Status and Proposal for Alternative Models." *Cancer* 124, no. 14 (2018): 2881–2889.

Carrera, P. M., et al. "The Financial Burden and Distress of Patients with Cancer: Understanding and Stepping-Up Action on the Financial Toxicity of Cancer Treatment." *CA,* January 16, 2018. https://doi.org/10.3322 /caac.21443.

Fojo, T., et al. "Unintended Consequences of Expensive Cancer Therapeutics— The Pursuit of Marginal Indications and a Me-Too Mentality That Stifles Innovation and Creativity: The John Conley Lecture." *JAMA Otolaryngology—Head & Neck Surgery* 140, no. 12 (2014): 1225–1236.

Krummel, M. F., and J. P. Allison. "CD28 and CTLA-4 Have Opposing Effects on the Response of T Cells to Stimulation." *Journal of Experimental Medicine* 182, no. 2 (1995): 459–465.

Davis, Daniel M. "The Rise of Cancer Immunotherapy: How Jim Allison Saved a Whole World." *Nautilus,* October 25, 2018.

Hutchinson, Lisa, and Rebecca Kirk. "High Drug Attrition Rates—Where Are We Going Wrong?" *Nature Reviews Clinical Oncology* 8, no. 4 (2011): 189–190.

Begley, G. C., and L. M. Ellis. "Raise Standards for Preclinical Cancer Research." *Nature* 483 (2012): 531–533.

Johnson, George. *The Cancer Chronicles: Unlocking Medicine's Deepest Mystery.* New York: Alfred A. Knopf, 2013.

Yong, Ed. "How to Fight Cancer When Cancer Fights Back." *Atlantic,* April 26, 2017.

Gilligan, A. M. "Death or Debt? National Estimates of Financial Toxicity in Persons with Newly-Diagnosed Cancer." *American Journal of Medicine* 131, no. 10 (2018): 1187–1199.

Baker, Monya. "1,500 Scientists Lift the Lid on Reproducibility: Survey Sheds Light on the 'Crisis' Rocking Research." *Nature,* May 25, 2016.

Cohen, J. D., et al. "Combined Circulating Tumor DNA and Protein Biomarker-Based Liquid Biopsy for the Earlier Detection of Pancreatic Cancers." *Proceedings of the National Academy of Sciences of the United States of America* 114, no. 38 (2017): 10202–10207.

Wang, Y., et al. "Detection of Tumor-Derived DNA in Cerebrospinal Fluid of Patients with Primary Tumors of the Brain and Spinal Cord." *Proceedings of the National Academy of Sciences of the United States of America* 112, no. 31 (2015): 9704–9709.

Bettegowda, C. "Detection of Circulating Tumor DNA in Early- and Late-Stage Human Malignancies." *Science Translational Medicine* 6, no. 224 (2014): 224ra24.

Vogelstein, Bert, Nickolas Papadopoulos, Victor E. Velculescu, Shibin Zhou, Luis A. Diaz, Jr., and Kenneth W. Kinzler. "Cancer Genome Landscapes." *Science* 339, no. 6127 (2013): 1546–1558.

"At the Forefront of Cancer Genetics, Bert Vogelstein, MD, Calls for Focus on Early Detection and Prevention." *ASCO Post,* June 3, 2017. www .ascopost.com/issues/june-3-2017-narratives-special-issue/at-the -forefront-of-cancer-genetics-bert-vogelstein-md-calls-for-focus-on-early -detection-and-prevention/.

DeVita, Vincent T., Jr., and Elizabeth DeVita-Raeburn. *The Death of Cancer.* New York: Sarah Crichton Books, 2015.

Ehrenreich, Barbara. *Natural Causes: An Epidemic of Wellness, the Certainty of Dying, and Killing Ourselves to Live Longer.* New York: Twelve, 2018.

CHAPTER 1: OMAR

Sullivan, Thomas. "A Tough Road: Cost to Develop One New Drug Is $2.6 Billion; Approval Rate for Drugs Entering Clinical Development Is Less Than 12 %." Policy and Medicine. www.policymed.com/2014/12/a-tough -road-cost-to-develop-one-new-drug-is-26-billion-approval-rate-for-drugs -entering-clinical-de.html.

DiMasi, J., et al. "Innovation in the Pharmaceutical Industry: New Estimates of R&D Costs." *Journal of Health Economics* 47 (2016): 20–33.

Wong, Chi Heem, Kien Wei Siah, and Andrew W. Lo. "Estimation of Clinical Trial Success Rates and Related Parameters." *Biostatistics* 20, no. 2 (2019): 273–286. https://doi.org/10.1093/biostatistics/kxx069.

Kim, Chul, and Vinay Prasad. "Cancer Drugs Approved on the Basis of a Surrogate End Point and Subsequent Overall Survival." *JAMA Internal Medicine* 175, no. 12 (2015): 1992–1994.

Maeda, Hiroshi, and Mahin Khatami. "Analyses of Repeated Failures in Cancer Therapy for Solid Tumors: Poor Tumor-Selective Drug Delivery, Low Therapeutic Efficacy and Unsustainable Costs." *Clinical and Translational Medicine* 7, no. 1 (2018): 11.

Kumar, Hemanth, Tito Fojo, and Sham Mailankody. "An Appraisal of Clinically Meaningful Outcomes Guidelines for Oncology Clinical Trials." *JAMA Oncology* 2, no. 9 (2016): 1238–1240.

Thomas, D. W., et al. *Clinical Development Success Rates, 2006–2015.* www .bio.org/sites/default/files/Clinical % 20Development % 20Success % 20 Rates % 202006-2015 % 20- % 20BIO, % 20Biomedtracker, % 20Amplion % 202016.pdf.

Philippidis, Alex. "Unlucky 13: Top Clinical Trial Failures in 2017." *Genetic Engineering & Biotechnology News.* www.genengnews.com/a-lists/unlucky -13-top-clinical-trial-failures-of-2017/.

Szabo, Liz. "Dozens of New Cancer Drugs Do Little to Improve Survival, Frustrating Patients." https://khn.org/news/dozens-of-new-cancer-drugs-do- -little-to-improve-survival-frustrating-patients/.

Rupp, Tracy, and Diana Zuckerman. "Quality of Life, Overall Survival, and Costs of Cancer Drugs Approved Based on Surrogate Endpoints." *JAMA Internal Medicine* 177, no. 2 (2017): 276–277. doi:10.1001 /jamainternmed.2016.7761.

Davis, C., C. Naci, E. Gurpinar, et al. "Availability of Evidence on Overall Survival and Quality of Life Benefits of Cancer Drugs Approved by the

European Medicines Agency: Retrospective Cohort Study of Drug Approvals from 2009–2013." *BMJ* (2017): 359.

Hall, Stephen S. *A Commotion in the Blood: Life, Death, and the Immune System.* New York: Henry Holt, 1997.

Sandomir, Richard. "Julie Yip-Williams, Writer of Candid Blog on Cancer, Dies at 42." *New York Times,* March 22, 2018. www.nytimes.com/2018/03 /22/obituaries/julie-yip-williams-dies-writer-of-candid-blog-on-cancer .html.

Yip-Williams, Julie. *The Unwinding of the Miracle: A Memoir of Life, Death, and Everything That Comes After.* New York: Random House, 2019.

Carrel, Alexis. "On the Permanent Life of Tissues Outside of the Organism." *Journal of Experimental Medicine* 15, no. 5 (1912): 516–528.

Friedman, David M. *The Immortalists: Charles Lindbergh, Dr. Alexis Carrel, and Their Daring Quest to Live Forever.* New York: Ecco/HarperCollins, 2007.

Hayflick, L. "Mortality and Immortality at the Cellular Level: A Review." *Biochemistry* (Moscow) 62, no. 11 (1997): 1180–1190.

Hayflick, L. "The Limited In Vitro Lifetime of Human Diploid Cell Strains." *Experimental Cell Research* 37, no. 3 (1965): 614–636.

Scherer, W. F., J. T. Syverton, and G. O. Gey. "Studies on the Propagation In Vitro of Poliomyelitis Viruses, IV: Viral Multiplication in a Stable Strain of Human Malignant Epithelial Cells (Strain HeLa) Derived from an Epidermoid Carcinoma of the Cervix." *Journal of Experimental Medicine* 97, no. 5 (1953): 695–710.

Macville, M., E. Schröck, H. Padilla-Nash, C. Keck, B. M. Ghadimi, D. Zimonjic, N. Popescu, and T. Ried. "Comprehensive and Definitive Molecular Cytogenetic Characterization of HeLa Cells by Spectral Karyotyping." *Cancer Research* 59, no. 1 (1999): 141–150.

Landry J. J., P. T. Pyl, T. Rausch, T. Zichner, M. M. Tekkedil, A. M. Stütz, A. Jauch, R. S. Aiyar, G. Pau, N. Delhomme, J. Gagneur, J. O. Korbel, W. Huber, and L. M. Steinmetz. "The Genomic and Transcriptomic Landscape of a HeLa Cell Line." *G3: Genes, Genomes, Genetics* 3, no. 8 (2013): 1213–1224.

Skloot, Rebecca. *The Immortal Life of Henrietta Lacks.* New York: Crown/Random House, 2010.

Ben-David, U., et al. "Genetic and Transcriptional Evolution Alters Cancer Cell Line Drug Response." *Nature* 560 (2018): 325–330.

Gillet, Jean-Pierre, Sudhir Varma, and Michael M. Gottesman. "The Clinical Relevance of Cancer Cell Lines." *Journal of the National Cancer Institute* 105, no. 7 (2013): 452–458.

Capes-Davis, A., G. Theodosopoulos, I. Atkin, H. G. Drexler, A. Kohara, R. A. MacLeod, J. R. Masters, Y. Nakamura, Y. A. Reid, R. R. Reddel, and R. I. Freshney. "Check Your Cultures! A List of Cross-Contaminated or Misidentified Cell Lines." *International Journal of Cancer* 127, no. 1 (2010): 1–8.

Wilding, Jennifer L., and Walter F. Bodmer. "Cancer Cell Lines for Drug Discovery and Development." *Cancer Research* (2014). doi:10.1158/0008 -5472.CAN-13-2971.

Kolata, Gina. "Hope in the Lab: A Special Report—A Cautious Awe Greets Drugs That Eradicate Tumors in Mice." *New York Times,* May 3, 1998.

"EntreMed Stock Rides Wave of Optimism About 2 Drugs." *Los Angeles Times,* May 5, 1998. www.latimes.com/archives/la-xpm-1998-may-05-fi -46397-story.html.

"Background on the History of the Mouse." National Human Genome Research Institute. December 2002. www.genome.gov/10005832/background-on -the-history-of-the-mouse/.

Ericsson, Aaron C., Marcus J. Crim, and Craig L. Franklin. "A Brief History of Animal Modeling." *Missouri Medicine* 110, no. 3 (2013): 201–205.

Pound, P., S. Ebrahim, P. Sandercock, M. B. Bracken, I. Roberts, and Reviewing Animal Trials Systematically (RATS) Group. "Where Is the Evidence That Animal Research Benefits Humans?" *BMJ* 328, no. 7438 (2004): 514–517.

Talmadge, J. E., et al. "Murine Models to Evaluate Novel and Conventional Therapeutic Strategies for Cancer." *American Journal of Pathology* 170, no. 3 (2007): 793–804.

Perlman, R. L. "Mouse Models of Human Disease." *Evolution, Medicine and Public Health* 2016, no. 1 (2016): 170–176.

Eruslanov, Evgeniy B., Sunil Singhal, and Steven Albelda. "Mouse Versus Human Neutrophils in Cancer—A Major Knowledge Gap." *Trends in Cancer* 3, no. 2 (2017): 149–160.

Day, C. P., G. Merlino, and T. Van Dyke. "Preclinical Mouse Cancer Models: A Maze of Opportunities and Challenges." *Cell* 163, no. 1 (2015): 39–53.

Shoemaker, R. H., A. Monks, M. C. Alley, D. A. Scudiero, D. L. Fine, T. L. McLemore, B. J. Abbott, K. D. Paull, J. G. Mayo, and M. R. Boyd. "Development of Human Tumor Cell Line Panels for Use in Disease-Oriented Drug Screening." *Progress in Clinical and Biological Research* 276 (1988): 265–286.

Monks, A., D. Scudiero, P. Skehan, R. Shoemaker, K. Paull, D. Vistica, C. Hose, J. Langley, P. Cronise, A. Vaigro-Wolff, et al. "Feasibility of a High-Flux Anticancer Drug Screen Using a Diverse Panel of Cultured Human Tumor Cell Lines." *Journal of the National Cancer Institute* 83 (1991): 757–766.

Monks, A., D. A. Scudiero, G. S. Johnson, K. D. Paull, and E. A. Sausville. "The NCI Anti-Cancer Drug Screen: A Smart Screen to Identify Effectors of Novel Targets." *Anti-Cancer Drug Design* 12 (1997): 533–541.

Grever, M. R., S. A. Schepartz, and B. A. Chabner. "The National Cancer Institute: Cancer Drug Discovery and Development Program." *Seminars in Oncology* 19 (1992): 622–638.

Seok, Junhee. "Genomic Responses in Mouse Models Poorly Mimic Human Inflammatory Diseases." *Proceedings of the National Academy of Sciences of the United States of America* 110, no. 9 (2013): 3507–3512.

Begley, C. G., and L. M. Ellis. "Drug Development: Raise Standards for Preclinical Cancer Research." *Nature* 483, no. 7391 (2012): 531–533.

Santarpia, L., et al. "Deciphering and Targeting Oncogenic Mutations and Pathways in Breast Cancer." *Oncologist* 21 (2016): 1063–1078.

DeVita, V. T., Jr., and E. Chu. "A History of Cancer Chemotherapy." *Cancer Research* 68 (2008): 8643–8653.

Sharpless, N. E., and R. A. Depinho. "The Mighty Mouse: Genetically Engineered Mouse Models in Cancer Drug Development." *Nature Reviews Drug Discovery* 5 (2006): 741–754.

Ben-David, Uri, et al. "Patient-Derived Xenografts Undergo Mouse-Specific Tumor Evolution." *Nature Genetics* 49, no. 11 (2017): 1567–1575.

Izumchenko, E., et al. "Patient-Derived Xenografts Effectively Capture Responses to Oncology Therapy in a Heterogeneous Cohort of Patients with Solid Tumors." *Annals of Oncology* 28, no. 10 (2017): 2595–2605.

Tentler, John J., et al. "Patient-Derived Tumour Xenografts as Models for Oncology Drug Development." *Nature Reviews Clinical Oncology* 9, no. 6 (2012): 338–350.

Willyard, Cassandra. "The Mice with Human Tumours: Growing Pains for a Popular Cancer Model." *Nature* 560, no. 7717 (2018): 156–157.

van der Worp, H. B., et al. "Can Animal Models of Disease Reliably Inform Human Studies?" *PLOS Medicine* 7, no. 3 (2010): e1000245.

Francia, Giulio, and Robert S. Kerbel. "Raising the Bar for Cancer Therapy Models." *Nature Biotechnology* 28 (2010): 561–562.

Ledford, Heidi. "Cancer-Genome Study Challenges Mouse 'Avatars.' Grafting Human Cancer Cells into Mice Alters Tumour Evolution." *Nature,* October 9, 2017.

"NCI Awards Champions Oncology $2M SBIR Grant for Prostate Cancer Research." Genome Web. www.genomeweb.com/business-policy-funding /nci-awards-champions-oncology-2m-sbir-grant-prostate-cancer-research# .XJvLfFVKjIU.

"Cancer Drug Benefits Are Overhyped." Dying for a Cure, June 5, 2016. http:// dyingforacure.org/blogs/cancer-drug-benefits-overhyped/.

Rubin, Eric H., and D. Gary Gilliland. "Drug Development and Clinical Trials—The Path to an Approved Cancer Drug." *Nature Reviews Clinical Oncology* 9 (2012): 215–222.

"Pharmaceutical Companies Acknowledge the Failure of Animal Models in Their Drug Development Process, and Write About This Openly in the Scientific Literature." For Life on Earth. www.forlifeonearth.org/wp -content/uploads/2013/05/Pharmaceutical-Company-Quotes2.pdf.

Pippin, John J. "The Failing Animal Research Paradigm for Human Disease." *Independent Science News,* May 20, 2014.

O'Rourke, Meghan. "Doctors Tell All—And It's Bad." *Atlantic,* November 2014.

Guwande, Atul. *Being Mortal.* New York: Metropolitan Books, 2014.

Cochran, Jack. *The Doctor Crisis.* New York: PublicAffairs, 2014.

Jauhar, Sandeep. *Doctored: The Disillusionment of an American Physician.* New York: Farrar, Straus and Giroux, 2015.

CHAPTER 2: PER

Buchanan, Mark. *Ubiquity: The Science of History . . . or Why the World Is Simpler Than We Think.* New York: Crown, 2001.

Bak, Per. *How Nature Works.* Oxford, UK: Oxford University Press, 1996.

Weinberg, R. *One Renegade Cell: The Quest for the Origins of Cancer.* New York: Basic Books, 1998.

Mehta, Suketu. "Fire in the Belly: A Batch of Chili Proves Life-Affirming in More Ways Than One." *Saveur,* September 27, 2010. www.saveur.com /article/Kitchen/Fire-in-the-Belly.

Gibbs, W. Wayt. "Untangling the Roots of Cancer." *Scientific American,* July 1, 2008. www.scientificamerican.com/article/untangling-the-roots-of-cancer -2008-07/.

Weinberg, Robert. "How Cancer Arises." *Scientific American,* September 1996. https://courses.washington.edu/gs466/readings/Weinberg.pdf.

Mukherjee, Siddhartha. *The Emperor of All Maladies: A Biography of Cancer.* New York: Scribner, 2010.

Danaei, G., S. Vander Hoorn, A. D. Lopez, C. J. Murray, and M. Ezzati. "Comparative Risk Assessment Collaborating Group (Cancers). Causes of Cancer in the World: Comparative Risk Assessment of Nine Behavioural and Environmental Risk Factors." *Lancet* 366, no. 9499 (2005): 1784–1793.

Mukherjee, Siddhartha. *The Gene: An Intimate History.* New York: Scribner, 2016.

zur Hausen, H. "Condylomata Acuminata and Human Genital Cancer." *Cancer Research* 36, no. 794 (1976).

Poiesz, B. J., F. W. Ruscetti, A. F. Gazdar, P. A. Bunn, J. D. Minna, and R. C. Gallo. "Detection and Isolation of Type C Retrovirus Particles from Fresh and Cultured Lymphocytes of a Patient with Cutaneous T-Cell Lymphoma." *Proceedings of the National Academy of Sciences of the United States of America* 77, no. 12 (1980): 7415–7419.

Gallo, R. C. "History of the Discoveries of the First Human Retroviruses: HTLV-1 and HTLV-2." *Oncogene* 24 (2005): 5926–5930.

Moore, Patrick S., and Yuan Chang. "Why Do Viruses Cause Cancer? Highlights of the First Century of Human Tumour Virology." *Nature Reviews Cancer* 10 (2010): 878–889.

Sansregret, Laurent, and Charles Swanton. "The Role of Aneuploidy in Cancer Evolution." *Cold Spring Harbor Perspectives in Medicine.* Published in advance, October 21, 2016. doi:10.1101/cshperspect.a028373.

Rous, P. "A Sarcoma of the Fowl Transmissible by an Agent Separable from the Tumor Cells." *Journal of Experimental Medicine* 13, no. 4 (1911): 397–399.

Rous, Peyton. "The Challenge to Man of the Neoplastic Cell." Nobel lecture, December 13, 1966. www.nobelprize.org/prizes/medicine/1966/rous/lecture/.

Kumar, Prasanna, and Frederick A. Murphy. "Francis Peyton Rous." *Emerging Infectious Diseases* 19, no. 4 (2013): 660–663. www.ncbi.nlm.nih.gov/pmc/articles/PMC3647430/.

Rubin, H. "The Early History of Tumor Virology: Rous, RIF, and RAV." *Proceedings of the National Academy of Sciences of the United States of America* 108 (2011): 14389–14396.

Weiss, R. A., and P. K. Vogt. "100 Years of Rous Sarcoma Virus." *Journal of Experimental Medicine* 208 (2011): 2351–2355.

Burkitt, D. "A Sarcoma Involving the Jaws in African Children." *British Journal of Surgery* 46, no. 197 (1958): 218–223.

Smith, Emma. "50 Years of Epstein-Barr Virus." Cancer Research UK. https://scienceblog.cancerresearchuk.org/2014/03/26/50-years-of-epstein-barr-virus/.

Javier, Ronald T., and Janet S. Butel. "The History of Tumor Virology." *Cancer Research* 68, no. 19 (2008): 7693–7706.

Bister, Klaus. "Discovery of Oncogenes: The Advent of Molecular Cancer Research." *Proceedings of the National Academy of Sciences of the United States of America* 112, no. 50 (2015): 15259–15260.

Lane, D., and A. Levine. "p53 Research: The Past 30 Years and the Next 30 Years." *Cold Spring Harbor Perspectives in Biology* 2, no. 12 (2010): a000893. doi:10.1101/cshperspect.a000893.

Donehower, Lawrence A. "Using Mice to Examine p53 Functions in Cancer, Aging, and Longevity." *Cold Spring Harbor Perspectives in Biology* 1, no. 6 (2009): a001081.

Lane, David P., Chit Fang Cheok, and Sonia Lain. "p53-Based Cancer Therapy." *Cold Spring Harbor Perspectives in Biology* 2, no. 9 (2010): a001222. doi:10.1101/cshperspect.a001222.

Bieging, Kathryn T., Stephano Spano Mello, and Laura D. Attardi. "Unravelling Mechanisms of p53-Mediated Tumour Suppression." *Nature Reviews Cancer* 14 (2014): 359–370.

Li, F. P., and J. F. Fraumeni. "Soft-Tissue Sarcomas, Breast Cancer, and Other Neoplasms: A Familial Syndrome?" *Annals of Internal Medicine* 71, no. 4 (1969): 747–752.

Hisada, M., J. E. Garber, F. P. Li, C. Y. Fung, and J. F. Fraumeni. "Multiple Primary Cancers in Families with Li-Fraumeni Syndrome." *Journal of the National Cancer Institute* 90, no. 8 (1998): 606–611.

Birch, J. M., A. L. Hartley, K. Tricker, J. Prosser, A. Condie, A. Kelsey, et al. "Prevalence and Diversity of Constitutional Mutations in the p53 Gene Among 21 Li-Fraumeni Families." *Cancer Research* 54, no. 5 (1994): 1298–1304.

Greicius, Julie. "And Yet, You Try: A Father's Quest to Save His Son." *Stanford Medicine: Diagnostics,* Fall 2016. https://stanmed.stanford.edu/2016fall/milan-gambhirs-li-fraumeni-syndrome.html.

Haase, Detlef. "TP53 Mutation Status Divides Myelodysplastic Syndromes with Complex Karyotypes into Distinct Prognostic Subgroups." *Nature,* January 2019. www.nature.com/articles/s41375-018-0351-2.

Martinez-Hoyer, Sergio, et al. "Mechanisms of Resistance to Lenalidomide in Del(5q) Myelodysplastic Syndrome Patients." *Blood* 126 (2015): 5228.

Abegglen, Lisa M., et al. "Potential Mechanisms for Cancer Resistance in Elephants and Comparative Cellular Response to DNA Damage in Humans." *JAMA* 314, no. 17 (2015): 1850–1860. doi:10.1001/jama.2015.13134.

Caulin, Aleah F., and Carlo C. Maley. "Peto's Paradox: Evolution's Prescription for Cancer Prevention." *Trends in Ecology & Evolution* 26, no. 4 (2011): 175–182. doi:10.1016/j.tree.2011.01.002.

Tollis, Marc, Amy M. Boddy, and Carlo C. Maley. "Paradox: How Has Evolution Solved the Problem of Cancer Prevention?" *BMC Biology* 15, no. 60 (2017).

Callaway, Ewen. "How Elephants Avoid Cancer: Pachyderms Have Extra Copies of a Key Tumour-Fighting Gene." *Nature,* October 8, 2015.

Armstrong, Susan. *P53: The Gene That Cracked the Cancer Code.* New York: Bloomsbury Sigma, 2016.

García-Cao, Isabel. "'Super p53' Mice Exhibit Enhanced DNA Damage Response, Are Tumor Resistant and Age Normally." *EMBO Journal* 21, no. 22 (2002): 6225–6235.

Hogenboom, Melissa. "The Animals That Don't Get Cancer." BBC, October 31, 2015. www.bbc.com/earth/story/20151031-the-animal-that-doesnt-get-cancer.

Tomasetti, Cristian, Lu Li, and Bert Vogelstein. "Stem Cell Divisions, Somatic Mutations, Cancer Etiology, and Cancer Prevention." *Science* 355, no. 331 (2017): 1330–1334.

Vogelstein, Bert, Nickolas Papadopoulos, Victor E. Velculescu, Shibin Zhou, Luis A. Diaz, Jr., and Kenneth W. Kinzler. "Cancer Genome Landscapes." *Science* 339, no. 6127 (2013): 1546–1558.

"New Study Finds That Most Cancer Mutations Are Due to Random DNA Copying 'Mistakes.'" Johns Hopkins Medicine, March 23, 2017. www.hopkinsmedicine.org/news/media/releases/new_study_finds_that_most_cancer_mutations_are_due_to_random_dna_copying_mistakes.

Yachida, S., S. Jones, I. Bozic, T. Antal, R. Leary, B. Fu, M. Kamiyama, R. H. Hruban, J. R. Eshleman, M. A. Nowak, V. E. Velculescu, K. W. Kinzler, B. Vogelstein, and C. A. Iacobuzio-Donahue. "Distant Metastasis Occurs Late During the Genetic Evolution of Pancreatic Cancer." *Nature* 467 (2010): 1114–1117.

Pienta, Ken, et al. "The Cancer Diaspora: Metastasis Beyond the Seed and Soil Hypothesis." *Clinical Cancer Research* 19, no. 21 (2013). doi:10.1158/1078 -0432.CCR-13-2158.

McGranahan, Nicholas, and Charles Swanton. "Clonal Heterogeneity and Tumor Evolution: Past, Present, and the Future." *Cell* 168 (2017): 631.

Giam, Maybelline, and Giulia Rancati. "Aneuploidy and Chromosomal Instability in Cancer: A Jackpot to Chaos." *Cell Division* 10 (2015): 3. doi: 10.1186/s13008-015-0009-7.

"How Well Do We Understand the Relation Between Incorrect Chromosome Number and Cancer?" EurekAlert! https://www.eurekalert.org/pub _releases/2017-01/cshl-hwd011117.php.

Sheltzer, J. M., et al. "Single-Chromosome Gains Commonly Function as Tumor Suppressors." *Cancer Cell* 31, no. 2 (2017): 240–255. doi:10.1016 /j.ccell.2016.12.004.

Ansari, David. "Pancreatic Cancer and Thromboembolic Disease, 150 Years After Trousseau." *Hepatobiliary Surgery and Nutrition* 4, no. 5 (2015): 325–335.

Campisi, Judith. "Aging, Cellular Senescence, and Cancer." *Annual Review of Physiology* 75 (2013): 685–705.

Lee, Seongju, and Jae-Seon Lee. "Cellular Senescence: A Promising Strategy for Cancer Therapy." *BMB Reports* 52, no. 1 (2019): 35–41.

Lan, Wei, and Ying Miao. "Autophagy and Senescence." *Senescence Signalling and Control in Plants* (2019): 239–253. https://doi.org/10.1016 /B978-0-12-813187-9.00015-9.

Franceschi, Claudio, and Judith Campisi. "Chronic Inflammation (Inflammaging) and Its Potential Contribution to Age-Associated Diseases." *Journals of Gerontology: Series A* 69, supplement 1 (2014): S4–S9.

Harley, Calvin B., and Bryant Villeponteau. "Telomeres and Telomerase in Aging and Cancer." *Current Opinion in Genetics & Development* 5, no. 2 (1995): 249–255.

Blackburn, Elizabeth, and Elissa Epel. *The Telomere Effect: A Revolutionary Approach to Living Younger, Healthier, Longer.* New York: Grand Central Publishing, 2017.

Steensma, D., et al. "Clonal Hematopoiesis of Indeterminate Potential and Its Distinction from Myelodysplastic Syndromes." *Blood* 126 (2015): 9–16.

Jaiswal, S., et al. "Age-Related Clonal Hematopoiesis Associated with Adverse Outcomes." *New England Journal of Medicine* 371 (2014): 2488–2498.

Bertamini, L., et al. "Clonal Hematopoiesis of Indeterminate Potential (CHIP) in Patients with Coronary Artery Disease and in Centenarians: Further Clues Linking CHIP with Cardiovascular Risk." *Blood* 130 (2017): 1144.

Thomas, Hugh. "Mutation and Clonal Selection in the Ageing Oesophagus." *Nature Reviews Gastroenterology & Hepatology* 16 (2019): 139.

Martincorena, I., et al. "Somatic Mutant Clones Colonize the Human Esophagus with Age." *Science* 362 (2018): 911–917.

Yokoyama, A., et al. "Age-Related Remodelling of Oesophageal Epithelia by Mutated Cancer Drivers." *Nature* 565 (2019): 312–317.

Malcovati, Luca, et al. "Clinical Significance of Somatic Mutation in Unexplained Blood Cytopenia." *Blood* 129 (2017): 3371–3378.

Fialkow, P. J., P. J. Martin, V. Najfeld, G. K. Penfold, R. J. Jacobson, and J. A. Hansen. "Evidence for a Multistep Pathogenesis of Chronic Myelogenous Leukemia." *Blood* 58 (1981): 158–163.

Gilliland, Gary D. "Nonrandom X-Inactivation Patterns in Normal Females: Lyonization Ratios Vary with Age." *Blood* 88, no. 1 (1996): 59–65.

Raza, Azra. "Consilence Across Evolving Dysplasias Affecting Myeloid, Cervical, Esophageal, Gastric and Liver Cells: Common Themes and Emerging Patterns." *Leukemia Research* 24, no. 1 (2000): 63–72.

CHAPTER 3: LADY N.

Montoro, Julia, Aslihan Yerlikaya, Abdullah Ali, and Azra Raza. "Improving Treatment for Myelodysplastic Syndromes Patients." *Current Treatment Options in Oncology* 19 (2018): 66. https://doi.org/10.1007/s11864-018-0583-4.

Fuchs, Ota, ed. *Recent Developments in Myelodysplastic Syndromes.* London: IntechOpen, 2019. doi:10.5772/intechopen.73936.

Platzbecker, U. "Treatment of MDS." *Blood* 133, no. 10 (2019): 1096–1107.

Ferrara. F., and O. Vitagliano. "Induction Therapy in Acute Myeloid Leukemia: Is It Time to Put Aside Standard 3 + 7?" *Hematological Oncology* (2019). doi:10.1002/hon.2615.

Cerrano, M., and R. Itzykson. "New Treatment Options for Acute Myeloid Leukemia in 2019." *Current Oncology Reports* 21, no. 2 (2019): 16. doi:10.1007/s11912-019-0764-8.

Buccisano, F. "The Emerging Role of Measurable Residual Disease Detection in AML in Morphologic Remission." *Seminars in Hematology* 56, no. 2 (2019): 125–130. doi:10.1053/j.seminhematol.2018.09.001.

Almeida, A., P. Fenaux, A. F. List, A. Raza, U. Platzbecker, and V. Santini. "Recent Advances in the Treatment of Lower-Risk Non-Del(5q) Myelodysplastic Syndromes (MDS)." *Leukemia Research* 52 (2017): 50–57. doi:10.1016/j.leukres.2016.11.008.

"Luspatercept—Acceleron Pharma/Celgene Corporation." Adis Insight. https://adisinsight.springer.com/drugs/800029519.

Fenaux, P. "Luspatercept for the Treatment of Anemia in Myelodysplastic Syndromes and Primary Myelofibrosis." *Blood* 133, no. 8 (2019): 790–794. doi:10.1182/blood-2018-11-876888.

Prasad, Vinay. "Do Cancer Drugs Improve Survival or Quality of Life?" *BMJ* 359 (2017). https://doi.org/10.1136/bmj.j4528.

Prasad, Vinay, et al. "The High Price of Anticancer Drugs: Origins, Implications, Barriers, Solutions." *Nature Reviews Clinical Oncology* 14 (2017): 381–390. www.nature.com/articles/nrclinonc.2017.31.

Keshavan, Meghana. "Did He Really Just Tweet That? Dr. Vinay Prasad Takes on Big Pharma, Big Medicine, and His Own Colleagues—With Glee." *Stat*, September 15, 2017.

"Exceptional Responders: Why Do Some Cancer Drugs Work for Them and Not Others?" Cancer Treatment Centers of America, March 8, 2018. www.cancercenter.com/community/blog/2018/03/why-do-some-cancer-drugs-work-for-them-and-not-others.

Milowsky, M. I., et al. "Phase II Study of Everolimus in Metastatic Urothelial Cancer." *BJU International* 112, no. 4 (2013): 462–470.

"NCI Sponsored Trials in Precision Medicine." Division of Cancer Treatment and Diagnosis. https://dctd.cancer.gov/majorinitiatives/NCI-sponsored_trials_in_precision_medicine.htm#h06.

West, Howard. "Novel Precision Medicine Trial Designs Umbrellas and Baskets." *JAMA Oncology* 3, no. 3 (2017): 423. doi:10.1001/jamaoncol.2016.5299.

Marquart, John, et al. "Estimation of the Percentage of US Patients with Cancer Who Benefit from Genome-Driven Oncology." *JAMA Oncology* 4, no. 8 (2018): 1093–1098. doi:10.1001/jamaoncol.2018.1660.

Prasad, Vinay. "Perspective: The Precision-Oncology Illusion." *Nature* 537 (2016): S63.

Kaiser, Jocelyn. "A Cancer Drug Tailored to Your Tumor? Experts Trade Barbs over 'Precision Oncology.'" *Science*, April 24, 2018. doi:10.1126/science.aat9794.

Harris, Lyndsay, et al. "Update on the NCI-Molecular Analysis for Therapy Choice (NCI-MATCH/EAY131) Precision Medicine Trial." *Pharmacogenetics, Pharmacogenomics, and Therapeutic Response* 17, supplement 1 (2018). doi:10.1158/1535-7163.TARG-17-B080.

Davis, C., et al. "Availability of Evidence of Benefits on Overall Survival and Quality of Life of Cancer Drugs Approved by European Medicines Agency: Retrospective Cohort Study of Drug Approvals, 2009–13." *BMJ* 359 (2017). https://doi.org/10.1136/bmj.j4530.

Drilon, A., T. W. Laetsch, S. Kummar, et al. "Efficacy of Larotrectinib in TRK Fusion–Positive Cancers in Adults and Children." *New England Journal of Medicine* 378 (2018): 731–739. doi:10.1056/NEJMoa1714448.

Broderick, Jason M. "FDA Approves Larotrectinib for NTRK+ Cancers." OncLive, November 26, 2018. www.onclive.com/web-exclusives/fda-approves-larotrectinib-for-ntrk-cancers.

Darwin, Charles. *On the Origin of Species.* Digireads.com.

Nowell, P. C. "The Clonal Evolution of Tumor Cell Populations." *Science* 194, no. 4260 (1976): 23–28.

Greaves, Mel, and Carlo C. Maley. "Clonal Evolution in Cancer." *Nature* 481 (2012): 306–313.

Janiszewska, Michalina, et al. "Clonal Evolution in Cancer: A Tale of Twisted Twines." *Cell Stem Cell* 16 (2015). https://doi.org/10.1016/j.stem.2014.12.011.

McGranahan, Nicholas, and Charles Swanton. "Clonal Heterogeneity and Tumor Evolution: Past, Present, and the Future." *Cell* 168, no. 4 (2017): 613–628.

Fidler, Isaiah J. "The Pathogenesis of Cancer Metastasis: The 'Seed and Soil' Hypothesis Revisited." *Nature Reviews Cancer* 3 (2003): 453–458.

Ribatti, D., et al. "Stephen Paget and the 'Seed and Soil' Theory of Metastatic Dissemination." *Clinical and Experimental Medicine* 6, no. 4 (2006): 145–149.

Fidler, Isiah J., et al. "The 'Seed and Soil' Hypothesis Revisited." *Lancet Oncology* 9, no. 8 (2008): 808.

Pienta, Ken, et al. "The Cancer Diaspora: Metastasis Beyond the Seed and Soil Hypothesis." *Clinical Cancer Research* 19, no. 21 (2013). doi:10.1158/1078-0432.CCR-13-2158.

Tiong, Ing S., et al. "New Drugs Creating New Challenges in Acute Myeloid Leukemia." *Genes, Chromosomes & Cancer* (2019). https://doi.org/10.1002/gcc.22750.

Kubal, Timothy Edward, et al. "Safety and Feasibility of Outpatient Induction Chemotherapy with CPX-351 in Selected Older Adult Patients with Newly Diagnosed AML." *Journal of Clinical Oncology* 36, supplement 15 (2018): e19013.https://ascopubs.org/doi/abs/10.1200/JCO.2018.36.15_suppl .e19013.

Levis, Mark. "Midostaurin Approved for FLT3-Mutated AML." *Blood* 129 (2017): 3403–3406.

CHAPTER 4: KITTY C.

Profiles in Science. The Mary Lasker papers. US National Library of Medicine.

Wallace, Langley Grace. "Catalyst for the National Cancer Act: Mary Lasker." Albert and Mary Lasker Foundation. December 15, 2016. www .laskerfoundation.org/new-noteworthy/articles/catalyst-national-cancer -act-mary-lasker/.

"National Cancer Act of 1971." National Cancer Institute. https://dtp.cancer .gov/timeline/noflash/milestones/M4_Nixon.htm.

Holford, T. R. "Tobacco Control and the Reduction in Smoking-Related Premature Deaths in the United States, 1964–2012." *JAMA* 311, no. 2 (2014): 164–171. doi:10.1001/jama.2013.285112.

Kolata, Gina. "Advances Elusive in the Drive to Cure Cancer." *New York Times,* April 23, 2009.

Leaf, Clifton. *The Truth in Small Doses: Why We're Losing the War on Cancer— And How to Win.* New York: Simon & Schuster, 2013.

Baker, Monya. "1,500 Scientists Lift the Lid on Reproducibility: Survey Sheds Light on the 'Crisis' Rocking Research." *Nature* 533 (2016): 452–454. www.nature.com/news/1-500-scientists-lift-the-lid-on-reproducibility -1.19970.

DeVita, Vincent T., Jr., and Edward Chu. "A History of Cancer Chemotherapy." *Cancer Research* 68, no. 21 (2008). doi:10.1158/0008-5472.CAN-07 -6611.

Gilligan, A. M. "Death or Debt? National Estimates of Financial Toxicity in Persons with Newly-Diagnosed Cancer." *American Journal of Medicine* 131, no. 10 (2018): 1187–1199.

Fojo, T., et al. "Unintended Consequences of Expensive Cancer Therapeutics—The Pursuit of Marginal Indications and a Me-Too Mentality That Stifles Innovation and Creativity: The John Conley Lecture." *JAMA Otolaryngology–Head & Neck Surgery* 140, no. 12 (2014): 1225–1236.

Marchetti, S., and J. H. M. Schellens. "The Impact of FDA and EMEA Guidelines on Drug Development in Relation to Phase 0 Trials." *British Journal of Cancer* 97 (2007): 577–581. www.nature.com/articles/6603925.

Kummar, Shivaani. "Compressing Drug Development Timelines in Oncology Using Phase '0' Trials." *Nature Reviews Cancer* 7 (2007): 131–139. www.nature.com/articles/nrc2066.

Murgo, J. A., et al. "Designing Phase 0 Cancer Clinical Trials." *Clinical Cancer Research* 14, no. 12 (2008).

Spector, Reynold. "The War on Cancer: A Progress Report for Skeptics." *Skeptical Inquirer,* January/February 2010.

Hitchens, Christopher. "Topic of Cancer." *Vanity Fair,* August 2010.

Adams, C. P., and V. V. Brantner. "Estimating the Cost of New Drug Development: Is It Really 802 Million Dollars?" *Health Affairs* (Millwood) 25, no. 2 (2006): 420–428.

CHAPTER 5: JC

"Donor Registry Data." US Department of Health and Human Services. https://bloodcell.transplant.hrsa.gov/research/registry_donor_data/index.html.

Koutsavlis, Ioannis. "Transfusion Thresholds, Quality of Life, and Current Approaches in Myelodysplastic Syndromes." *Anemia,* 2016. doi:10.1155/2016/8494738.

Black Bone Marrow.com. http://blackbonemarrow.com/.

Poynter, J. N., M. Richardson, M. Roesler, C. K. Blair, B. Hirsch, P. Nguyen, A. Cioc, J. R. Cerhan, and E. Warlick. "Chemical Exposures and Risk of Acute Myeloid Leukemia and Myelodysplastic Syndromes in a Population-Based Study." *International Journal of Cancer* 140, no. 1 (2017): 23–33. doi:10.1002/ijc.30420.

Murphy, T., and K. W. L. Yee. "Cytarabine and Daunorubicin for the Treatment of Acute Myeloid Leukemia." *Expert Opinion on Pharmacotherapy* 18, no. 16 (2017): 1765–1780. doi:10.1080/14656566.2017.1391216.

Steele, John. "The Man Who Would Tame Cancer: Patrick Soon-Shiong Is Opening a New Front in the War on the Deadly Disease." *Nautilus,* January 28, 2016.

Raza, A., et al. "Apoptosis in Bone Marrow Biopsy Samples Involving Stromal and Hematopoietic Cells in 50 Patients with Myelodysplastic Syndromes." *Blood* 86, no. 1 (1995): 268–276.

Raza, A., et al. "Novel Insights into the Biology of Myelodysplastic Syndromes: Excessive Apoptosis and the Role of Cytokines." *International Journal of Hematology* 63, no. 4 (1996): 265–278.

Raza, A., et al. "Thalidomide Produces Transfusion Independence in Long Standing Refractory Anemias of Patients with Myelodysplastic Syndromes." *Blood* 98, no. 4 (2001): 958–965.

Raza, A., and N. Galili. "The Genetic Basis of Phenotypic Heterogeneity in Myelodysplastic Syndromes." *Nature Reviews Cancer* 12, no. 12 (2012): 849–859. doi:10.1038/nrc3321.

CHAPTER 6: ANDREW

Wen, P. Y., and S. Kesari. "Malignant Gliomas in Adults." *New England Journal of Medicine* 359 (2008): 492–507.

Stewart, L. A. "Chemotherapy in Adult High-Grade Glioma: A Systematic Review and Meta-Analysis of Individual Patient Data from 12 Randomised Trials." *Lancet* 359 (2002): 1011–1018.

Kübler-Ross, Elisabeth. *On Death and Dying.* New York: Scribner, 1997.

Izard, Jason, and D. Robert Siemens. "What's in Your Toolkit? Guiding Our Patients Through Their Shared Decision-Making." *Canadian Urological Association Journal* 12, no. 10 (2018): 294–295.

Hagedoorn, Mariët, Ulrika Kreicbergs, and Charlotte Appel. "Coping with Cancer: The Perspective of Patients' Relatives." *Acta Oncologica* 50, no. 2 (2011): 205–211.

Wohlfarth, Philipp, et al. "Chimeric Antigen Receptor T-Cell Therapy—A Hematological Success Story." *Memo* 11, no. 2 (2018): 116–121. doi:10.1007/s12254-018-0409-x.

Titov, Aleksei, et al. "The Biological Basis and Clinical Symptoms of CAR-T Therapy-Associated Toxicities." *Cell Death & Disease* 9 (2018): article 897.

Fried, Shalev, et al. "Early and Late Hematologic Toxicity Following CD19 CAR-T Cells." *Bone Marrow Transplantation,* 2019. https://doi.org/10.1038/s41409-019-0487-3.

Brudno, Jennifer N., and James N. Kochenderfer. "Chimeric Antigen Receptor T-Cell Therapies for Lymphoma." *Nature Reviews Clinical Oncology* 15 (2018): 31–46.

Mahadeo, K. M. "Management Guidelines for Paediatric Patients Receiving Chimeric Antigen Receptor T Cell Therapy." *Nature Reviews Clinical Oncology* 16 (2019): 45–63.

Hoos, A. "Development of Immuno-Oncology Drugs—From CTLA4 to PD1 to the Next Generations." *Nature Reviews Drug Discovery* 15, no. 4 (2016): 235–247.

Coulie, P. G., B. J. Van den Eynde, P. van der Bruggen, and T. Boon. "Tumour Antigens Recognized by T Lymphocytes: At the Core of Cancer Immunotherapy." *Nature Reviews Cancer* 14, no. 2 (2014): 135–146.

Schmidt, Charles. "The Struggle to Do No Harm in Clinical Trials: What Lessons Are Being Learnt from Studies That Went Wrong?" *Nature*, December 20, 2017.

Maude, S. L., et al. "Tisagenlecleucel in Children and Young Adults with B-Cell Lymphoblastic Leukemia." *New England Journal of Medicine* 378, no. 5 (2018): 439–448.

Editorial. "CAR T-Cell Therapy: Perceived Need Versus Actual Evidence." *Lancet Oncology* 19, no. 10 (2018): 1259.

Osorio, Joana. "Cancer Immunotherapy Research Round-Up: Highlights from Clinical Trials." *Nature*, December 20, 2017.

Barreyro, L., T. M. Chlon, and D. T. Starczynowski. "Chronic Immune Response Dysregulation in MDS Pathogenesis." *Blood* 132, no. 15 (2018): 1553–1560.

Almasbak, Hilde, et al. "CAR T Cell Therapy: A Game Changer in Cancer Treatment." *Journal of Immunology Research*, 2016. doi:10.1155/2016/5474602.

Sun, Shangjun, et al. "Immunotherapy with CAR-Modified T Cells: Toxicities and Overcoming Strategies." *Journal of Immunology Research*, 2018. doi:10.1155/2018/2386187.

Doudna, Jennifer A., and Samuel H. Sternberg. *A Crack in Creation: Gene Editing and the Unthinkable Power to Control Evolution.* Boston: Houghton Mifflin Harcourt, 2017.

Haapaniemi, Emma, Sandeep Botla, Jenna Persson, Bernhard Schmierer, and Jussi Taipale. "CRISPR–Cas9 Genome Editing Induces a p53-Mediated DNA Damage Response." *Nature Medicine*, 2018. doi:10.1038/s41591-018-0049-z.

Shin, Ha Youn, et al. "CRISPR/Cas9 Targeting Events Cause Complex Deletions and Insertions at 17 Sites in the Mouse Genome." *Nature Communications* 8 (2017): article 15464.

Kosicki, Michael, et al. "Repair of Double-Strand Breaks Induced by CRISPR–Cas9 Leads to Large Deletions and Complex Rearrangements." *Nature Biotechnology* 36 (2018): 765–771.

CHAPTER 7: HARVEY

Weir, Hannah K., et al. "The Past, Present, and Future of Cancer Incidence in the United States: 1975 Through 2020." *Cancer* 121, no. 11 (2015): 1827–1837. doi:10.1002/cncr.29258.

By the Numbers: NCI Budget Breakdown, FY 2018. doi:10.1158/2159-8290 .CD-NB2019-002.

Aparicio, Samuel, and Carlos Caldas. "The Implications of Clonal Genome Evolution for Cancer Medicine." *New England Journal of Medicine* 368 (2013): 842–851. doi:10.1056/NEJMra1204892.

Walter, M. J., et al. "Clonal Architecture of Secondary Acute Myeloid Leukemia." *New England Journal of Medicine* 366 (2012): 1090–1098.

Ruiz, C., E. Lenkiewicz, L. Evers, et al. "Advancing a Clinically Relevant Perspective of the Clonal Nature of Cancer." *Proceedings of the National Academy of Sciences of the United States of America* 108 (2011): 12054–12059.

Cohen, Jon. "'It's Sobering': A Once-Exciting HIV Cure Strategy Fails Its Test in People." *Science,* July 25, 2018. doi:10.1126/science.aau8963.

Crowley, E., et al. "Liquid Biopsy: Monitoring Cancer-Genetics in the Blood." *Nature Reviews Clinical Oncology* 10 (2013): 472–484.

Bleyer, Archie, and H. Gilbert Welch. "Effect of Three Decades of Screening Mammography on Breast-Cancer Incidence." *New England Journal of Medicine* 367, no. 21 (2012): 1998–2005.

Miller, Anthony B., et al. "Twenty Five Year Follow-Up for Breast Cancer Incidence and Mortality of the Canadian National Breast Screening Study: Randomised Screening Trial." *British Medical Journal* 348 (2014): 366.

Fagin, Dan. *Toms River: A Story of Science and Salvation.* Washington, DC: Island Press, 2014.

Ilic, D., M. Djulbegovic, J. H. Jung, et al. "Prostate Cancer Screening with Prostate-Specific Antigen (PSA) Test: A Systematic Review and Meta-Analysis." *BMJ* 362 (2018): k3519.

Loud, Jennifer, and Jeanne Murphy. "Cancer Screening and Early Detection in the 21st Century." *Seminars in Oncology Nursing* 33, no. 2 (2017): 121–128.

Adami, Hans-Olov, et al. "Towards an Understanding of Breast Cancer Etiology." *Seminars in Cancer Biology* 8, no. 4 (1998): 255–262.

Esserman, Laura J. "Overdiagnosis and Overtreatment in Cancer: An Opportunity for Improvement." *JAMA* 310, no. 8 (2013): 797.

Autier, P., and M. Boniol. "Effect of Screening Mammography on Breast Cancer Incidence." *New England Journal of Medicine* 368 (2013): 677–679. https://citeseerx.ist.psu.edu/viewdoc/download?doi = 10.1.1.691.3537 &rep = rep1&type = pdf.

Das, Srustidhar, and Surinder K. Batra. "Understanding the Unique Attributes of MUC16 (CA125): Potential Implications in Targeted Therapy." *Cancer Research,* 2015. doi:10.1158/0008-5472.CAN-15-1050.

Leaf, Clifton. *The Truth in Small Doses: Why We're Losing the War on Cancer—And How to Win.* New York: Simon & Schuster, 2013.

Adami, Hans-Olov, et al. "Time to Abandon Early Detection Cancer Screening." *European Journal of Clinical Investigation,* December 19, 2018. https://onlinelibrary.wiley.com/doi/full/10.1111/eci.13062.

Kopans, D. B. "Breast Cancer Screening: Where Have We Been and Where Are We Going? A Personal Perspective Based on History, Data and Experience." *Clinical Imaging* 48 (2018): vii–xi.

Malvezzi, M., et al. "European Cancer Mortality Predictions for the Year 2019 with Focus on Breast Cancer." *Annals of Oncology,* March 19, 2019. https://doi.org/10.1093/annonc/mdz051.

Malvezzi, M., et al. "European Cancer Mortality Predictions for the Year 2018 with Focus on Colorectal Cancer." *Annals of Oncology* 29, no. 4 (2018): 1016–1022.

Prasad, V. "Why Cancer Screening Has Never Been Shown to 'Save Lives'—And What We Can Do About It." *BMJ* 352 (2016). https://doi.org/10.1136/bmj.h6080.

Narod, S. A., et al. "Why Have Breast Cancer Mortality Rates Declined?" *Journal of Cancer Policy* 5 (2015): 8–17. https://doi.org/10.1016/j.jcpo.2015.03.002.

Colantonio, S., et al. "A Smart Mirror to Promote a Healthy Lifestyle." *Biosystems Engineering* 138 (2015): 33–43.

Iverson, N. M., et al. "In Vivo Biosensing Via Tissue Localizable Near Infrared Fluorescent Single Walled Carbon Nanotubes." *Nature Nanotechnology* 8 (2013): 873–880.

Gambhir, Sanjiv Sam. "Toward Achieving Precision Health." *Science Translational Medicine* 10, no. 430 (2018): 3612. doi:10.1126/scitranslmed.aao3612.

Wong, D. "Saliva Liquid Biopsy for Cancer Detection." Paper presented at the American Association for the Advancement of Science 2016 Annual Meeting, Washington, DC, February 11–15, 2016.

Johnson, J. "Intelligent Toilets, Smart Couches and the House of the Future," *Financial Post,* June 6, 2012. http://business.financialpost.com/uncategorized/intelligent-toilets-smart-couches-and-the-house-of-the-future.

Wang, Lulu. "Microwave Sensors for Breast Cancer Detection." *Sensors* 18, no. 2 (2018): 655. https://doi.org/10.3390/s18020655.

Hsu, Jeremy. "Can a New Smart Bra Really Detect Cancer?" *Live Science,* October 17, 2012.

Kahn, N., et al. "Dynamic Nanoparticle-Based Flexible Sensors: Diagnosis of Ovarian Carcinoma from Exhaled Breath." *Nano Letters* 15, no. 10 (2015): 7023–7028.

Czernin, Johannes, and Sanjiv Sam Gambhir. "Discussions with Leaders: A Conversation Between Sam Gambhir and Johannes Czernin." *Journal of Nuclear Medicine* 59, no. 12 (2018): 1783–1785. doi:10.2967/jnumed.118.221648.

Vermesh, Ophir, et al. "An Intravascular Magnetic Wire for the High-Throughput Retrieval of Circulating Tumour Cells In Vivo." *Nature Biomedical Engineering* 2, no. 9 (2018): 696–705.

Ferrari, E., et al. "Urinary Proteomics Profiles Are Useful for Detection of Cancer Biomarkers and Changes Induced by Therapeutic Procedures." *Molecules* 24, no. 4 (2019): 794. https://doi.org/10.3390/molecules24040794.

Colditz, Graham A., Kathleen Y. Wolin, and Sarah Gehlert. "Applying What We Know to Accelerate Cancer Prevention." *Science Translational Medicine,* 4, no. 127 (2012): 127rv4.

Wan, J. C., et al. "Liquid Biopsies Come of Age: Towards Implementation of Circulating Tumour DNA." *Nature Reviews Cancer* 17 (2017): 223–238.

Bianchi, D. W. "Circulating Fetal DNA: Its Origin and Diagnostic Potential—A Review." *Placenta* 25, supplement (2004): S93–S101. https://doi.org/10.1016/j.placenta.2004.01.005.

Jahr, S., et al. "DNA Fragments in the Blood Plasma of Cancer Patients: Quantitations and Evidence for Their Origin from Apoptotic and Necrotic Cells." *Cancer Research* 61 (2001): 1659–1665.

Thierry, A. R., et al. "Clinical Validation of the Detection of KRAS and BRAF Mutations from Circulating Tumor DNA." *Nature Medicine* 20 (2014): 430–435.

Ding, L., M. C. Wendl, J. F. McMichael, and B. J. Raphael. "Expanding the Computational Toolbox for Mining Cancer Genomes." *Nature Reviews Genetics* 15, no. 8 (2014): 556–570.

Murtaza, M., et al. "Non-Invasive Analysis of Acquired Resistance to Cancer Therapy by Sequencing of Plasma DNA." *Nature* 497 (2013): 108–112.

Siravegna, Giulia, et al. "Integrating Liquid Biopsies into the Management of Cancer." *Nature Reviews Clinical Oncology* 14 (2017): 531–548.

Taylor, D. D., and C. Gercel-Taylor. "MicroRNA Signatures of Tumor-Derived Exosomes as Diagnostic Biomarkers of Ovarian Cancer." *Gynecologic Oncology* 110 (2008): 13–21.

Yuan, Zixu. "Dynamic Plasma MicroRNAs Are Biomarkers for Prognosis and Early Detection of Recurrence in Colorectal Cancer." *British Journal of Cancer* 117 (2017): 1202–1210.

Hinkson, I., IV, et al. "A Comprehensive Infrastructure for Big Data in Cancer Research: Accelerating Cancer Research and Precision Medicine." *Frontiers in Cell and Developmental Biology,* September 21, 2017. https://doi .org/10.3389/fcell.2017.00083.

Philippidis, Alex. "Next-Gen Diagnostics: Thermo Fisher Scientific, University Hospital Basel Partner to Develop, Validate NGS Cancer Diagnostics." *Clinical OMICs* 4, no. 3 (2017). https://doi.org/10.1089/clinomi.04 .03.17.

BloodPac: Blood Profiling Atlas in Cancer. www.bloodpac.org.

Liu, M. C., et al. "Plasma Cell-Free DNA (cfDNA) Assays for Early Multi-Cancer Detection: The Circulating Cell-Free Genome Atlas (CCGA) Study." *Annals of Oncology* 29, supplement 8 (2018): mdy269.048. https:// doi.org/10.1093/annonc/mdy269.048.

Sallam, Reem M. "Proteomics in Cancer Biomarkers Discovery: Challenges and Applications." *Disease Markers,* 2015. http://dx.doi.org/10.1155/2015/321370.

Taylor and Gercel-Taylor. "MicroRNA Signatures."

Peng, Liyuan. "Tissue and Plasma Proteomics for Early Stage Cancer Detection." *Molecular Omics* 14 (2018): 405–423. doi:10.1039/C8MO00126J.

Tajmul, M. D., et al. "Identification and Validation of Salivary Proteomic Signatures for Non-Invasive Detection of Ovarian Cancer." *International Journal of Biological Macromolecules* 108 (2018): 503–514.

Simpson, R. J., S. S. Jensen, and J. W. Lim. "Proteomic Profiling of Exosomes: Current Perspectives." *Proteomics* 8 (2008): 4083–4099.

Chen, Ziqing, et al. "Current Applications of Antibody Microarrays." *Clinical Proteomics* 15, no. 7 (2018). https://doi.org/10.1186/s12014-018-9184-2.

Halvaei, S. "Exosomes in Cancer Liquid Biopsy: A Focus on Breast Cancer." *Nucleic Acid* 10 (2018): 131–141.

Xu, Rong, et al. "Extracellular Vesicles in Cancer—Implications for Future Improvements in Cancer Care." *Nature Reviews Clinical Oncology* 15, no. 10 (2018): 617–638.

Valentino, A., et al. "Exosomal MicroRNAs in Liquid Biopsies: Future Biomarkers for Prostate Cancer." *Clinical and Translational Oncology* 19 (2017): 651–657.

Rajagopal, C., and K. B. Harikumar. "The Origin and Functions of Exosomes in Cancer." *Frontiers in Oncology*, March 20, 2018. https://doi.org/10.3389/fonc.2018.00066.

Rani, S., et al. "Isolation of Exosomes for Subsequent mRNA, MicroRNA, and Protein Profiling." *Methods in Molecular Biology* 784 (2011): 181–195.

Liu, F., U. Demirci, and S. S. Gambhir. Exosome-Total-Isolation-Chip (Ex-oTIC) Device for Isolation of Exosome-Based Biomarkers. US patent application 16/073,577, filed 2019.

Alix-Panabieres, C., and K. Pantel. "Circulating Tumor Cells: Liquid Biopsy of Cancer." *Clinical Chemistry* 59 (2013): 110–118.

Green, B. J., et al. "Beyond the Capture of Circulating Tumor Cells: Next-Generation Devices and Materials." *Angewandte Chemie International Edition* 55 (2016): 1252–1265. https://onlinelibrary.wiley.com/doi/full/10.1002/anie.201505100%4010.1002/%28ISSN%291521-3773. Microfluidics.

Vona, G., et al. "Isolation by Size of Epithelial Tumor Cells: A New Method for the Immunomorphological and Molecular Characterization of Circulating Tumor Cells." *American Journal of Pathology* 156, no. 1 (2000): 57–63.

Paterlini-Brechot, Patrizia, and Naoual Linda Benali. "Circulating Tumor Cells (CTC) Detection: Clinical Impact and Future Directions." *Cancer Letters* 253, no. 2 (2007): 180–204.

Hood, Leroy, and Stephen H. Friend. "Predictive, Personalized, Preventive, Participatory (P4) Cancer Medicine." *Nature Reviews Clinical Oncology* 8 (2011): 184–187.

Cohen, J. D., et al. "Combined Circulating Tumor DNA and Protein Biomarker-Based Liquid Biopsy for the Earlier Detection of Pancreatic Cancers." *Proceedings of the National Academy of Sciences of the United States of America* 114, no. 38 (2017): 10202–10207. https://doi.org/10.1073/pnas.1704961114.

Wang, Qing, et al. "Mutant Proteins as Cancer-Specific Biomarkers." *Proceedings of the National Academy of Sciences of the United States of America* 108, no. 6 (2011): 2444–2449. https://doi.org/10.1073/pnas.1019203108.

Lennon, A. M., et al. "The Early Detection of Pancreatic Cancer: What Will It Take to Diagnose and Treat Curable Pancreatic Neoplasia?" *Cancer Research* 74, no. 13 (2014): 3381–3389.

Moses, H., III, E. R. Dorsey, D. H. Matheson, and S. O. Thier. "Financial Anatomy of Biomedical Research." *JAMA* 294, no. 11 (2005): 1333–1342.

Claridge, Laura. *Emily Post: Daughter of the Gilded Age, Mistress of American Manners.* New York: Random House, 2008.

AFTERMATH: GIVE SORROW WORDS

Kübler-Ross, Elisabeth, and David Kessler. *On Grief and Grieving: Finding the Meaning of Grief Through the Five Stages of Loss.* New York: Scribner, 2005.

Robinson, Katherine. "Robert Frost: 'The Road Not Taken.' Our Choices Are Made Clear in Hindsight." Poetry Foundation, May 27, 2016. www.poetryfoundation.org/articles/89511/robert-frost-the-road-not-taken.

"Fairfield Minuteman Archives, Feb 12, 2004, p. 40." Newspaper Archive. https://newspaperarchive.com/fairfield-minuteman-feb-12-2004-p-40/.

Lang, Joel. "Barbara Griffiths: Downsizing Gives Artist Pause to Ponder Her Life and Her Art." *CT Post,* August 14, 2016. https://www.ctpost.com/living/article/Barbara-Griffiths-Downsizing-gives-artist-pause-9141213.php.

Sontag, Susan. *Illness As Metaphor.* New York: Farrar, Straus and Giroux, 1978.

Adams, Lisa Bonchek. *Persevere: A Life with Cancer.* Lancaster, PA: Bonchek Family Foundation, 2017.

EPILOGUE: THE DAWN HAS ALREADY ARRIVED

Weinberg, Robert A. "Coming Full Circle—From Endless Complexity to Simplicity and Back Again." *Cell* 157, no. 1 (2014): 267–271.

Fojo, Tito, and Christine Grady. "How Much Is Life Worth: Cetuximab, Non–Small Cell Lung Cancer, and the $440 Billion Question." *JNCI: Journal of the National Cancer Institute* 101, no. 15 (2009): 1044–1048. https://doi.org/10.1093/jnci/djp177.

Yachida, S., S. Jones, I. Bozic, T. Antal, R. Leary, B. Fu, M. Kamiyama, R. H. Hruban, J. R. Eshleman, M. A. Nowak, V. E. Velculescu, K. W. Kinzler, B. Vogelstein, and C. A. Iacobuzio-Donahue. "Distant Metastasis Occurs

Late During the Genetic Evolution of Pancreatic Cancer." *Nature* 467 (2010): 1114–1117.

Desai, Pinkal, et al. "Somatic Mutations Precede Acute Myeloid Leukemia Years Before Diagnosis." *Nature Medicine* 24 (2018): 1015–1023.

Ehrenreich, Barbara. "Pathologies of Hope." *Harper's,* February 1, 2007. http://barbaraehrenreich.com/hope/.

Ibn Abi Talib, Ali. *Nahjul Balagha: Peak of Eloquence.* India: Alwaaz International, 2010.

Credits

Photo Credits

Text Credits

Page 21: Excerpted from "Eye Bank" by Ahmad Faraz. Translated into English by Anjuli Fatima Raza Kolb and published in English first at Guernica, June 6, 2018. Used with permission of Guernica and Ms. Kolb.

Page 59: "Miss Gee" Copyright 1940 and © renewed 1968 by W. H. Auden from COLLECTED POEMS by W. H. Auden. Used by permission of Random House, an imprint and division of Penguin Random House LLC. All Rights Reserved.

Page 122: ("My life had stood a loaded gun" J 754/F 764—Lines 1–4) and page 225 ("After great pain a formal feeling comes" J 341/F 372—Lines 1–4): THE POEMS OF EMILY DICKINSON: READING EDITION, edited by Ralph W. Franklin, Cambridge, Mass.: The Belknap Press of Harvard University Press, Copyright © 1998, 1999 by the President and Fellows of Harvard College. Copyright © 1951, 1955 by the President and Fellows of Harvard College. Copyright © renewed 1979, 1983 by the President and Fellows of Harvard College. Copyright © 1914, 1918, 1919, 1924, 1929, 1930, 1932, 1935, 1937, 1942 by Martha Dickinson Bianchi. Copyright © 1952, 1957, 1958, 1963, 1965 by Mary L. Hampson.

Pages 209–210: "When I Die" by Lisa Bonchek Adams is taken from the book *Persevere: A Life with Cancer* published by the Bonchek Family Foundation, 2017. The poem is quoted with permission granted from the Bonchek Family Foundation.

Page 256: "Funeral Blues" Copyright 1940 and © renewed 1968 by W. H. Auden from COLLECTED POEMS by W. H. Auden. Used by permission of Random House, an imprint and division of Penguin Random House LLC. All Rights Reserved.

Index

Page numbers in *italics* indicate illustrations.

Reading Group
Guide for
The First Cell

Q&A

1. What made you decide to become an oncologist?

I cannot recall any particularly noteworthy natural gifts that would explain a career in oncology except for having an inquisitive nature. As a child, I spent long summer afternoons in Karachi, following ants. As a teenager, I was obsessed with evolutionary biology. I am certain that had I gone to school in this country, I would have become a field biologist. Growing up in Pakistan, however, my only entry into science was through medical school, which is what I did, with the full intention of coming to the United States upon graduation and pursuing a PhD program. However, my curiosity abruptly changed to wonder as I began interacting with patients. It was love at first sight. While curiosity seeks explanations for things, wonder creates a sense of awe by turning the known on its head. Patients did that for me. Those medical school clinical rotations left no question in my mind that patient-related issues would be the driving force for all my future endeavors. Why oncology?

Because as my medical studies progressed, I witnessed firsthand the violence and cruelty of cancer, especially ghastly in Pakistan because patients often presented with advanced stages of the disease, something I have not seen since coming to America. These appalling, hideous monstrosities sticking out of gaunt, skeletal, wasted bodies seemed to mock at our ignorance and provided an electric shock to my system. The unspeakable suffering, especially of the older, often impoverished, villagers, who had traveled miles and miles to seek a cure, inspired me to dedicate my life to cancer treatment and research. The dual emotional and intellectual challenges gripped my heart, seized my imagination with such potency that by the time I was twenty, I was fully committed to oncology. I was never interested in research purely for the sake of research; I was interested only in research that would help my patients. I have never looked back.

2. When and how did you decide to write this book?

Dorothy Parker once said that if you have any young friends who aspire to become writers, the second greatest favor you can do for them is to present them with copies of *The Elements of Style*. The first greatest, of course, is to shoot them now, while they're happy. I never imagined myself as a writer. What forced me to pick up the pen was not just our staggering failure to deal effectively with cancer but the unspeakable tragedy of Andrew, my daughter Sheherzad's best friend. Andrew had been in and out of our home since both were fifteen. Cancer is called a silent killer for a good reason. By the time Andrew developed symptoms, his violently invasive brain tumor had already grown into a nine-centimeter monstrosity. The sheer ferocity of Andrew's vicious tumors, coupled with the utter powerlessness of the entire cancer enterprise to help this poor twenty-two-year-old young man at any level, hit me physically like a slap in the face. How would I tell his family, his friends, *him*, that his only choice from the moment of diagnosis was to die of the cancer or die of the treatment? On one hand, I was astounded by the lack of progress in the field, evidenced by the unqualified, categorical, disgraceful failure of all of us functioning as his oncologists. On the other, I cringed when accosted by the absurd hype around advances in "biologic understanding" of cancer in animals and a few new targeted and immune therapies, called "game changers," which benefited only a handful of patients. This dual affront added insult to injury. It forced me to survey the field with uncompromising honesty and rip off the blinders, first from my own eyes, and then from the eyes of the public. *The First Cell* is the result.

3. Why do you study myelodysplastic syndromes (MDS)?

My quest to understand MDS was the direct result of a soul-shaking experience with my thirty-four-year-old patient JC (Chapter 5). I started my career in medicine in the United States in 1977 by studying and treating acute myeloid leukemia (AML). As I watched the dizzying, disorienting malevolence visited upon JC by her leukemia, it became clear to me that using the awful chemotherapy, even if curative for a few patients, should not be our best hope for AML. What could be a better solution? The answer came to me like a flash. Stop AML before it becomes AML. JC, like many other patients, gave a history of having low blood counts for months, sometimes years, prior to the diagnosis of leukemia. This earlier form of leukemia, or pre-leukemia, called myelodysplastic syndromes (MDS), I reasoned, had to be the right place to restart. Perhaps, we could intercept the disease at the MDS stage, when it would be less complicated and easier to treat. Perhaps, we could arrest its evolution to AML altogether. Soon, it became apparent that MDS itself can be highly malignant, and it took many more years of trial and error before we realized that the disease needs detection at an even earlier stage than MDS. I am confident that by using the most sophisticated technology to study the painstakingly collected Tissue Repository, the biomarkers and footprints of the earliest form of the disease will be traceable. Then we will finally reveal what makes some individuals, even healthy ones, susceptible to MDS. Monitoring individuals for the appearance of the first cell could then target such healthy but

high-risk individuals. Every type of cancer would need to be subjected
to the same exercise; identify high-risk populations through careful
study of tissue samples (like mutations in BRCA genes, which make
women susceptible to breast and ovarian cancers) and attempt to catch
and kill cancers at inception.

**4. How has being the wife of a cancer patient had an impact on
your approach to treating your patients?**
The experience forced me to revise my perception of reality in unexpected ways and to acknowledge my growing confusions. The war on
cancer is very confusing. It is a war for the body, on the body, and by
the body. Harvey taught me not to become emotionally involved with
patients because feelings clouded judgment. I always questioned his
advice because patients demand an emotionally invested, empathetic
doctor. Why would I go through years of hard work in medicine to
remain detached, dispassionate, distanced from my patients? But even
I was taken aback when Harvey named me as his primary oncologist.
Another issue was dealing with the simultaneous existence of hope
and despair throughout his illness. I resorted to Freud who pointed
out that normally, it is hope that gives subject to action. When there is
no hope, hopelessness becomes a form of action. Ultimately, the only
consolation is that there is no consolation. This served as a remarkable
revision of the reality principle because once there is no hope one is
forced to go on living day to day. As Harvey faced mortality head-on,
the words meant to empower patients and their families—war, battle,
fight, magic bullets—ended up detracting from the profound human
experience.

**5. What does it mean "to do no harm" when the medication
available to you is often harmful and fruitless?**
While almost all drugs come with attendant toxicities, the question for
cancer patients is a greater challenge because radiation and chemotherapies kill cancer cells along with normal cells, indiscriminately causing

life-threatening and extraordinarily painful side effects. Paradoxically, these very poisons offer the only glimmer of hope for prolonging survival. The justification for our actions can be traced back to *Summa Theologica*, where Thomas Aquinas states the Principle of Double Effect: "Nothing hinders one act from having two effects, only one of which is intended, while the other is beside the intention." As long as good is the intent, the possibility of a harmful side effect, even death, is acceptable.

6. There are 3.5 million papers on cancer. There is a staggering disconnect between great scientific insights and translation to improved therapy. What are we doing wrong?
I call it the CRUSH syndrome. C stands for **C**omplexity of cancer that begins in a single cell, but following Darwinian principles, evolves into thousands of daughter cells, each carrying the founder mutations as well as new passenger mutations. The end result is that by the time this silent killer becomes clinically apparent, the tumor has acquired tremendous heterogeneity. Many daughter cells with new mutations acquire the ability to metabolize drugs differently and thus escape elimination. If the treatment manages to kill the dominant clone and produces a response, the response will last only as long as it takes the next surviving cell to expand its clone and form a new tumor, once again carrying thousands of potential new cancers within it. In other words, cancer is not just complex; it is a rapidly evolving, moving target. We are trying to address this complexity with **R**eductionist strategies, hoping to find one abnormality that can be targeted with a magic bullet. The **U**ltra-hype accorded every little step, be it associated with prolonging survival by weeks in humans or be it just an animal study, is the main reason our public is lulled into thinking that a cure for cancer is just around the bend. Then there are the **S**implistic, archaic methods of performing clinical trials using agents brought to the bedside through even more simplistic, reductionist animal models. Finally, the **H**igh cost (42 percent of newly diagnosed cancer patients lose every penny of their life savings and become financially ruined

by year 2+ for very little improvement in survival) has brought the healthcare system to the verge of a fiscal collapse. In fact, 45 percent of women with advanced stage breast cancer are currently being hounded by collection agencies. It is simply unconscionable. This **CRUSH** syndrome is why the results of millions of publications fail to translate into improved treatment outcome. The whole paradigm of doing things is sclerotic and unsupportable for long.

7. What advice do you have for patients with advanced cancer, their families, and those who want to go into the healthcare profession?

The best piece of advice is imparted by Antonio Gramsci in the *Prison Notebooks*: pessimism of the intellect and optimism of will. See the facts for what they are, not as you may want them to be, and instead of being broken, have more confidence in your capacity to see things through, to overcome the odds. The simultaneous existence of despair and hope, of pessimism and optimism; one realistic, the other brightening the darkest of times with resilience.

Many of my patients say something to the effect that they are not afraid of dying but of death. What is the actual experience of death? A surprisingly reassuring answer comes from the great French Renaissance writer Michel de Montaigne. In his essay on death, after he had a brutal fall from his horse and a near-death experience, Montaigne tells us calmly, "If you don't know how to die, don't worry; Nature will tell you what to do on the spot, fully and adequately. She will do this job perfectly for you; don't bother your head about it."

DISCUSSION QUESTIONS

1. Many of us have had cancer or know someone who has had cancer. What impact has cancer had on your life?
2. Have you, or has someone you know, benefited from early cancer detection?

3. What does the principle "to do no harm" mean to you?

4. Have you ever had to make healthcare decisions for a loved one with late-stage cancer? If so, how did you weigh the potential benefits of aggressive cancer treatments against the likely harms?

5. If your life has been touched by cancer, what advice do you have for patients, their families, or healthcare professionals?

6. Has there been a figure in your life—a family member, a friend, a medical professional, or even a stranger—who has changed your attitude toward cancer treatment?

7. Have you ever had to navigate the exorbitant price of cancer treatment? Did that change your ideas about the American healthcare system?

8. What steps do you think are necessary for transforming the conversation around cancer treatment? How do you think you can help?

FURTHER READING

Gawande, Atul. *Being Mortal: Medicine and What Matters in the End*. New York: Metropolitan Books, 2014.

Kalanithi, Paul. *When Breath Becomes Air*. New York: Random House, 2016.

Marsh, Henry. *Do No Harm: Stories of Life, Death, and Brain Surgery*. London: Macmillan, 2015.

Mukherjee, Siddhartha. *The Emperor of All Maladies: A Biography of Cancer*. New York: Simon & Schuster, 2010.

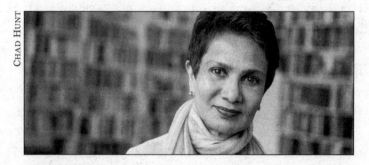

AZRA RAZA is the Chan Soon-Shiong Professor of Medicine and director of the MDS Center at Columbia University. In addition to publishing widely in basic and clinical cancer research, Raza is also the coauthor of *Ghalib: Epistemologies of Elegance* and the coeditor of the highly acclaimed website 3QuarksDaily.com. She and her daughter, Sheherzad, live in New York City. Her website is https://azraraza.com.